METANARRATIVES OF DISABILITY

This book explores multiple metanarratives of disability to introduce and investigate the critical concept of assumed authority and the normative social order from which it derives.

The book comprises 15 chapters developed across three parts and, informed by disability studies, is authored by those with research interests in the condition on which they focus as well as direct or intimate experiential knowledge. When out and about, many disabled people know only too well what it is to be erroneously told the error of our/their ways by non-disabled passers-by, assumed authority often cloaked in helpfulness. Showing that assumed authority is underpinned by a displacement of personal narratives in favour of overarching metanarratives of disability that find currency in a diverse multiplicity of cultural representations – ranging from literature to film, television, advertising, social media, comics, art, and music – this work discusses how this relates to a range of disabilities and chronic conditions, including blindness, autism, Down syndrome, diabetes, cancer, and HIV and AIDS.

Metanarratives of Disability will be of interest to all scholars and students of disability studies, medical sociology, medical humanities, education studies, cultural studies, and health.

David Bolt is Professor of Disability Studies and Director of the Centre for Culture and Disability Studies at Liverpool Hope University, United Kingdom.

Autocritical Disability Studies

Series Editor: David Bolt, Liverpool Hope University, UK.

This new book series represents both a contribution to, and a departure from, the academic field of critical disability studies. According to some concerns about that field, disability is the start but never the finish, there is insufficient engagement with the ethical and political issues faced by disabled people, and the work is too insensitive to individual experiences. Such concerns are addressed boldly in the new series via a formal coupling of critical disability studies with the research method of autoethnography.

The qualitative method of autoethnography acknowledges a researcher's individual experience in the most explicit of ways, from the very start of the process to the finished product that reaches publication. Whereas most traditional research methods claim, or at least aspire to, objectivity, autoethnography owns its subjectivity as paramount. This being so, when academic authors/editors have direct or at least intimate individual experience of disability, the subjectivity of their books can predicate a shift in typology from critical disability studies to what the new series terms autocritical disability studies.

In encouraging textual and theoretical work, the series also introduces autocritical discourse analysis and autocritical disability theory to formalize the ethical and epistemological importance of disability experience in many aspects of critical studies. The key point about the books sought for the series, then, is precisely that the individual experience of disability is recognized and positioned as both start and finish.

The book series editor, Professor David Bolt, encourages expressions of interest from potential monograph authors and volume editors.

Metanarratives of Disability
Culture, Assumed Authority, and the Normative Social Order
Edited by David Bolt

For a full list of titles in this series, please visit: https://www.routledge.com/Autocritical-Disability-Studies/book-series/ASHSERADS

METANARRATIVES OF DISABILITY

Culture, Assumed Authority, and the Normative Social Order

Edited by David Bolt

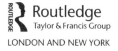

Routledge
Taylor & Francis Group

LONDON AND NEW YORK

First published 2021
by Routledge
2 Park Square, Milton Park, Abingdon, Oxon OX14 4RN

and by Routledge
605 Third Avenue, New York, NY 10158

Routledge is an imprint of the Taylor & Francis Group, an informa business

British Library Cataloguing-in-Publication Data
A catalogue record for this book is available from the British Library

Library of Congress Cataloging-in-Publication Data
Names: Bolt, David, editor.
Title: Metanarratives of disability : culture, assumed authority, and the normative social order / edited by David Bolt.
Description: Milton Park, Abingdon, Oxon ; New York, NY : Routledge, 2021. | Series: Autocritical disability studies | Includes bibliographical references and index.
Identifiers: LCCN 2020053522 (print) | LCCN 2020053523 (ebook) | ISBN 9780367523190 (paperback) | ISBN 9780367523206 (hardback) | ISBN 9781003057437 (ebook)
Subjects: LCSH: People with disabilities.
Classification: LCC HV1568 .M485 2021 (print) | LCC HV1568 (ebook) | DDC 305.9/08--dc23
LC record available at https://lccn.loc.gov/2020053522
LC ebook record available at https://lccn.loc.gov/2020053523

ISBN: 978-0-367-52320-6 (hbk)
ISBN: 978-0-367-52319-0 (pbk)
ISBN: 978-1-003-05743-7 (ebk)

Typeset in Bembo
by Deanta Global Publishing Services, Chennai, India

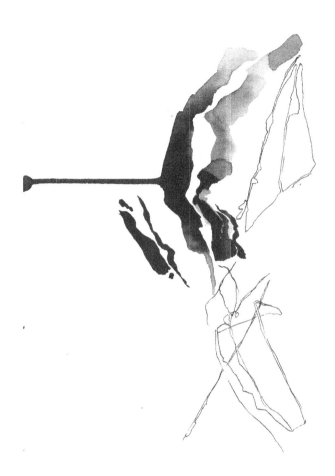

TRACK AND TRACE (V): OUR PATHS CROSS; WE DO NOT TOUCH.

Artwork by Claire Penketh

Description: Two characters extend from the top right-hand corner, across and into the centre of the page. They are uneven in tone, shifting from light to dark. The space between them varies and at different points they all but touch. At a midpoint, the left-hand mark shoots off at a near right angle. Beneath this spill are smaller disconnected brush marks. Below and to the side of the main protagonists are finer lines. Passing over and under one another, they trace uneven triangular and rectangular forms. The lines appear to cross yet touch nothing but the surface of the paper.

In loving memory of my dad and with eternal thanks to my mum
— David Bolt

CONTENTS

CONTRIBUTORS

Owen Barden is Associate Professor of Disability Studies at Liverpool Hope University in the United Kingdom. He completed his EdD at the University of Sheffield in 2011.

David Bolt is Personal Chair at Liverpool Hope University, the United Kingdom. He holds a PhD from the University of Staffordshire.

Helen Davies is Senior Lecturer in English Literature at the University of Wolverhampton in the United Kingdom. She completed her PhD at Leeds Beckett University in 2010.

Bianca C. Frazer is Postdoctoral Research Associate in Disability and Human Development at the University of Illinois at Chicago, the United States. She completed her PhD at the University of Colorado at Boulder in 2019.

Devon Healey is SSHRC Postdoctoral Fellow at York University in Canada. She completed her PhD at the University of Toronto in 2019.

Hemachandran Karah is Assistant Professor of English at the Indian Institute of Technology, Madras, India. He completed his PhD at Cambridge University in 2011.

Angela J. Kim is Doctoral Candidate at the University of Southern California, the United States. She completed her MA in 2021.

Danielle Kohfeldt is Assistant Professor of Community Psychology at California State University Long Beach, the United States. She completed her PhD at the University of California Santa Cruz in 2014.

Dana Combs Leigh is Doctoral Candidate at the University of Portsmouth, the United Kingdom. She completed her MA in 2019.

Sonya Freeman Loftis is Professor of English at Morehouse College, the United States. She holds a PhD from the University of Georgia.

Nicola Martin is Professor of Social Justice and Inclusive Education at London South Bank University, the United Kingdom. She holds a PhD from the University of Derby.

Katharine Martyn is Principal Lecturer and Disability Liaison Tutor at the University of Brighton, the United Kingdom. She completed her PhD in 2015.

Gregory Mather is pursuing MSc in Human Factors Psychology at California State University Long Beach, the United States. He completed his BSc at James Madison University in 2019.

Rod Michalko is (retired) Professor of Disability Studies at the University of Toronto in Canada. He holds a PhD from the University of British Columbia.

Alexis Padilla is Independent Researcher at the Phillips Theological Seminary, the United States. He completed his PhDs at the University of New Mexico in 1995 and 2018.

Claire Penketh is Associate Professor of Disability Studies at Liverpool Hope University, the United Kingdom. She completed her PhD at Goldsmiths College, University of London in 2010.

Erin Pritchard is Lecturer in Disability Studies at Liverpool Hope University, the United Kingdom. She completed her PhD at Newcastle University in 2014.

Annette Thompson is intern and service user at the University of Brighton, the United Kingdom. She completed her LLM at Birkbeck College, University of London in 2013.

Brenda Tyrrell is Doctoral Candidate at Miami University, the United States. She completed her MA at Iowa State University in 2017.

Steven J. Walden is Lecturer in Learning Disabilities Nursing at the University of South Wales, the United Kingdom. He completed his PhD at Cardiff University in 2017.

Heather R. Walker is Social Scientist at the University of Utah, the United States. She completed her PhD at the University of Illinois Chicago in 2019.

ACKNOWLEDGEMENTS

The editor thanks everyone who has made the idea of this volume a reality, from Claire Jarvis, Catherine Jones, and all involved at Routledge to Claire Penketh, who created the powerful and indeed beautiful artwork, Track and Trace (V): Our Paths Cross; We Do Not Touch, and the chapter authors Devon Healey, Rod Michalko, Alexis Padilla, Hemachandran Karah, Katharine Martyn, Annette Thompson, Angela J. Kim, Owen Barden, Steven J. Walden, Sonya Freeman Loftis, Helen Davies, Erin Pritchard, Danielle Kohfeldt, Gregory Mather, Heather R. Walker, Bianca C. Frazer, Nicola Martin, Brenda Tyrrell, and Dana Combs Leigh.

Given the interdisciplinary roots of the volume, broader thanks are due to Elizabeth J. Donaldson, Julia Miele Rodas, and everyone responsible for the Palgrave Macmillan/Springer Literary Disability Studies book series; as well as to Robert McRuer and all involved with Bloomsbury's *A Cultural History of Disability*. Similar thanks are of course due to Liverpool University Press and the extensive list of people who have made the *Journal of Literary and Cultural Disability Studies* a field-defining periodical, including editorial board members such as Rachel Adams, Susan Anderson, Clare Barker, Tammy Berberi, James Berger, Michael Berube, Stella Bolaki, Lucy Burke, Fiona Kumari Campbell, Simone Chess, Johnson Cheu, G. Thomas Couser, Michael Davidson, Lennard J. Davis, Helen Deutsch, Nirmala Erevelles, Jim Ferris, Anne Finger, Chris Foss, Ann Fox, Maria Frawley, Chris Gabbard, Rosemarie Garland-Thomson, Alice Hall, Beth Haller, Martin Halliwell, Diane Price Herndl, Martha Stoddard Holmes, Joyce Huff, Chloë Hughes, Jonathan Hsy, Merri Lisa Johnson, Alison Kafer, Deborah Kent, Georgina Kleege, Christopher Krentz, Miriamne Ara Krummel, Petra Kuppers, Stephen Kuusisto, Cynthia Lewiecki-Wilson, Rebecca Mallett, Susannah Mintz, David T. Mitchell, Stuart Murray, Catherine Prendergast, Margaret Price, Ato Quayson, Carrie Sandahl, Ralph Savarese, David Serlin,

Margrit Shildrick, Sharon L. Snyder, Tanya Titchkosky, Hannah Tweed, and Cynthia Wu.

As the institutional base of the volume, Liverpool Hope University must be credited. Everyone at this institution is due thanks and so cannot be named individually, but the School of Social Science has to be mentioned via Michael Lavalette, Amy Scott, Rhona O'Brien, Michael Brennan, Scott Massie, Lauren Whiston, Wendy Coxshall, Susan Creaney, and many others. Most obviously, thanks are due to everyone who has contributed to the work of the Centre for Culture and Disability Studies since its foundation in 2009, including core members such as Ana Bê, Leah Burch, Marie Caslin, Ria Cheyne, David Feeney, Manel Herat, Alan Hodkinson, Jennifer Hough, Dominika Kurek-Chomycz, Elizabeth Mitchell, Amy Redhead, Doris Rohr, Irene Rose, and Laura Waite, along with recurrent visitors such as Emmeline Burdett, Lisa Davies, Pauline Eyre, Cath Nichols, Sue Smith, Alex Tankard, David Doat, Harriet Dunn, Nina Michelle Worthington, Gesine Wegner, and many others.

On a still more personal level, the editor acknowledges that much gratitude is due to those who have been employed as academic support workers, from Sarah Cooper and Jane Goetzee at the University of Staffordshire to Tom Coogan, Heather Cunningham, Pippa Leddra, Heidi Mapley, Suzi Angus, and Holly Lightburn at Liverpool Hope University. These people have all been a pleasure to know and deserve every success in their subsequent ventures. Particular thanks are now due to the wonderful Kay Ross, who has taken up the post at the most difficult of times and yet approaches it with much appreciated cheer, as well as the requisite efficiency and reliability.

Finally, given that this volume is in part a product of the COVID-19 lockdowns, far from forgetting what happens when isolation becomes essential rather than incidental, the editor is keen to extend extra special thanks to Nisha Bolt, Stephen Bolt, and Ella Houston, as well as to Turgut Olgun, Andranik Naira Tigran, Karen White, Lorraine Case, and everyone else at Childwall's Eton Place and Boss Burgers, who week after week and month after month ensured that food, medication, technology, and other key provisions arrived as and when required. This community of family and friends proved paramount rather than merely nice in the editing of the present volume.

PROLOGUE

The inequity of the normative social order is divisive and profound. When out and about, many disabled people know only too well what it is to be erroneously told the error of our ways by passers-by, a primary example of normative arrogance cloaked in helpfulness and often accompanied by virtue signalling. Although support, assistance, and indeed helpfulness are all sometimes desired if not required, these things are distinct from the 'assumed authority' (Bolt, 2014, 9, 99) so widespread in its diminishment of agency that it even extends into the workplace, home, and so on. The trouble is that, in this divisive social order, benefiting from the knowledge of a colleague thereby becomes a matter of inclusion; enjoying the company of a friend becomes complicated by notions of duty; and sexual attraction becomes haunted by the spectre of charity. The other problem is that, amid this reframing, the non-disabled person is elevated to a level from which it is easier to grasp at opportunities and relationships that may be more pertinent to a disabled counterpart, meaning the latter becomes reduced to a stepping stone in the advancement of the former. In effect, everything from meritocracy to desirability is trumped by the received wisdom of the normative social order from which a sense of entitlement surely grows. This edited volume demonstrates that, although apparently automatic, the assumed authority is underpinned by a displacement of personal narratives in favour of overarching metanarratives of disability that find currency in a diverse multiplicity of cultural representations – ranging from advertising to comics, drama to film, novels to soap opera, social media to television, and so on. In so doing, the volume locates and reads social attitudes to disability in a cultural landscape.

The metanarrative of disability has its deepest theoretical roots in French philosophy. A cultural classic, *The Postmodern Condition* (Lyotard, 1984) identifies metanarratives in relation to a problematic universality that explains, and thus excludes, all personal narratives. Characteristic of modernity, these metanarratives organize and legitimize culture and politics by 'positing an origin (God) or an end (universal emancipation) that can supposedly organize a story without becoming part of it' (Macey, 2001, 167). When applied to the metanarrative of disability, in the terms of the tripartite model (i.e. normative positivisms, non-normative negativisms, and non-normative positivisms), both origin and end can be understood as normative positivisms (i.e. an indifference to the pros and cons of disability). Disability thereby becomes a product of its own exclusion, as the metanarrative effectively organizes and legitimizes social attitudes – and, by extension, actions.

Culturally informed engagements with social encounters can be traced back over half a century to classic work on stigma (Goffman, 1963; Hunt, 1966) and still resonate in what is sometimes termed critical disability theory. Most obviously relevant to the present volume are a couple of contributions to the first and second editions of *The Routledge Handbook of Disability Studies* (Bolt, 2012; Bolt, 2020), which invoke the metanarrative of disability alongside the concept of normative reductionism derived from *Extraordinary Bodies* (Garland-Thomson, 1997). This being so, the subject position of a so-called normal person is termed the normate, the reason being that, in social encounters, most destructive to the potential for continuing relations is such a person's assumption that a disability cancels out other qualities – reduces the complex disabled person to one attribute (Garland-Thomson, 1997). The metanarrative of disability (Bolt, 2012; Bolt, 2020) extends this model of social friction by adding that normate reductionism simultaneously initiates a grand expansion into the realms of myths, tropes, stereotypes, and other aspects of the cultural imagination. Personal narratives are displaced in favour of an overarching metanarrative of disability largely defined by non-disabled people.

In critical responses to culturally informed engagements with social encounters, the generalized conception of a metanarrative of disability is often productive, for it acknowledges a community of experience from which to draw, but the present volume deals with specifics. That is to say, over the past decade or so, many disabled people and other interested parties have discussed the manifestation of received notions in the social setting, critical conversations that have been assisted by the concept of the metanarrative of disability (Mapley, 2016; Burch, 2018; Cheyne, 2019). However, it can be useful to focus on a particular condition when illustrating or exploring the metanarrative. This specificity is demonstrable in a related monograph in David T. Mitchell and Sharon L. Snyder's Corporealities series (Bolt, 2014), where it is posited that the complex person who has a visual impairment is reduced to that impairment but also keyed to the metanarrative of blindness (i.e. a vast array of received notions and universals about 'the blind'). The present volume begins by deepening this foundational concept, reconsidering and reworking it from international perspectives far beyond the British base of the original, taking the literary starting point to a much broader cultural context.

Following a kind of deductive logic that traces the metanarrative from general disability to blindness, in particular, numerous foci become of obvious interest.

Judging by previously published work on condition-specific representation (e.g. Krentz and Sanchez, 2021; Coogan, 2014), consideration of the metanarrative of Deafness would be a clear line of progression, as would the metanarrative of scoliosis – if and when we start to move the focus away from the senses. The reception and perception of such non-normative bodies, as well as minds, helpfully termed bodyminds (Price, 2015; Schalk, 2018), are considered in the present volume via the metanarratives of mental illness, Obsessive Compulsive Disorder (OCD); learning disability; autism; Down syndrome; and dwarfism. All of these conditions are historically, or at least recently, acknowledged as factors in the disability experience.

More than expanding the scope of the metanarrative of blindness in relation to a selection of bodies and minds typically rendered beyond the normative divide, the present volume continues this expansion in relation to conditions that may be unnoticeable for some time but can involve an emerging identification with disability. Again, numerous other conditions could and should be included in the broader discourse, a couple of obvious examples being multiple sclerosis and consumption (Krummel, 2001; Tankard, 2018), but those on which the present volume's focus falls are chronic pain, diabetes, cancer, HIV and AIDS, sarcoidosis, and arthritis. After all, as increasingly recognized in the progressive field of disability studies (e.g. Patsavas, 2014; Price, 2015; Bê, 2016; Gould, 2017; Sheppard, 2020), such chronic conditions must also be recognized as aspects of the disability experience.

All in all, in this volume, multiple metanarratives of disability are illustrated to investigate the critical concept of assumed authority and the normative social order from which it derives. The metanarratives of disability thereby deconstruct to reveal, among others, self-other, adult-child, person-animal, strong-weak, rational-irrational, sexual-asexual, respected-ridiculed, and productive-unproductive binaries. The investigation is interdisciplinary in its crossing of lines among education, the humanities, the social sciences, and medicine, for the authors and analyses represent all of these schools. Most importantly, although this is an academic volume, it is far from irrelevant to practice; it is by no means premised on a false dichotomy of theory and reality. Not only are the authors researchers in the field, but it is also the case that most have direct or intimate experience of the conditions under discussion. Indeed, a guiding principle of this edited volume is that authors recognize their experience at the very epistemological level of their methodology, the aim being to herald formal advancement from critical theory and critical disability theory to autocritical disability theory.

References

Bê, A. (2016) Disablism in the lives of people living with a chronic illness in England and Portugal. *Disability and Society* 31 (4): 465–480.

Bolt, D. (2012) Social encounters, cultural representation and critical avoidance, in N. Watson, A. Roulstone, and C. Thomas (eds.), *Routledge Handbook of Disability Studies*. Abingdon: Routledge.

Bolt, D. (2014) *The Metanarrative of Blindness: A Re-Reading of Twentieth-Century Anglophone Writing.* Ann Arbor: University of Michigan Press.

Bolt, D. (2020) The metanarrative of disability: Social encounters, cultural representation and critical avoidance, in N. Watson and S. Vehmas (eds.), *Routledge Handbook of Disability Studies* (2nd edition). Abingdon: Routledge.

Burch, L. (2018) 'You are a parasite on the productive classes': Online disablist hate speech in austere times. *Disability and Society* 33 (3): 392–415.

Cheyne, R. (2019) *Disability, Literature, Genre: Representation and Affect in Contemporary Fiction.* Liverpool: Liverpool University Press.

Coogan, T. (2014) The 'hunchback': Across cultures and time, in D. Bolt (ed.), *Changing Social Attitudes Toward Disability: Perspectives from Historical, Cultural, and Educational Studies.* Abingdon: Routledge.

Garland-Thomson, R. (1997) *Extraordinary Bodies: Figuring Physical Disability in American Culture and Literature.* New York: Columbia University Press.

Goffman, E. (1963) *Stigma: Notes on the Management of Spoiled Identity.* Middlesex: Penguin.

Gould, D. (2017) 'I am/in pain': The form of suffering in David Wolach's *Hospitalogy* and Amber DiPietra and Denise Leto's *Waveform. Journal of Literary and Cultural Disability Studies* 11 (2): 169–185.

Hunt, P. (1966) *Stigma: The Experience of Disability.* London: Geoffrey Chapman.

Krentz, C. and Sanchez, R. (2021) Representations of deafness in literature and culture. *Journal of Literary and Cultural Disability Studies* 15 (2).

Krummel, M. (2001) Am I MS?, in J. C. Wilson and C. Lewiecki-Wilson, *Embodied Rhetorics: Disability in Language and Culture.* Carbondale: Southern Illinois University Press.

Lyotard, Jean-Francois. (1984) *The Postmodern Condition: A Report on Knowledge*, tr. Geoffrey Bennington and Brian Massumi. Manchester: Manchester University Press.

Macey, D. (2001) *The Penguin Dictionary of Critical Theory.* London: Penguin.

Mapley, H. (2016) 'Culture as pharmakon': Representation, social encounters, and discourses of disability. *Considering Disability Journal* 1 (3 and 4): 1–24.

Patsavas, A. (2014) Recovering a cripistemology of pain: Leaky bodies, connective tissue, and feeling discourse. *Journal of Literary and Cultural Disability Studies* 8 (2): 203–218.

Price, M. (2015) The bodymind problem and the possibilities of pain. *Hypatia* 30 (1): 268–284.

Schalk, S. (2018) *Bodyminds Reimagined: Disability, Race, and Gender in Black Women's Speculative Fiction*, Durham: Duke University Press.

Sheppard, E. (2020) Chronic pain as emotion. *Journal of Literary and Cultural Disability Studies* 14 (1): 5–20.

Tankard, A. (2018) *Invalid Lives.* London: Palgrave Macmillan/Springer.

PART I

International developments of the foundational concept

1

THE METANARRATIVE OF BLINDNESS IN NORTH AMERICA

Meaning, feeling, and feel

Devon Healey and Rod Michalko

Preliminary discussion

This chapter explores the metanarrative of blindness in contemporary Western culture. Zygmunt Bauman (2001, 1) tells us that all words have a meaning and some also have a 'feel'; *blindness* is one such word. The meaning of blindness cannot be separated from its feel, nor can its feel be separated from its meaning. The two comingle and live together in the single word *Blind*. The word itself almost forces a meaning and a feel into the world. It comes with a narrative, one replete with a feel of meaning and a meaningful feel. The word itself evokes a feeling in us connected to its meaning, and this feel comes to us automatically, naturally. It comes to us, too, as the authoritative voice of what blindness *is*. This voice is, of course, the voice of culture, and it tells the story of blindness, the metanarrative of what perception *is*, and of what it *means* to perceive. The voice of culture almost always speaks the meaning and feel of blindness in terms of its opposite, sight; and, it speaks blindness as though it were the opposite of sight, the lack of sight, as sight gone missing.

Methodological discussion

Our critical approach to the metanarrative is to explore the connection between the meaning of blindness and its feel through comparative analyses of two representations of blindness. We make use of the film *Scent of a Woman*[1] to reveal the ocular normative (Bolt, 2014) formation of blindness in contemporary Western

---

1 All quotations are taken from our viewing of the film, *Scent of a Woman*. Quotations are also taken from our listening to the audio recording of a live performance of the play, *Weights*. We are responsible for any inaccuracies in the transcription of quotations used in this chapter.

culture. Al Pacino, a sighted actor, plays Lieutenant Colonel Frank Slade, a blind character in this Hollywood film. *Scent of a Woman* is a cinematic portrayal of blindness and, like most of these portrayals, relies entirely on the ocular-centric (Levin, 1997) version of sight as the only legitimate way of being in the world and the ocular normative version of blindness as a severely limited way of being in the world. This film, set in New York City in the early 1990s, depicts blindness as the worst possible thing that can happen. Yet worse still is the fact that blindness happened to a white, middle-class military man. Conventional versions of masculinity, race, sight, and blindness intersect in this film. Blindness is shown to be a way of life not worthy of living, through the tacit invocation of the metanarrative of blindness as pity, tragedy, loss, and so on. We use this film as a backdrop to the version of blindness presented in the play *Weights*, written and performed by Lynn Manning.

It is crucial to note that a key feature of our methodology is our experience of blindness. This allows us to explore representations through the epistemological position of the experience of blindness. We treat blindness not as a lack of perception but as itself a perception that reveals an episteme particular to the experience. One of us is totally blind; the other, legally blind. These two experiences of blindness generate a further particularity of expression and a further epistemological positioning. This allows us to attend to language and to examine how it creates meanings of blindness in relation to sight. Dian Million (2014) puts it this way: 'I try to work with an attention to language – to listen for the way that people make meanings from the various meanings that are "always-already" available and the way they reach to move beyond these meanings' (41). She calls this methodological process 'languaging' (Million, 2014, 41). Our method, at the bottom, may also be understood as languaging – as an analysis of the language and thus the meaning and place of blindness in the world and its creative potential for making new meanings of and, places for, blindness.

Analytical discussion 1

A tale of two blindnesses

At age 23, in October 1978, Lynn Manning became blind. Like Al Pacino in *Scent of a Woman*, Manning's blindness came in extremely traumatic and even dramatic circumstances. Unlike Pacino's, Manning's blindness was real. Pacino's blindness came to him in the script of a Hollywood film; Manning's came to him in his life. Whether revealed in fiction or in non-fiction, blindness comes to us in a neatly wrapped but unrecognizable package of the life-world (Husserl, 1970; Schutz, 1967), of a world we have in common, a common-sense world. The life-world, with its assumed authority, presents blindness to us as though it were a 'natural condition' – understood as the result of the 'natural condition' of sight-gone-wrong. This authority is comprised of a plethora of implicated assumptions and presuppositions regarding what blindness *is*, its negative influence on people, what to do about such an influence, and how to live with it if nothing can be done to remove it. Both film and play rely upon the assumed authority of blindness for their production. They re-present versions of this authority in the presentation of blindness to their audiences.

What does each of these representations *do* with the assumed authority of blindness? Do they merely imitate it, or do they change it? How does each contribute to the sustaining of this authority? And finally, do both or either unsettle this assumed authority?

With these questions in mind, we analyze the circumstances of blindness in each portrayal, including the extreme trauma. Like blindness, this trauma relies upon an aspect of the assumed authority of the normative order. This authority intersects gender (specifically, masculinity) and race to produce the trauma socially. Both *Scent of a Woman* and *Weights* are set in the United States: the former, as we have said, in New York City in the early 1990s, and the latter in Los Angeles in the late 1970s.

Pacino plays his 'military man' character to its stereotypical hilt. This is understandable since the Colonel's blindness occurred in the midst of this stereotype. He was drunk and, as a way to show off his masculine military courage, juggled live grenades. Predictably, one exploded in his face, blinding him, perhaps the film's attempt to inflict a dent in the 'military man's' sense of courage and masculinity. Whether this attempt succeeded is doubtful since the assumed authority of the normative order's version of blindness intersecting with masculinity and the stereotype of the 'military man' orients the film from beginning to end.

The most striking difference between Manning's and the Colonel's onset of blindness is that the former is real. Manning was a 23-year-old Black man living in Los Angeles. Just before his blindness, his life began taking a turn for the better. He was the second oldest of nine children. Although his first few years of life were happy and he experienced family bliss, it did not last long. His parents began to drink heavily and have violent arguments. Manning and his siblings were relegated to the bedroom where they could hear their parents fight. 'Our new knowledge of the violent possibilities', he says in *Weights*, 'caused the nights to fall with ominous swiftness. Sleep for me came through quiet rocking and prayers to God that I'd awaken in the morning and find that it had been all one long bad dream' (Manning, 2000).

The nightmare culminated with Manning's mother stabbing his father and the two separating. His mother continued to drink heavily, resulting in the family living in 'squalor' and 'abject poverty' (Manning, 2000). It did not take long for the state to remove Manning and his siblings from their home, to place them in foster care. None of the children ever returned home. Manning moved from foster home to foster home, from school to school, until he eventually secured a 'good job' (Manning, 2000) in the same boys home in which he was detained from time to time when he was a juvenile. Manning's father taught him to draw when he was a child and he pursued this love in adulthood. He began painting on canvas and was an aspiring artist. The 'universe', as he put it, 'was turning in my favor' (Manning, 2000). It was then that Murphy's law (i.e. anything that can go wrong will go wrong) kicked in.

Manning went to his favourite Hollywood bar to celebrate his good fortune. He was provoked into a fight that ended badly and he was shot in the head. The bullet severed his optic nerve and left him blind in both eyes. Manning's understanding of blindness, however, began much earlier.

Guided by Murphy's law, Manning prepared for the most difficult of fates for a visual artist. 'What's the worst possible thing that can happen to you?' he asked himself. 'To go blind', was his answer (Manning, 2000). With this in mind he began preparing for blindness; tying his shoes, using the telephone, washing dishes – he did these things in the dark or with his eyes closed. This was Manning's version of blindness. It was simply not seeing; it was the lack of sight, and it was doing things that sighted people did, but doing them without sight. He did not want blindness to 'catch' him 'off guard' (Manning, 2000). It was five years later (i.e. half a decade after he began to prepare for blindness) that the worst thing happened: he became blind. But, his experience of blindness was not the blindness for which he had prepared. Instead of not seeing, *he was seeing*. Yet, he was seeing sights that he had not seen before: 'colour and geometric shapes' (Manning, 2000).

With this experience, and 'cruising on pain killers' as he lay on his hospital bed (Manning, 2000), he became anxious regarding the cause of his blindness. One aspect of the taken-for-granted character of blindness, an authoritative sensibility that comes to us automatically, is that it indicates something wrong and that it is caused by something, something external to itself. Manning wondered whether he had subconsciously brought on his blindness, if he was subconsciously fulfilling his own 'orbit prophecy' (Manning, 2000). He knew that despite seeing colours and geometric shapes on his mental canvas, that this was, nonetheless, blindness. 'But', then again, he wondered, 'is this blindness or madness?' (Manning, 2000). He concluded he could 'handle' blindness as long as he did not bring it on himself, as long as his blindness was not 'hysterical blindness' (Manning, 2000).

'Something akin to joy surges through me', was Manning's response when the doctor informed him that he would be blind for the rest of his life and that it was a gunshot wound that caused his blindness. He was not 'mad'. 'You do understand what I am telling you, Mr. Manning?' was the doctor's response to Manning's expression of joy at the news. The doctor informed his mother and sister that his reaction to being told that he would be totally blind for the rest of his life was 'abnormal' and that he would 'bear close watching for a while' (Manning, 2000). This made his hospital visitors both sad and cautious around him, so Manning spent most of his time 'trying to cheer them up', which was understood as 'more abnormal behaviour' on his part (Manning, 2000).

But, as he says, 'loss has been an integral part of our family history' (Manning, 2000). The assumed authority of the normative order that surrounds blindness in our culture frames it as a loss, a devastating one at that. Like any loss, blindness framed as such generates the implicit requisite of grieving. Celebrating blindness, feeling it as 'akin to joy', according to the metanarrative, could be understood as nothing other than a sign of mental health deterioration brought on by the shock following the devastating loss. Manning's response to blindness did not rely on this metanarrative resulting in his being psychologized as not accepting his loss, his blindness. This is why the necessity of grieving comes with the prerequisite of the metanarrative of loss, one that is ubiquitous in *Scent of a Woman*.

Unlike Manning's prior knowledge of, and preparation for the possibility of, blindness and his subsequent joy in being blind, Lieutenant Colonel Frank Slade is portrayed in *Scent of a Woman* as a man encumbered with, and by, blindness. The assumed authority of this film relies upon the tropes of loss and tragedy. The loss of one's sight and the tragic life of blindness in a world of sights to be seen is what grounds both the meaning and the feel of blindness.

Colonel Slade is committed to ending his life, as a life in blindness is one that, to him, is not worth living. He laments, 'What life? I got no life! I'm in the dark here! You understand? I'm in the dark!' (*Scent of a Woman*, 1992). The cultural understanding of blindness as darkness is one that haunts both sighted and blind people alike. The being of blindness has been narrated as though the person who is blind is in a constant state of vulnerability, trapped in a world cloaked by the unknown and unrecognizable darkness that is blindness. There must, however, be a glimmer of hope, some semblance of resilience within the blind character – otherwise, why watch? And so, the metanarrative of blindness becomes the story of the resilience, not of people but of the senses.

There are the sounds of movement, the smell of freshly baked bread, and of course, the scent of a woman. There are the memories hidden deep within the body – muscle memory – to do, to dance, to drive. The heightened abilities of 'the blind' to tap into a world unknown to those with sight, these are the gifts from, and of, darkness that work to make the metanarrative of blindness not desirable but at least palatable. Pacino's character knows the exact brand of perfume a woman is wearing from a distance; he can dance the tango with skill and grace with no more than the 'coordinates' of an unknown dancefloor; he can sense the physicality of someone in the room, 'Don't shrug [...] I'm blind [...] save your body language'; and drive a Ferrari so well that he is able to fool a police officer into thinking he is sighted (*Scent of a Woman*, 1992). The height-ened senses of blindness portrayed in this film serve as the reason for Colonel Slade to keep living. It is not blindness that is explored or appreciated; it is the remaining senses that dull the pain of blindness.

The metanarrative's understanding of blindness permeates our social imagi-nary such that Pacino's portrayal of blindness is not merely box office worthy, there is no question of whether people will pay to watch blindness portrayed onscreen, but also Academy Award winning; the very portrayal of blindness garners accolades. Ironically, the portrayal of sight by blind people also garners accolades. And yet, unlike Pacino in his portrayal of blindness, no blind person has ever won an Oscar for their portrayal of sight. Most interestingly, blind people do not play blind people on the silver screen; sighted people do. Perhaps, blind people play sighted people on the biggest stage of all – the stage of everyday life (Healey, 2019). *Scent of a Woman* may be 'seen' as a feature film-long lament, a lament of the loss of sight with no 'light' at the end of the grieving tunnel. This is why it is conventionally understood that blindness *must* be grieved and not merely lamented if any 'progress' is to be made.

Analytical discussion 2

Loss

Loss, a key aspect of the metanarrative of blindness, is revealed vividly in *Weights* in the words of a rehabilitation councillor, herself legally blind: 'I'm really surprised to see you here so soon after your accident, Mr. Manning. It's only been, what, three weeks?' (Manning, 2000). He explains that he wants to 'take control' of his life 'as quickly as possible' to which the councillor says,

> Mr. Manning, after a loss such as yours there is a grieving process that occurs. There are phases you have to go through. This usually takes several months, with some people it can take years.
>
> *(Manning, 2000)*

Any deviation from the metanarrative's ascription of loss requires some sense to be made of that deviation. One of the more common ways to make sense of such deviation is to frame it within the concept of lack of information. Manning could not have been aware of how devastating a loss the onset of his blindness was and that he was required to grieve. He complicated the situation still further by suggesting that he did not have to grieve the loss, that he already accepted his blindness – more abnormal behaviour on his part. This, of course, did not deter the councillor, who informed him that 'he has to come to terms with losing his sight' (Manning, 2000).

The exchange portrayed by Manning in *Weights* demonstrates just how authoritative and how assumed the metanarrative of blindness as loss is in our culture. Equally as important, it demonstrates how such a narrative orientates the lives of some blind people and is sustained *by* those lives. This is not surprising since most disabled people come from non-disabled families (Zola, 1993, 167). Most of us grow up with the implicit and powerful understanding that the world is 'sighted' and, for anyone who is not, there remain the related traces of cure, acceptance, and rehabilitation culminating in a 'normal life' and being 'just like everyone else', with the emphasis on 'like' (Stiker, 2019, 16). After all, this metanarrative generates blind people as reasonable facsimiles of sighted people, but only facsimiles and hopefully reasonable ones at that. The closer a blind person resembles a sighted person, the more they fit in and, belong to, the presumptive 'sighted world'.

Once Manning realized he would not get rehabilitation services before he grieved the loss of his sight, he asked the councillor what he could expect in terms of a career after rehabilitation. She told him there were many vocational possibilities, and the most promising one was operating his own retail snack franchise. His response to this career possibility traversed the disability-race intersection: 'I may be new to this blind thing, but this feels awfully close to being offered my own shoe-shine stand' (Manning, 2000).

Manning told the councillor that his aspiration was to go to college with the aim of becoming a writer. Given that the councillor's orientation to blindness was fuelled by the taken-for-granted assumption that blindness was a technical problem in need of technical solutions, her response was predictable: 'Mr. Manning, careers in the arts are something we really do like to discourage' (Manning, 2000). Disabled or not, the 'failure rates' were 'phenomenal' and it was her job to steer him towards 'the best possibilities for success' (Manning, 2000).

Manning's orientation to blindness, new as it was to him, was not fuelled by this orientation. His orientation did not give way to the metanarrative's ascription of pity, or psychological grieving and acceptance, nor did it generate an understanding of blindness as merely and only a technical problem. He had 'dreams' away from which people had been steering him for most of his life, and he was 'not going to let that happen again' (Manning, 2000). 'You may not want to believe me, but the grieving process is real', were the last words the rehabilitation councillor spoke to him (Manning, 2000).

Treating blindness as a technical problem in need of technical solutions is an implicit assumption tacitly evoked not only by sighted people but by blind people as well, as attested to by the rehabilitation councillor. The need to cultivate a utilitarian orientation to life is something possessed by everyone. How to get through life, to achieve success; how to do whatever it is we do within the normative order of specific cultural and societal structures formed within local and global contexts are key features of human life. Blindness, however, brings these features to a pedestrian level while simultaneously framing them in an arcane orientation.

How do you get to point A from point B when blind? How do you wash dishes? How do you sort your money and where do you get money in the first place? All of these activities, and many more like them, typically taken for granted by sighted people, are almost violently extracted from the taken-for-granted realm of the life-world by blindness. Even the thought of becoming blind often jerks people from the relative safety of sight, in particular from the taken-for-granted apparatus of functioning sight that allows for the assumed way of doing the ordinary things of ordinary life. Blindness brings this ordinariness to conciseness revealing, often in an astonishing and bewildering way, the unsettling character of a life stripped of its taken-for-granted nature. Perhaps, it is this life we grieve when we go through the grieving process that blindness is said to inevitably bring.

Manning tells his mother and his sister of his interview with the rehabilitation councillor. They encourage him to take her advice and pursue a practical vocation rather than a career as a writer. He becomes frustrated with this response and says 'screw Mrs. Herferd. I got to do for my damn self. I am the one who is blind here. I'm the one who's got to live with this shit' (Manning, 2000).

The expression of frustration shown by Manning is not surprising. Frustration is often interpreted as a reasonable, if not inevitable, expression of 'coming to terms' with blindness and accepting its limitations. Within an ocularnormative social order, blindness is a limiting condition requiring a practical response as a way to mitigate the inevitability of blindness as a limiting condition.

This metanarrative of blindness includes the concept of 'help'. We can do for our 'damn self' when the condition of life is that of the normative able body (McRuer, 2017), but not when this normative order goes wrong. The normative body, mind, and senses bring with them 'normal limitations', limitations that we take for granted and with which we 'come to terms' in the same way. For this, help is not required. In contrast, the disappearance of these normative structures simultaneously disappears any semblance of 'normal limitations' and brings to the fore with shocking suddenness the debilitating feel of 'abnormal limitations'. It is the devastation of this state of affairs that requires coming to terms with and, for this, we cannot do for our 'damn self', and so help is needed. But first, the traumatic loss of 'normal limitations' must be grieved. We must come to terms with the 'fact' for our 'damn self' under these conditions.

Even though Manning did not understand his blindness as solely a technical problem, he did know that, like all other ways of experiencing the world, blindness too required its own set of techne in order to allow it to explore its experiential and horizons of creative possibility. For this, he searched for a source that would give him the techniques to accomplish the mundane everyday tasks for which he once prepared – washing dishes, tying his shoes – not in the dark but in his blindness, and he now added to his list 'how to get from point A to point B and how to figure out where the hell you are once you get there', how to live alone in his own apartment, and, perhaps most importantly, how to write (Manning, 2000). Mrs. Herferd, the rehabilitation councillor, was not willing to provide Manning with these techniques given her particular way of understanding blindness; but the same was not true of the Brail Institute, a rehabilitation centre for blind people in Los Angeles.

Analytical discussion 3

Putting techne in its place and the making of a different blindness

At the Brail Institute, Manning found the techniques for which he was searching (i.e. orientation and mobility, the use of a white cane, typing, and brail); learned techniques for doing everyday tasks; and was then prepared to move with his blindness from the realm of techne into that of creative perceptual possibilities. He began to describe the 'feel' of blindness, a feel that went beyond blindness understood as solely a technical problem and beyond its accompanying metanarrative of blindness as living 'with this shit'. After a few orientation and mobility lessons, for example, he was thrilled 'just to be able to dictate something as simple as my own pace' (Manning, 2000). Conceiving of blindness in relation to 'pace' and dictating this pace marks the beginning of the removing of blindness from the pace of sight and permitting it a 'freedom of movement' (Michalko and Titchkosky, 2020, 71), a freedom typically understood as the feature loss in the loss of sight. So deeply is such a loss felt in accordance with the metanarrative of blindness that any freedom and pace that blindness has is also lost to any possible conception or perception of it. The only choice this metanarrative offers blindness is to follow, as best as it can, in the movement of sight and to provide it with the technologies to keep up with the pace of sight, again, as best it can.

Following is an oppressive, if all too familiar, phenomenon making up a large part of the experience of marginalized groups (Ahmed, 2006; Sharpe, 2016). Linda Martin Alcoff (2006) explores the converse of following. Social identities often precede those of us who are marginalized:

> As we move through the myriad of social settings that make up our world, we find ourselves already known and our identities already defined in those settings. They await us as though anticipating our arrival and yet surprised as though not expecting us to show up.
>
> *(Alcoff, 2006, 193)*

Our blindness, as we have shown, is often defined within the metanarrative's strands of grief, pity, dependence, and so on. We are known through this structure and the subsequent interpretation of us with its practices and interactions that orient the treatment of us are direct results of this metanarrative of blindness. Those who typically populate these structures and institutions of our society know blindness and thus know us long before we make our way on the scene. They know, too, and all too well, whether we fit in and belong to these institutions and whether or not we are part of that population. Equally as important, they know, and have always known, precisely what role blindness plays in their population, since they have already written the script.

Assumed authority represents an enactment of such metanarrative structures. Not only do sighted others automatically know us before we make an appearance in their midst, they also know this with authority; their knowledge is authoritative and surpasses the knowledge that is ours – the knowledge of the world we bring when we enter their lives. These settings are, after all, built by, and for, those who are sighted, and part of this construction includes the exclusion of the distortion that is blindness. As Tanya Titchkosky puts it, we are 'included as an excludable type' (Titchkosky, 2008, 46). Our exclusion is all but certain; our inclusion remains always-already precarious. The former marks our existential state of being; the latter hinges upon our capacity to follow 'in the wake' of sight (Sharpe, 2016, 13).

In *Weights*, Manning depicts alternative narratives of blindness to the one held by sight and sketches some of the possibilities of such alternatives. He begins his narrative restructuring epistemologically, with knowledge and knowing. His restructuring is not, however, strictly an epistemological matter. Knowledge and knowing are now wrapped, for him, in the ontology of blindness: 'A whole new way of knowing the world was opening up to me' (Manning, 2000). This way of knowing opened up as Manning began to move in the world after learning the technique of moving with a white cane. Not only did he make the 'dorky' rhythm of white cane use look 'cool', but he began to 'dictate' his own 'pace' (Manning, 2000). He began to experience moving *in* blindness and not merely *with* it as it follows the wake of sight. Learning to move and know in this way started something far beyond technique. This way of being blind is not a derivative of the typical metanarrative of blindness. Instead, it represents the beginning of carving out a blind identity at our own pace and crossing over the turbulence of the path sight leaves in its wake. It is, as Manning suggests, to experience the world through the body. He begins experiencing the world through his body, his nose, his ears, his pores, and in this new way of knowing the world, the world 'came closer' to him (Manning, 2000). He said that the world he was now experiencing, now that he was blind, was not anywhere near its 'former infinity' (Manning, 2000). Blindness brought the world to him; he was more intimate with the world.

'In the absence of that vastness, that visual feast', Manning 'came to recognize the overwhelming distraction that sight had been' (Manning, 2000). Blindness is not merely the absence of sight as it is typically posited. It is the absence of the 'vastness', the absence of a veritable 'feast' of visuality. It is almost as though sight is imposing itself onto the world and into its inhabitants; as though it is forcing its way into our understanding and knowledge not only of the world but of ourselves; sight has positioned itself as the 'master' of our sensorium and of our way of experiencing. Manning's personal narrative offers a counternarrative to this 'vastness' and 'visual feast' understood as mastery; he offers a narrative of blindness that 'sees' the distraction from intimacy that is sight. Coming to know the world more intimately through the body, Manning askes in *Weights*, 'who knew such sensory lushness existed in this more immediate realm?'; he answers, 'Blind people knew. Blind people had to have known all along' (Manning, 2000).

The world Manning was discovering in his blindness, the one that came to him through his blindness – its lushness, its intimacy – was not the only version of blindness he was discovering. He was discovering sight's conception of blindness as well: 'Coming to terms with my blindness was a challenge. Coming to terms with other people's perception of it was something else' (Manning, 2000). He began to realize that 'living with this shit' included the challenge of living with other people's perception of the experience, the metanarrative of blindness. He soon began to realize that his blindness was not the only one with which he had to live.

Despite his six-foot-two, 220-pound stature, people would try to 'help' him up curbs and onto busses: 'All they managed to do is throw me off my balance and make me look as clumsy as they assumed I was in the first place' (Manning, 2000). Clumsiness, weakness, and groping are not essential features of blindness, nor are they the essential qualities of blind people. The 'groping blind' (Bolt, 2014, 14) is a social invention, a creation of a metanarrative of blindness enacted as such. Who knew blind people groped? Sighted people knew. Sighted people had to have known all along. Groping, then, is but one feature of one blindness among many with which we live as our blindness brings the world closer to us.

Much of our life in blindness is presented to us as knowledge and its lack by the taken-for-granted world and the assumed authority of its knowledge. Moving through the world of a kaleidoscope of meanings and feels of blindness, we navigate not merely the material world but the world of the kaleidoscope[2] of blindness as well. The white cane, as Manning discovered, might help us navigate the material world, but it acts in an almost magical way to bring the world's sense of blindness to our attention. Manning speaks of this in *Weights* through a poem titled 'The Magic Wand':

> My final form is never my choosing
> I only wield the wand
> You are the magicians.
>
> *(Manning, 2000)*

Disability studies, activism, and the arts have shown us, time and time again, that disabled people move through a world full of barriers. The world is largely inaccessible to us insofar as it has been and, continues to be, created by and for those who understand themselves as non-disabled. Perhaps, the most solid and impenetrable of these barriers is the one of which Manning speaks; the many blindnesses of the world act to generate both an identity and a place for blind people. The form of these identities and places are 'never [our] choosing'. Our blindness does act like a magic wand and the 'sighted world' with its people are the magicians. Not only do they magically create our final form, they also magically disappear the social processes of interpretation that leads to this 'final form'. *Sight is truly magical.*

What is astonishing in its paradox is that we, blind people ourselves, harbour remnants of the magic of sight within. We, too, make something with the wands we wield. We, too, harbour many blindnesses in our wands. Ocularcentrism and ocularnormativity are inescapable. This is exemplified in Manning's characterization

---

2 Stephen Kuusisto in, *Planet of the Blind* (1998, 13) makes use of the concept 'kaleidoscope' as a way to describe what he sees in his blindness. His use of this concept is visual in character and follows the ocular sense of it. We, in contrast, use 'kaleidoscope' as a synesthesia to depict the plethora of meanings and feels that accompany blindness as it moves through the meanings with which culture endows it.

of a personal encounter he had with his writing teacher, Meghan, at the Brail Institute: 'I don't know how to read this woman. I can't see her mouth, her eyes, her body language. I can't read anything beyond the touch of those few fingers, such weight they have' (Manning, 2000). He is lost in his attempt to read this woman. Reading requires sight; reading print and reading people take on a surprising similarity when the metanarrative of blindness presents sight as the quintessential path to knowledge. Harbouring this narrative, blind people sometimes fear misreading a situation, making a mistake, as though mistakes are not part of the lives of sighted people. And yet, blindness ironically magnifies our mistakes. As Manning says, he fears coming across as 'the needy blind dude' (Manning, 2000).

Manning's discovery of a more intimate world in his blindness is the other side of this fear and his writing becomes a way for him to explore *both* sides. As he wakes up on the first morning of life in his new apartment, he says, 'I start a pot of coffee brewing; splash water on my face; feed a blank page into the typewriter and begin to write' (Manning, 2000). This is a sharp contrast to Lieutenant Colonel Slade driving a Ferrari.

Concluding discussion

Rather than a discussion, we conclude with a blind awakening, a poem depicting waking with blindness at the end of *Weights*:

> Eyes wide and unshielded from glare.
> Undistracted by colour and contrast.
> Unified in shadow.
> It is then that the imagination can reach up into itself and grasp the universe.
>
> *(Manning, 2000)*

In this chapter, we attempt to depict meanings and feels of blindness as they are lived and experienced by blind people. We attempt, too, an exploration of dramatic expressions of blindness, one fictional, the other 'real'. This is our way to demonstrate our life in blindness as we live it in the midst of the meanings and feels of blindness available to us in the world. And like Million (2014) suggests, we attempt to demonstrate the possibility that we might 'reach to move beyond these meanings' (41) and feels; to allow 'the imagination [to] reach up into itself and grasp the universe' (Manning, 2000). There is something exhilarating about two blind authors writing together and reaching up with the imagination of blindness to explore new possibilities for the ways blindness can mean and feel.

References

Ahmed, S. (2006) Orientations: Toward a queer phenomenology, *GLC: A Journal of Lesbian and Gay Studies* 12 (4): 543–574.

Alcoff, L. M. (2006) *Visible identities: Race, gender and the self*, New York: Oxford University Press.

Bauman, Z. (2001) *Community: Seeking safety in an insecure world*, Cambridge: Polity.

Bolt, D. (2014) *The metanarrative of blindness: A re-reading of twentieth-century Anglophone writing*, Ann Arbor: University of Michigan Press.

Scent of a Woman (1992) Film. Directed by Martin Brest, Universal Pictures.

Healey, D. (2019) *Blindness in V acts: Disability studies as critical creative inquiry*, [Doctoral dissertation, University of Toronto]. ProQuest Dissertations Publishing.

Husserl, E. (1970) *Introduction to phenomenological philosophy*, Transl. D. Carr, Evanston: Northwestern University Press.

Kuusisto, S. (1998) *Planet of the blind*, New York: Dial Press.

Levin, D. M. (1997) *Signs of vision: The discursive construction of sight in the history of philosophy*, Cambridge: MIT Press.

Manning, L. (2000 [revised unpublished script 2007]). *Weights*. Written and Performed by Lynn Manning; Off Broadway Premiere by *Theatre by the blind*, 2004.

McRuer, R. (2017) Compulsory able-bodiedness and queer/disabled existence, in, L. J. Davis (Ed.), *The disability studies reader* (5th ed.), New York: Routledge.

Michalko, R., and Titchkosky, T. (2020) Blindness: A cultural history of blindness, in, D. T. Mitchell and S. L. Snyder (Eds.), *A cultural history of disability in the 20th century*, New York: Bloomsbury.

Million, D. (2014) There is a river in me: Theory from life, in, A. Simpson and A. Smith (Eds.), *Theorizing native studies*, Durham: Duke University Press.

Schutz, A. (1967) *The phenomenology of the social world*, Evanston: Northwestern University Press.

Sharpe, C. (2016) *In the wake: On blackness and being*, Durham: Duke University Press.

Stiker, H. J. (2019) *A history of disability*, Trans. W. Sayers, Ann Arbor: University of Michigan Press.

Titchkosky, T. (2008) 'To pee or not to pee?' Ordinary talk about extraordinary exclusions in a university environment, *Canadian Journal of Sociology* 3 (1): 37–60.

Zola, I. K. (1993) Self, identity and the naming question: Reflections on the language of disability, *Social Science and Medicine* 36 (2): 167–173.

2

THE METANARRATIVE OF BLINDNESS IN THE GLOBAL SOUTH

A LatDisCrit counterstory to the bittersweet mythology of blindness as giftedness

Alexis Padilla

Preliminary discussion

Through the universalizing gaze of Western, Eurocentric cultural representations, being blind in the Global South might seem very much like being blind in the Global North. After all, the 'impairment' is conceived as the same. Yet, somehow, using a similar universalizing representation of blind professionals in the Global South is not as common. The unstated assumption in the background of Eurocentric, colonializing representations is that blind professionals in the Global South are either non-existent or an unusual extension of class privilege (Teklu, 2007).

This chapter describes a metanarrative of blindness which has unique representational features insofar as it (1) relates and reflects events that take place in the Global South and (2) keeps in mind Global North readership as its addressee, particularly in terms of representational tropes and hidden assumptions that may filter their interpretational stance for this unique metanarrative. In parallel, the chapter pursues a critical hermeneutics (Morrow, 1994; Roberge, 2011) reading of the reifying representational and discursive symbolism embedded in my 1980s nickname as El Libro Gordo de Petete (hereafter, ELGP), alluding to a television series with the same name which aired in Latin America and Spain (and which now sells as a children's series in several collectible comic books; see ELGP, 2011, for a sample episode from the original television series).

There is another point to clarify here. Bolt (2014) warns about the complex contours of the word *blind* as an identitarian-designating concept. Omansky's (2011) emancipatory research volume, which aims to elevate the grey zone occupied by the ontological realities and experiential layers of understanding unique to 'legally blind' individuals in the United States goes in a similar, although qualitatively different, direction. Despite these cautionary indications, and respecting their epistemological and axiological value, I opt to use the word *blind*, especially since the Global South's designations and categorizations to which I have been exposed for decades in Latin America rely on this nomenclature.

The meritocratic ambiguities embedded in the counterstory and metanarrative of blindness central to this chapter go way beyond mere unintentional misrepresentations. Their bittersweet characterization of blindness as giftedness, as a super-brain mythology of sorts, stems from a paradoxical generalized conviction on the part of sighted individuals about the inability of the blind to know so many 'real' things of life precisely because they lack the ocularcentric power inherent to 'normal' folks. There is in fact a popular saying highly diffused throughout Latin America and Spain: 'el que no sabe es como el que no ve' (whose equivalent in English would be the one who does not know is like the one who does not see). Its implication, of course, is that not seeing or not seeing well is tantamount to not knowing, to ignorance of the things that really matter. In this sense, these representational mythologies permeate the micro and macropolitical spheres of what certain thinkers (Maldonado-Torres, 2007; Wynter, 2003) call the coloniality of being, knowledge, and power (see also Quijano, 1992, 2000, for a political philosophy perspective on these notions coming from Latin America).

It is thus fitting for me to end this preliminary discussion with a word on LatDisCrit. In my last doctoral dissertation (Padilla, 2018), where I was exploring issues of intersectional agency, I came up with the term *LatDisCrit*. Through it, I pursue (Padilla, Forthcoming) a critical merging of the literature strands associated with LatCrit (Bernal, 2002; Dávila and de Bradley, 2010; Solórzano and Bernal, 2001; Valdes, 1999, 2000; Yosso, 2000) and DisCrit (Annamma, Connor, and Ferri, 2013, 2016; Annamma, Ferri, and Connor, 2019). Both literature strands stress the significance of looking critically at the interplay of race/ethnicity, diasporic cultures, historical sociopolitics, and disability in relation to the multiple possibilities of Global South and Global North Latinx identities. Most of the works are carried out in Global North contexts. Nevertheless, Global South epistemologies are an important part of the emerging political embodiments enacted through LatDisCrit as a paradigm. This is especially evident among decolonial Latinx and intersectionally grounded critical feminist political philosophers (Alcoff, 2009; Calderón, 2014; Castro-Gómez, 2002, 2007; Mignolo, 2000; Mignolo and Tlostanova, 2006; Mignolo and Walsh, 2018; Saldívar, 1991 and 2012; Sandoval, 2000; Wynter, 2003).

Methodological discussion

This chapter builds on the idea of assumed authority as an extension of nor-mate reductionism (Garland-Thomson, 1997; Bolt, 2012; Bolt, 2014; Bolt, 2020). On the basis of my firsthand experiential reflection as a blind Latinx non-white scholar and activist born and raised in the Global South, yet residing and struggling for more than three decades in the Global North, I expand on the general argumentation presented in this edited volume to the effect that this reductionism derives from culturally filtered representations of extraordinary bodies and disabling constructions of their social beings. In my case, I target Global South higher education contexts of representational reductionism for disabled people. Overarching dynamics in these contexts are so pervasive that they stifle whatever meagre meritocratic prospects disabled people could realistically aspire to in settings where corruption is rampant, classist colonialist linking mechanisms and cast-like exclusionary modes of stratification are prevalent (Aramayo, 2005; Bustos García, 2014; Ferrante and Dukuen, 2017; Ferrante and Joly, 2017; Lajous Vargas, 2019; Miguez, 2013; Miguez, Piñato and Machado, 2013).

Methodologically speaking, one of the most important features of critical race theory, and LatCrit in particular, is counterstorytelling (Yosso, 2006). This mode of counter-narrative constitutes both a methodological and an epistemological component. It simultaneously aims to disrupt dominant, normalizing narratives as well as establishing generalizable metatheoretical concepts or frameworks of relevance for situated emancipatory resistance in conjunction to subaltern actors. Among certain Latinx circles, counterstories are also called testimonios (Flores and García, 2009). In the words of Moraga (2011), testimonios are theory in the flesh, that is, they give a tangible sense of existential embodiment to conceptual and metatheoretical explorations.

It is thus true that the chapter is closely tied to autobiographical elements. However, these elements are articulated as reflexive, metatheoretical testimonies. In the past (Padilla, 2018), I formulated counterstories through the pseudonym *Arturo*. I employed Arturo in the critical hermeneutics of cultivating what Ricoeur (1981) and others characterize as distanciation. Arturo represented a 'distanciation alter ego, a textual means to read through critical hermeneutics events which I have experienced firsthand but whose analysis is tackled … in terms of Ricoeur's … assertion that authors are the first interpreters of their text' (Padilla, 2018, 9).

Since most of the events in this chapter's counterstory go back almost 40 years, there is already a strong element of distanciation. Hence, I have opted to use the first-person autobiographical tone ubiquitous in this edited volume. My analysis centres, however, on elevating the normalizing features of meritocratic representational ambiguities which permeate the chain of events and the organizational culture of 'myths and ceremonies' (as characterized in Meyer and Rowan's 1978 classical sociological piece) in the Global South context of higher education institutions at stake in the metanarrative of blindness I analyze.

On the other hand, as mentioned in the previous section, there is a discursive element as well, which links my analysis with the cultural sociology tradition (Alexander, 2003; Alexander, Giesen and Mast, 2006) and the critical hermeneutics heritage of Paul Ricoeur. Methodology-wise, it is worth mentioning with respect to Ricoeur's contribution, his core idea that social action itself can and should be analyzed as a text (Ricoeur, 1971, 1974). For my purposes, this means that even the organizational and macro-sociological components, which seem to occupy a peripheral place in the flow of my counterstory, acquire special significance as paratextual ingredients for its overall understanding and explanation.

Analytical discussion 1

The 1980s higher education context for disabled people in Venezuela

Since the late 1930s, it was an 'urban legend' of Venezuelan democracy that Arturo Uslar Pietri, then minister of education, had coined the phrase *sowing oil*. Nonetheless, it was not until the oil nationalization process of the 1970s that resources were substantially transferred into education and health to engender a snowball trickling effect that would allow disabled people from working-class families like myself to go to university and graduate with professional degrees. Although, it must be said that this process of shifting public investments was at the time indirect, driven by a rhetoric of developmentalist modernism.

Only a few blind folks, or disabled people for that matter, got to this higher learning stage. For them, especially blind people, law proved to be the most permeable degree. This was true only for males and exclusively in the provincial context of a couple of historical 'autonomous' (public entities which, at that time, held the highest quality indicators in the Venezuelan and international rankings) universities in the western part of the country.

I met disabled individuals in Caracas during the 1980s who had to drop out of their higher education options altogether. They did so despite having circumvented a complicated and highly selective process to get into the Universidad Central de Venezuela. There was a crucial problem which worked in combination with the intrinsic demands of the curriculum and the already biased institutional-environmental barriers in place. For materially deprived disabled folks, and lower-class blind individuals, in particular, it was necessary to master unique notetaking and relational skills that would allow them to get access to books and reliable readers which, of course, were not and have never been provided in Latin American university contexts. One needs to keep in mind that this is the pre-screen reader period. In those years, I became aware of a single privileged disabled person in Venezuela who owned advanced reading technology. Needless to say, at the time, this kind of technology was merely experimental and highly ineffective. Yet, to avoid expanding further into relational abstractions, I explore in this section, and the following, my personal experience with Roman Law I. This was one of the most dreadful filtering courses in the first year of my undergraduate legal studies.

It was April 1982. I was 16 at the time, new to the university town of Mérida from Barinas, the same state that a couple of decades later would brew for the world the infamous quasi-dictatorial/populist figure of Hugo Chávez Frías. The

Universidad de los Andes, where my law school was embedded, was two centuries old and had more than 30,000 students. When exams took place, which was the only occasion when classes were at their full capacity, there could be close to 200 students in the room. Most students in the Roman Law I crowd doubled my age; some of them tripled it.

Having been warned about the dreadful nature of the course, I dived into studying it. Several of the folks who were repeating the course, often for the third or fourth time, owned the required and recommended books. Hence, I did not have to worry about buying them, which would have been financially impossible since, as everybody knows both in the Global North and in the Global South, law and medicine books are usually among the most expensive on the market. These older individuals came to me because they had seen my performance in other courses. Yet, they came above all because they had a firm conviction, which they repeated to me with too much frequency: as a blind person, my brain would 'compensate' for the missing sense, a 'guaranteed' sign of special giftedness as far as 'intelligence' is concerned.

It is paramount to observe with great attention the representational implications of this kind of assumed authority in action. As seen below, this was a discursive fabrication, to use Popkewitz's (2004) terminology, which ended up constituting a poisoned double-edged sword.

Analytical Discussion 2

Labouring pains giving birth to the myth of ELGP

By the time I turned 17 in July 1982, my studying efforts were so focused, so determined, so much of a full-time obsession that my roommates claimed I would say a bunch of things in Latin while sleeping. I had already observed countless students go through the interrogation process, and here the word has all its cross-examination weight. Questions were so random that even students who had read the materials did not know how to anticipate a thematic focus. But the worst part was the ridiculing. Not knowing the answer, which was the most common occurrence, was met with name calling, 'funny' remarks for the class to 'enjoy', and so forth. It was truly a nightmare.

I would take braille notes frantically. I would catch every legend, every anecdote, every possible thing I could be asked about, reading those notes over and over, along with diving into multiple textbook reading sessions with several study groups in parallel. And one random day it just happened. I do not know how early or late it was in the flow of the academic year. I just know that it suddenly and ineluctably happened.

I do not have a remote recollection of what the professor asked that day. It just was a bursting into words. Being the right words, as they apparently were, the professor kept asking more and more questions to which I gave oral answers. At some point, the cross-examination stopped. The man simply exclaimed with a performative gesture: 'the Bible has spoken'. I guess that was the moment when the ELGP myth was born.

By the time the Roman Law I course was over, more than 95% of its students had failed. My final grade was 16 on a scale of 20 points, which, in the Venezuelan university system, constituted the threshold grade to earn the privilege not to have to take a final exam.

The mantra in this professor's performative torture was to repeat in a loud voice to class after class that 20 was for the Romans; after all they embodied the genius which created Roman law. The book deserved a grade of 19, since it had some imperfections. The professor deserved a grade of 18. Later the man would confide that a grade of 16 was unprecedented for him.

Yet, there was something incomplete, something rather uneventful about the whole ordeal. For students in the class, it was a natural thing, something to be expected, that I would achieve a high passing grade, despite their personal acquaintance with the difficulties involved in the process. Even the word *achieve* feels inappropriate since the mechanical nature with which they awaited the chain of events had an announced rhythm, a sense of almost boring ableist predictability.

Marcia Rioux (1997, 102) says that ways of looking at 'disability, of developing research questions, of interpreting research results … and of putting policies and programs in place are as much about ideology as they are about fact'. On the other hand, in his semiological treatise on mythologies, Barthes, being concerned with the resistance of those who seek to expose the falsehood in ideological myths, puts it this way:

> The mythologist is condemned to live in a theoretical sociality … to be in society is, at best, to be truthful … His connection with the world is of the order of sarcasm … The havoc which he wreaks in the language of the community is absolute for him, it fills his assignment to the brim: he must live this assignment without any hope of going back … Utopia is an impossible luxury for him: he greatly doubts that tomorrow's truths will be the exact reverse of today's lies … The mythologist is not even in a Moses-like situation: he cannot see the Promised Land. For him, tomorrow's positivity is entirely hidden by today's negativity. All the values of his undertaking appear to him as acts of destruction.
>
> *(Barthes, 1972, 156)*

There is therefore in the myths of normalizing ideologies a post-truth kind of vitality. Going against them, as they get expressed acritically over and over through the mechanisms of assumed authority, feels very much like a vaie enterprise. I still remember the many times I tried to dissuade these older students of the nonsensical nature of their idea of magic intelligence in the blind. I stressed countless times that believing something like that was tantamount to erasing one's effort to learn, to be prepared, to be ahead of the game. It was all to no avail. The myth was already inoculated; the metanarrative, firmly in place. Better still, at least for the purposes of hegemonic normalizing ideologies, it was a helpful tool to nullify merits, to dehumanize through an abstract utilitarian medicalizing gaze any trace of a unique sense of personhood with which to contend. Was it perhaps also a way to justify their own unsuccessful encounter with the interrogation monster in Roman Law I?

There is a reifying word game embedded in my ELGP nickname. I was not Petete. I was the book, the thing, the non-human part of the television series. In the video episode on snow (ELGP, 2011), one can observe Petete opening the conversation, drawing, playing, being somebody lively. When the book appears, the deep voice in the background lets the spectator know that some kind of dead, almost sacred knowledge was going to be imparted. You had to get ready to receive it, to be immersed in its trans-human, all-knowing substance.

Therefore, looking at the matter in retrospect, I now realize that being the 'Bible' who speaks in an oracular manner was by no means good. For one thing, it was not natural. Additionally, being the Bible had a fricking, alienating feel about it, a heavy sense of abnormality. That was the whole problem. The whole affair was no longer about a regular student who was meeting class responsibilities with a lot of effort. It was wrapped in an abnormal spirit. It had the aura of a non-human energy which flowed on its own and whose personhood was absent. By way of the myth itself, it was being thrown away, trampled over, fully denied. I, my sense of self, my most basic sense of dignity as a disabled student, all of that was suddenly and forever gone.

Analytical discussion 3

Fast-forwarding and unveiling the anti-meritocratic realities hidden behind the myth of ELGP

It was 1991. My wife and I were sitting at the graduate scholarship office for the Universidad de los Andes. Having graduated Magna Cum Laude in 1987, I was starting courses towards my first doctoral degree in the Department of Sociology at the University of New Mexico in Albuquerque, USA. As an honours student, I was entitled to full doctoral funding through the 'High Performance Scholarship' programme. I was there to sign the corresponding paperwork. After signing, I still remember the sincere words of that programme's director, Professor Josefina de Corredor, in the presence of my wife: 'You deserve this. You've earned it. You don't have to thank me for anything'.

Since it was conceived as a faculty recruitment mechanism, the terms of the High-Performance Scholarship arrangement were such that the recipient was obliged to work for the Universidad de los Andes at least twice the amount of time for which the doctoral funding was provided. The university, in turn, guaranteed faculty hiring, under the terms of established contests for concrete faculty openings. The deal seemed straightforward, and so it was when candidates were not disabled or perceived to be a threat to the institutional sense of ritualized homogeneity which served as the foundation to securing embodied sameness, the epitome of material, and ideological normality.

Five years later, by 1996, the School of Criminology had been opened. The new school was embedded within the Universidad de los Andes as a third departmental unit in the Faculty of Legal, Political, and Criminological Sciences. This undergraduate criminology school was the first of its kind in Latin America since all the institutions that held criminological studies throughout the region at the time were operating at the graduate level.

The school opened a Credential Contest for a faculty person to teach the criminal justice sequence at the rank of assistant professor, and I applied. The amount of information on the events that unfolded is overwhelming. There was substantial press coverage at the local and national level, especially for an event of this kind. Who cares about low-ranking university faculty hiring? A lot of people did in this case. As a matter of fact, even drunken fellows, I mean perfect strangers would stop me in the street to offer words of support.

As it turned out, the Universidad de los Andes law school from which I had graduated with Honours in 1987 now was refusing to accept my credentials for this teaching position. Their sole reason, which was shamelessly exhibited throughout their documents, was that I was blind.

Due to this intense press coverage, a lawyer from the Latin American Blind Union (ULAC for its initials in Spanish) contacted me. They were offering to mediate, and I gave my assent for them to mediate in the matter. To my knowledge, it did not seem that ULAC representatives were paid any attention by university authorities either. Why should one be surprised by this outcome? After all, were they not blind as well? They could not be viewed in this instance as valid, respectable interlocutors.

The foregoing may seem digressional. However, I offer it here in the spirit of critical hermeneutics, whose emphasis on strict ideological scrutiny is extremely important (Geuss, 1981; Thompson, 1984). Echoing Steven Meyers' (2014, 2016, 2019a, 2019b) targeted work on the disempowering consequences for grassroots activism through the process of homogenizing Disabled Persons' organizations (DPOs) in the era of the United Nations Convention on the Rights of Persons with Disability (CRPD), I noticed at the time that, even though nothing like CRPD was in place or loosely on the horizon, the sense of agency for local grassroots disability organizations in Venezuela and throughout Latin America was already severely undermined. I remember vividly the hesitancy and the blunt fear with which the president of our tiny local association of the blind spoke on my case when approached by the press. It was way beyond proportion for her. When accepting to preside us, nothing like this was on her radar. How could it be? How could she be prepared for an event of this sort? Why was she not given in advance the option to refuse such a demanding responsibility for her in the provincial context of that university town? There, her family ties could be negatively impacted for whatever comment she would make. It was by no means a minor concern.

Regarding ULAC, the truth is that small grassroots organizations like ours had no say whatsoever in its ongoing operations or its four-year pronouncements at the regional conventions. We were invisible to them. To me, even at that time, it was clear that, if things went well with my case, they were likely to take the credit. Hence, they had a great deal to win and nothing to lose.

Finally, it is crucial to stress that by no means was ableism the only evil afflicting Venezuelan autonomous universities at the time. Overall, they were and remain highly politicized. Party systems have penetrated their operations through an electoral set of mechanisms by which university presidents, deans, and all the rest of the administrative apparatus are subject to ritualized voting cycles which involve students, faculty, and, more recently, even janitorial personnel. Instead of incentivizing democratizing dynamics, this creates clientelist arrangements by which each faculty position gets preassigned since it constitutes a voting element that can tip the election in one direction or another. As a disabled figure outside their political game, I was disposable. Therefore, the dehumanizing nature of the myths I described above was only a portion of the explanation for the outrageous behaviour they displayed.

Knowing in advance what they wanted to do with my Opposition Contest, the ultimate one, the one that in 1998 would determine whether I could become a tenured faculty, in 1997, they instigated a student uprising targeting me. The corresponding machinations were led at the time by an individual who has occupied in the past two decades ministerial and vice-presidential roles in the Chávez/Maduro quasi-dictatorial regimes. It is my understanding that the United States Department of Justice has a pending case against him and several other members of these regimes involving very serious criminal charges. Unfortunately, this is the kind of axiological milieu one is likely to encounter in this Global South higher education context – indeed a pitiful picture for rights-based strategies to offer hopes of ever being successful in achieving transformational social justice.

Concluding Discussion

It was Thursday night. On July 30, 1987, the University Paraninfo, where commencement ceremonies were held, was full beyond capacity. The only thing that mattered to me at that crucial moment was that my mother and grandmother were there. They had endured so much before I could get to that instance. They had not witnessed the university graduation of anybody else in our family. Hence, this was a big deal for them.

Right then and there, in front of me, handing me the diploma was the famous Perucho, a university president who won election after election at the Universidad de los Andes in the 1970s and 1980s. The standing ovation was so long that I could not tell how much it lasted. Yet, like most things in this chapter's counterstory, the ritualized noise of the moment proved to be an ephemeral chimera, an ableist fiasco. Many of those same actors would soon be playing a role as perpetrators or accomplices in the events of 1996 and 1998. Their external expressions of 'admiration' were at last disclosed as yet another masquerade in the mythologies of assumed authority.

The dehumanizing representational features of ELGP I describe throughout this chapter show that normate ideologies of ableism do not work in isolation. They operate in tandem with a myriad of ideological features of the coloniality of power, knowledge, and being (Calderón, 2014; Maldonado-Torres, 2007; Mignolo and Walsh, 2018; Quijano, 2000; Saldívar, 2012; Sandoval, 2000; Wynter, 2003). Above all, one must realize that their horrifying hegemonic enactments are not exclusive to the Global South. The LatDisCrit paradigm creates epistemological and axiological ways to expose the ontological and material precarity features of these mythologies in action. LatDisCrit's epistemological and axiological avenues bridge, in multifaceted ways, Global North and Global South contexts. The counterstory power of LatDisCrit can help awaken cross-Latinx and radical solidarity mechanisms for multiple types of subaltern subjects to resist together, disrupt, and undo the semiotic codes sustaining these mythologies as well as their tangible exclusionary consequences in the Global North as much as in the Global South (Padilla, 2018, Forthcoming).

Finally, from the discussions in this chapter, it is evident that rights-based approaches by themselves are not enough for pandisability and intersectional subaltern emancipatory purposes. A plethora of discursive, materialist, situationally, and culturally grounded frameworks are necessary in a well-articulated combination unique to each context and strongly grounded in metatheoretical and strategic sophistication (Bell, 2011; Iverson, 2012; Obourn, 2020; Piepzna-Samarasinha, 2018). For instance, one of the first ableist moves in trying to block my entry into the faculty ranks of the university was to claim the incapacitation rules that have come down to us from Roman times through the Napoleonic civil code, which frames the underlying assumptions in the great majority of Latin American legal systems. Under those rules, the default assumption is that blind, deaf, and other disabled people are incapable of exercising any activity, especially lawyering, which involves representing other people's interests (De Vries, 1965; Merryman, 1978). In the case of Venezuela, to be 'able' to practice law, these categories of disabled individuals must undergo a judicial process of approval called 'habilitación'. Habilitación is not required from other categories of individuals to practice law and is therefore discriminatory, particularly after CRPD has come into effect. Such rules have obviously not been derogated because they embody the spirit of the prevailing belief system of hegemonic normalizing ideologies.

Even if these rules were removed, the status quo of legal practices would most likely be similar. Much more is needed. Above all, a critical assessment of ableism and disableism as hegemonic manifestations of assumed normate authority is indispensable, keeping in mind that the situation in Global North contexts is not substantially better and requires concerted collective action with a wide array of subaltern allies. Why, for example, has the United States not ratified CRPD after almost two decades of its promulgation by the United Nations? The reason is that failing to do so has served to perpetuate, within the American context under an aura of apparent legitimacy, systemic discriminatory and exclusionary practices. These practices encompass areas such as education (Connor, 2019), employment (Mason, 2004) and so forth. In short, the road ahead of us is long and arduous (Pothier, 1992; Wildeman, 2016, 2020). We must approach the journey in the Global North and in the Global South with a strong pandisability sense of radical emancipatory solidarity, which embraces creatively the causes of other intersectionally grounded subaltern decolonial groups.

References

Alcoff, L. M. (2009) Comparative Race, Comparative Racisms, in J. J. E. Gracia (ed) *Race or Ethnicity? On Black and Latino Identity*, Ithaca: Cornell University Press.

Alexander, J. C. (2003) *The Meanings of Social Life: A Cultural Sociology*, New York: Oxford University Press.

Alexander, J. C., Giesen, B., and Mast, J. L. (eds). (2006) *Social Performance: Symbolic Action, Cultural Pragmatics and Ritual*, New York: Cambridge University Press.

Annamma, S. A., Connor, D. J., and Ferri, B. A. (2013) Dis/Ability Critical Race Studies (DisCrit): Theorizing at the Intersections of Race and Dis/Ability, *Race, Ethnicity and Education* 16 (1): 1–31.

Annamma, S. A., Connor, D. J., and Ferri, B. A. (2016) Introduction: A Truncated Genealogy of DisCrit, in D. J. Connor, B. A. Ferri, and S. A. Annamma (eds) *DisCrit: Disability Studies and Critical Race Theory in Education*, New York: Teachers College Press.

Annamma, S. A., Ferri, B. A., and Connor, D. J. (2019) Cultivating and Expanding Disability Critical Race Theory (DisCrit), in K. Ellis, R. Garland-Thomson, M. Kent, and R. Robertson (eds) *Manifestos for the Future of Critical Disability Studies*, New York: Routledge.

Aramayo, M. (2005) *Universidad y Discapacidad*, Caracas: Cátedra Libre de la Discapacidad, Universidad Central de Venezuela.

Barthes, R. (1972) Myth as a Semiological System, in R. Barthes (ed) *Mythologies*, A. Layers, Trans, New York: Hill and Wang.

Bell, C. (2011) *Blackness and Disability: Critical Examinations and Cultural Interventions*, East Lansing: Michigan State University Press.

Bernal, D. D. (2002) Critical Race Theory, LatCrit Theory, and Critical Race-Gendered Epistemologies: Recognizing Students of Color as Holders and Creators of Knowledge, *Qualitative Inquiry* 8 (1): 105–26.

Bolt, D. (2012) Social Encounters, Cultural Representation and Critical Avoidance, in N. Watson, A. Roulstone, and C. Thomas (eds) *Routledge Handbook of Disability Studies*, Abingdon: Routledge.

Bolt, D. (2014) *The Metanarrative of Blindness: A Re-Reading of Twentieth-Century Anglophone Writing*, Ann Arbor: University of Michigan Press.

Bolt, D. (2020) The Metanarrative of Disability: Social Encounters, Cultural Representation and Critical Avoidance, in N. Watson and S. Vehmas (eds) *Routledge Handbook of Disability Studies*, 2nd edition, Abingdon: Routledge.

Bustos García, B. A. (2014) El 'Boteo' en las Calles como Práctica Contradiscursiva: Análisis de Narrativas Identitarias de Personas Ciegas, *Revista de Ciencias Sociales* 27 (35): 33–48.

Calderón, D. (2014) Anticolonial Methodologies in Education: Embodying Land and Indigeneity in Chicana Feminisms, *Journal of Latino/Latin American Studies* 6: 81–96.

Castro-Gómez, S. (2002) The Social Sciences, Epistemic Violence and the Problem of the 'Invention of the Other', *Nepantla: Views from the South* 3 (2): 269–85.

Castro-Gómez, S. (2007) The Missing Chapter of Empire: Postmodern Reorganization of Coloniality and Post-Fordist Capitalism, *Cultural Studies* 21 (2–3): 428–48.

Connor, D. J. (2019) Why Is Special Education So Afraid of Disability Studies?, *Journal of Curriculum Theorizing* 34 (1): 10–23.

Dávila, E. R., and de Bradley, A. A. (2010) Examining Education for Latinas/os in Chicago: A CRT/LatCrit Approach, *Educational Foundations* 24 (1): 39–58.

De Vries, H. P. (1965) *The Law of the Americas: An Introduction to the Legal Systems of the American Republics*, Dobbs Ferry: Oceana Publications.

El Libro Gordo de Petete [ELGP]. (2011) La Nieve. Available from https://www.you tube.com/watch?v=qGfAqXTlqig

Ferrante, C., and Dukuen, J. (2017) Discapacidad y Opresión: Una Crítica desde la Teoría de la Dominación de Bourdieu, *Procesos De Cambio* 40 (6): 151–60.

Ferrante, C., and Joly, E. (2017) Begging and Disability: A Paradigmatic Way to Earn One's Living, in S. Grech and K. Soldatic (eds) *Disability in the Global South: The Critical Handbook*, Cham: Springer.

Flores, J., and García, S. (2009) Latina Testimonios: A Reflexive, Critical Analysis of a 'Latina Space' at a Predominantly White Campus, *Race Ethnicity and Education* 12 (2): 155–72.

Garland-Thomson, R. (1997) *Extraordinary Bodies: Figuring Physical Disability in American Culture and Literature*, New York: Columbia University Press.

Geuss, R. (1981) *The Idea of a Critical Theory: Habermas and the Frankfurt School*, New York: Cambridge University Press.

Iverson, S. V. (2012) Constructing Outsiders: The Discursive Framing of Access in University Diversity Policies, *The Review of Higher Education* 35 (2): 149–77.

Lajous Vargas, A. (2019) *La Sociedad Civil vs. la Corrupción*, Ciudad de México: Penguin Random House Grupo Editorial.

Maldonado-Torres, N. (2007) On the Coloniality of Being: Contributions to the Development of a Concept, *Cultural Studies* 21 (2–3): 240–70.

Mason, M. G. (2004) *Working against Odds: Stories of Disabled Women's Work Lives*, Boston: Northeastern University Press.

Merryman, J. H. (1978) *Comparative Law: Western European and Latin American Legal Systems: Cases and Materials*, Indianapolis: Bobbs-Merrill.

Meyer, J. W., and Rowan, B. (1978) Institutionalized Organizations: Formal Structure as Myth and Ceremony, in W. W. Powell and P. J. DiMaggio (eds) *The New Institutionalism in Organizational Analysis*, Chicago: University of Chicago Press.

Meyers, S. (2014) Disabled Persons Associations at the Crossroads of Two Organizational Environments: Grassroots Groups as Part of an International Movement and a Local Civil Society, *Research in Social Science and Disability: Environmental Contexts and Disability* 8: 3–31.

Meyers, S. (2016) NGO-ization and Human Rights Law: The CRPD's Civil Society Mandate, *Laws: Special Edition on Disability Human Rights Law* 5 (2): 1–14.

Meyers, S. (2019a) *Civilizing Disability Society: The Convention on the Rights of Persons with Disabilities Socializing Grassroots Disabled Persons' Organizations in Nicaragua*, New York: Cambridge University Press.

Meyers, S. (2019b) Misrecognising Persons with Disabilities in the Global South: The Need for a Comparative Disability Studies Framework, in K. Ellis, R.

Garland-Thomson, M. Kent, and R. Robertson (eds) *Interdisciplinary Approaches to Disability: Looking towards the Future*, New York: Routledge.

Mignolo, W. D. (2000) *Local Histories/Global Designs: Coloniality, Subaltern Knowledges and Border Thinking*, Princeton: Princeton University Press.

Mignolo, W. D., and Tlostanova, M. (2006) Theorizing from the Borders. Shifting to Geo-and Body-Politics of Knowledge, *European Journal of Social Theory* 9 (2): 205–21.

Mignolo, W. D., and Walsh, C. E. (2018) *On Decoloniality: Concepts, Analytics, Praxis*, Durham: Duke University Press.

Miguez, M. N. (2013) Ensayo sobre Presencias\Ausencias en torno a la Relación Discapacidad – Trabajo en Francia y Uruguay, Crítica Contemporánea, *Revista de Teoría Política* 3: 1–21.

Miguez, M. N., Piñato, C., and Machado, R. (2013) Discapacidad y Trabajo: Una Mirada desde la Ideología de la Normalidad, *Revista Regional de Trabajo Social* 59 (3): 34–41.

Moraga, C. L. (2011) *A Xicana Codex of Changing Consciousness: Writings, 2000–2010*, Durham: Duke University Press.

Morrow, R. A. (1994) *Critical Theory and Methodology*, Thousand Oaks: SAGE.

Obourn, M. W. (2020) *Disabled Futures: A Framework for Radical Inclusion*, Philadelphia: Temple University Press.

Omansky, B. (2011) *Borderlands of Blindness*, Boulder: Lynne Rienner Publishers.

Padilla, A. (2018) Race, Disability, and the Possibilities of Radical Agency: Toward a Political Philosophy of Decolonial Critical Hermeneutics in Latinx Discrit. Doctoral Dissertation, Albuquerque: University of New Mexico.

Padilla, A. (Forthcoming) *Disability, Intersectional Agency and Latinx Identity: Theorizing LatDisCrit Counterstories*, Abingdon: Routledge.

Piepzna-Samarasinha, L. L. (2018) *Care Work: Dreaming Disability Justice*, Vancouver: Arsenal Pulp Press.

Popkewitz, T. (2004) The Alchemy of the Mathematics Curriculum: Inscriptions and the Fabrication of the Child, *American Educational Research Journal* 41 (1): 3–34.

Pothier, D. (1992) Miles to Go: Some Personal Reflection on the Social Construction of Disability, *Dalhousie Law Journal* 14 (3): 526–543.

Quijano, A. (1992) Colonialidad y Modernidad/ Racionalidad, in H. Bonilla (ed) *Los Conquistados: 1492 y la Población Indígena de las Américas*, Quito: Libri Mundi/Tercer Mundo.

Quijano, A. (2000) Colonialidad del Poder, Eurocentrismo y América Latina, in E. Lander (ed) *La Colonialidad del Saber: Eurocentrismo y Ciencias Sociales, Perspectivas Latinoamericanas*, Buenos Aires: Clacso.

Ricoeur, P. (1971) The Model of the Text: Meaningful Action Considered as a Text, *Social Research* 38: 529–62.

Ricoeur, P. (1974) *The Conflict of Interpretations: Essays in Hermeneutics*, Evanston: Northwestern University Press.

Ricoeur, P. (1981) What Is a Text? Explanation and Understanding, in J. B. Thompson (ed and trans) *Hermeneutics and the Human Sciences: Essays on Language, Action, and Interpretation*, Cambridge: Cambridge University Press.

Rioux, M. H. (1997) Disability: The Place of Judgement in a World of Fact, *Journal of Intellectual Disability Research* 41: 102–11.

Roberge, J. (2011) What Is Critical Hermeneutics? *Thesis Eleven* 106 (1): 5–22.

Saldívar, J. D. (1991) *The Dialectics of Our America*, Durham: Duke University Press.

Saldívar, J. D. (2012) *Trans-Americanity: Subaltern Modernities, Global Coloniality, and the Cultures of Greater Mexico*, Durham: Duke University Press.

Sandoval, C. (2000) *Methodology of the Oppressed*, Minneapolis: University of Minnesota Press.

Solórzano, D., and Bernal, D. D. (2001) Examining Transformational Resistance through a Critical Race and Latcrit Theory Framework: Chicana and Chicano Students in an Urban Context, *Urban Education* 36 (3): 308–42.

Teklu, A. A. (2007) The Voices of Ethiopian Blind Immigrants and Their Families: Facing the Challenges of Life in Canada. Doctoral Dissertation, Victoria: Department of Curriculum and Instruction, University of Victoria.

Thompson, J. B. (1984) *Studies in the Theory of Ideology*, Cambridge: Polity Press.

Valdes, F. (1999) Afterword, Theorizing 'OutCrit' Theories: Coalitional Method and Comparative Jurisprudential Experience – RaceCrits, QueerCrits and LatCrits, *University of Miami Law Review* 53: 1265–1306.

Valdes, F. (2000) Race, Ethnicity, and Hispanismo in a Triangular Perspective: The 'Essential Latina/o' and LatCrit Theory, *UCLA Law Review* 48: 1–41.

Wildeman, S. (2016) Agonizing Identity in Mental Health Law and Policy (Part II): A Political Taxonomy of Psychiatric Subjectification, *Dalhousie Law Journal* 39 (1): 147–94.

Wildeman, S. (2020) Disabling Solitary: An Anti-Carceral Critique of Canada's Solitary Confinement Mitigation, in C. Spivakovsky, L. Steele, and P. Weller (eds) *The Legacies of Institutionalisation: Disability, Law and Policy in the 'Deinstitutionalised' Community*, Oxford: Hart.

Wynter, S. (2003) Unsettling the Coloniality of Being/Power/Truth/Freedom. Towards the Human, after Man, Its Overrepresentation: An Argument, *The New Centennial Review* 3 (3): 257–337.

Yosso, T. J. (2000) A Critical Race and LatCrit Approach to Media Literacy: Chicana/o Resistance to Visual Microagressions. Unpublished Doctoral Dissertation, University of California, Los Angeles.

Yosso, T. J. (2006) *Critical Race Counterstories along the Chicana/Chicano Educational Pipeline*, New York: Routledge.

3

THE METANARRATIVE OF BLINDNESS IN INDIA

Special education and assumed knowledge cultures

Hemachandran Karah

Preliminary discussion

Schools for the blind in India deeply influence the career choices of their pupils; they do this via a metanarrative that establishes a natural (or otherwise) connection between blindness and several disciplines. The metanarrative commands assumed authority over blind people, especially within locations where they come into contact with disciplinary formations at the cutting edge. For example, the following impressions shape blind people's mobility across the social sciences, the humanities, and the sciences:

1. Fieldworks entail visual engagements, and therefore social sciences cannot take blind people that far.
2. Due to its interpretative verbiage, humanities may remain forever a natural home for the blind.
3. Sciences are hard for blind people since they will be required to gather an observational eye for precision and mechanical objectivity.

No doubt, ocularnormativism (Bolt, 2014) drives such impressions. All the same, a stamp of authenticity by special schools pushes such normative leanings into assumptions of authority – namely, an assortment of unwritten rules and practical decisions that shape blind people's life courses across knowledge domains. In this chapter, I look back at moments of authenticity-making during my stay in an Indian blind school. The metanarrative generated by such schools prior to globalization of the 1990s still shapes, almost automatically, blind people's disciplinary mobility. This is certainly true for my generation.

Methodological discussion

A little bit of a flashback: during the early 1990s, a dozen of us parted our ways from a blind school in Chennai (known those days as Madras). At the time, we were told that we were ambassadors of our school and the blind community at large – that the sighted world would judge us based on how we conducted ourselves. In a sense, we were soldiers who were required to defend our school, the blind community, and by extension, our own performative selves. Flashforward three decades: I am writing now about the assumed authority of special education. I am in touch with some of my classmates, immediate seniors, and juniors; many of them for the first time after my schooling. It is sad that we could not keep in touch. In our respective ways, we were soldiering on, fighting the scopic in multifarious ways and registers. An ambitious meeting is ruled out these days due to COVID-19 lockdown. Hence, we decided to make contact via telephone conversations. Even on the telephone, class differences between us become apparent, but still we connect fondly, bound by what I call *cohort consciousness.*

In order to explain, I should point out that I seek recourse to autoethnography as a collective enterprise. Autoethnography may not always concern one person's individual immersion into a social milieu; it may involve a collectivity such as one particular generation of students (e.g. my cohort from St. Louis Institute for Deaf & the Blind). However miniscule it is, this collectivity is what I rely on for exploring the metanarrative of blindness and its assumed authority over our disciplinary journeys. I could have named the collectivity *cohort memory*, but *cohort consciousness* is better since it is true to our sense of oneness. My cohort is heavily influenced by a broader cosmology such as blind psychology. Methodologically, I explore the workings of blind psychology amid our cohort for traces of the metanarrative of blindness and assumed authority. To explore an archive of examples of the metanarrative, I rely on biographical sketches, sayings, and conversational memories.

It is useful for me to begin with cohort consciousness (CC) and its intrinsic link with my autoethnography. Broadly, cohort consciousness is a collectivity that one willingly entertains on account of a shared past. Military cadets, classmates, hostelites, yoga mates, and many such formations build a bonding that often is self-referential about their grouping. Such a bonding is also super-conscious of their original context of becoming (e.g. time, place, and particular mode of institutional affiliation). Also, no matter the size of the grouping, cohorts are acutely aware of their unique legacy, and what that means to them for life. This way, as we, the pass outs of the 1990s from St Louis, look back on our formation, and its bearing on our current lives, some sentiments keep bouncing back.

The first such sentiment and enduring collective belief is that we are all 'chronic overcomers'. If there were a space in which we could thrive at the other side, and perhaps beyond the scopic, it must have been our school for the blind.

St Louis school for the blind and the deaf had four raised walls. It housed a society of blind boys and teachers who were routinely told that the outside world was fiercely sighted. Within those four walls, we were imparted skills that were supposed to be useful in the sighted world. As a preparation for scopic mobility, we were trained well in a number of disciplines, habits, and visual protocols. We were also exposed to rigorous Physical Education Training (PET) so that we were as good as the sighted. When we left the school, all social interactions outside seemed to be test cases of what we learnt within the four walls concerning scopic survival. Some of us survived such tests very well; others did not. As amateur blind survivors of the scopic during the 1990s, we know how our schooling is part of our muscle memory, no matter how strong or weak it is now. By *muscle memory* I mean compulsive reflexes that concern one or other aspect of our scopic engagements. These reflexes just made one point clear: we should be as good as the sighted. I am sure there are generations of blind students who literally walked out into the scopic with such reflexes; so did we; but we stepped out into a world order that was already a notch closer to globalization. One of the features of globalization involves a permanent break with the idea that spectacle can be rendered static. Globalization inaugurates what Guy Debord calls 'An unceasing flow of the spectacle' (Debord, 2012). During globalization, the spectacle multiplies, often inducing newer flows of commodities, visual cultures, disciplines, and ideologies. We were not really ready for this. Our special education training was primarily geared for binary thinking. That is to say, the scopic comes with two modes of engagement: the sighted and the blind way of doing things. Our entire focus, we were told, should have been invested in overcoming the inferior shade of this binary. The passage of time has somewhat, but not entirely, lessened our commitment to the business of overcoming.

Our cohort consciousness is also strung together by our messy formation. When any adults are with favourite classmates from school, they may end up talking about a game in which they did something spectacular. So do we converse about many a tiny thing. We drift into conversations on our messy formation. For a starter, we mimic our school teachers and their endless commandments. Stories of childhood antics, volleyball matches, boy talk, and the rest follow. I am pretty sure we become aware of our individual differences. Equally, in the distance we look like haptic extensions of each other, and not really as Hem, Jayachandran, Durai, Karthik, Rambabu, and Anburajan. We can locate with some exactitude who was next to whom amid a row of desks in the classroom, the never-ending row of beds in the dormitory, the shoulder-to-shoulder group formations for an evening stroll, and the eager volleyball gangs on either side of the net. These haptic geographies seem as formidable now as they were in those days. All in all, our lives at the school seem now like pre-adult selves in incubation for the sighted world outside.

Cohort consciousness is certainly not my invention. As a method of exploring collective memory, concepts such as *generation* and *cohort* are in active circulation. Barry Schwartz, for example, identifies individuals as primary carriers and agents of memory. As carriers, individuals form divergent collectivities, where memories in transmission undergo some kind of mutation (Corning and Schuman, 2015). Schwartz also acknowledges the idea that individual memory collectives are shaped by larger archives of memory that surround them in real life. In some sense, our cohort consciousness is very much like collective memory as envisaged by Schwartz. Our formations, for example, are all in our individual muscle memory. But they attain a fuller meaning via our overcoming strategies as much as a public projection of them in equal measure.

Now that I have acknowledged the pivotal role of cohort consciousness for my autoethnographic dip into collective memories of our blind school, I must also name the special cosmology that animates the same from all directions: *blind psychology*. Why do I call it cosmology? First and foremost, blind psychology is a climate of opinions. In this capacity, blind psychology hosts special attitudes, customs, rituals, and practices of learning linked to blind children (i.e. it is part of the metanarrative of blindness). Thomas Cutsforth (1893–1962) made foundational contributions to special education – more particularly to the psychology of the blind. Cutsforth argues for an emancipatory model of special education. Emancipation comes with true self-expression. Blind children will never experience the thrill of self-expression until they are artificially trained to please the sighted. According to Cutsforth, undue emphasis on familiarity with colours, shades, sizes, landscaping, looks, and so on undermines the inner resources of blind pupils. Instead of a preparation for the sighted world, blind children should be taught to draw on their inner resources and capabilities. For example, they can be taught to draw wholesomely on sensory resources other than sight.

Cutsforth does not stop there. He introduces frameworks such as verbalism and blindism, which do the rounds as parts of the metanarrative of blindness. Verbalism is word-mindedness. It demonstrates a tendency to treat words as substitutes for objects that they are supposed to represent. Cutsforth offers an example of a blind child who is heavily influenced by verbalism. This child learns the distinction between a rooster and a fire engine by their sounds, plus the pair of English words that represent the same. The child can never know the difference between the two until taken tactually closer to them, which is surely an exaggeration (i.e. the child may not be as withdrawn and apperceptive as made out to be). Nevertheless, Cutsforth gets the larger picture right about the evils of special education pedagogy that holds the pleasure of the other as an inviolable norm (i.e. a tendency to prepare blind clients only from the point of view of expectations by the sighted majority). Verbalism is an undue emphasis on words, and words alone. For example, a special education teacher who is fond of verbalism may train her or his pupil in a capacity to describe colours and landscapes. Such a training without any meaningful exploration of something like touch and hearing may potentially undermine a blind child's resources from within. Within such a scheme of things, *blindism* emerges more or less as a generic term. It refers to involuntary acts that are deemed undesirable, and yet found among blind children. They include self-stimulation, rocking, mimicry, unusual haptic curiosity, and much more (Cutsforth, 1951). Again, Cutsforth may sound harsh and unscrupulous, but he has a larger point to make: blind children need care, support, and guidance to learn socially acceptable modes of living, learning, moving, and speaking. Special education can offer such a holding environment for systematic learning.

This indeed happens, for the most part, but all in the name of blind psychology. Because it works like a cosmology, special education for the blind does not remain as a mere technical expertise. In fact, wherever blind people seek assistance by way of accessibility, accommodation, and specialist training, they find themselves inadvertently drifting into blind psychology. Blind adults, children, parents, teachers, educationists, and so on work and flourish within the system. That said, Cutsforth did not found the cosmos of blind psychology. On the contrary, his grand thesis on the psychology of the blind is symptomatic of its overreach as a grand metanarrative cluster. Irrespective of the popularity of Cutsforth, blind psychology as a special cosmos is characterized by essentialism. It is for this reason that perceived deficits of blind children seem inherent and irremediable. My fellow cohort Mr Anburajan puts this very candidly:

> All that is considered blind psychology is nothing but a collection of perceived deficits among blind children and adults alike. I haven't heard anyone say anything positive at all in the name of blind psychology.
>
> *(Anburajan, 2020a)*

Here Anburajan is talking about a strand of blind psychology that is charged with negative aspects of the metanarrative of blindness.

Blind psychology is not a cosmology that can be forcefully kept inside special schools such as St Louis. Naturally, the many aspects of the metanarrative of blindness do not always stay intramurally there; they spill over into society. Equally, they can originate outside the special schools as well. Such symbiotic outflows and inflows render a sense of authenticity (plus assumed authority) to the metanarrative of blindness. This is how metanarratives, in general, gain legitimacy, validation, and authority.

Formation questions, for example, are crucial to special education settings. At the outset I must mention that formation questions are self-referential in nature; they do not require one-to-one answers. Special education strives for the formation of meaningful personhoods and skillsets among people with disabilities. Such a striving becomes nothing less than a mission when it is exclusively made for disabled children. Either way, the keyword that drives special education is *formation*, however messy it may seem. It is unsurprising that St Louis now seems like our place of incubation. For example, how we handle family life, professions, recreation, culture, and so on somehow seem to be linked to our early formation. That way, a personal wanting in any of these domains runs the risk of being treated as a symptom of a sketchy formation. I am sure that we six are a diverse lot, and there is nothing common among us excepting blindness tied by a cohort consciousness. Also, we all realize that certain formation questions continue to haunt us today, although we became vaguely familiar with them via our teachers in our school in the name of blind psychology. Some of these questions include:

> In what way is a blind child's cognition different? How does blindness affect interpersonal relationships? Are some knowledge systems and disciplines more accessible to blind children than others? Are blind children given to self-eroticism or egocentrism? Does blindness stunt one's sexuality? Can a blind child understand anything about visual reality?

These questions are meant to drive the special education mission in favour of affirmative action and a pedagogy of care. They are also meant to aid a wholesome specialist training. The problem is that such questions already are shaped by multiple crooked cuts long before they are picked up and finetuned by the special education system. For example, families may discover one or other of these formation questions convenient in making sense of (and therefore reaffirm the perceived deficits of) a blind relative. Special education settings borrow these questions from the mainstream so that they can fix formational anomalies among blind children (to nip them in the bud, as it were). Such a system of finetuning establishes some kind of narrative looping between social expectations and how they are formatively managed by specialist institutions. Such narrative loops also assume authority by the fact that they are given a stamp of authenticity by special education settings. In addition, formational perfectionism is an incessant ideology. Special schools can keep their pupils interlocked into it via instructions concerning fields of knowledge.

At St Louis, we were taught English, Tamil, science, mathematics, history, and geography. At that time, we never knew that these disciplines belong to one or other of the three cultures of knowledge: the humanities, the social sciences, and the sciences. All the same, we knew by intuition (and not by reasoning) that only one of these knowledge cultures was suitable for us. Careers in language studies, history, philosophy, and music seemed appropriate. We could forget about the social sciences and the sciences. They were reserved for sighted folks outside the raised walls. Such a deep sense of intuition, practicality, and disciplinary persuasion are influential now as they were then.

To make sense of our adaptation into, and lacking thereof across all the three cultures of knowledge, I make use of Jerome Kagan's observations concerning their reasons of being. Kagan's tripartite classification of knowledge mentioned above rests on the principle that all the three forms of knowledge distinguish themselves from each other based on how they relate to, and define the following key variables: primary materials, specialist vocabulary, historical legacy, autonomy, ethics, political influence, contribution to national economy, and beauty (Kagan, 2009). When we passed out of the school, Kagan's variables did not seem as important as the notion of practical wisdom, which actually prompted us to choose one or other field of knowledge. Our teachers at St Louis were of the opinion that it was not practicable for us to pursue certain disciplines. What is practicality then? In special school settings like ours, blind students learn a score of what is locally labelled as 'practical things' concerning what works, and what does not in the sighted world. Blind young adults keep perfecting and, when necessary, altering such a know-how as they go on to discover a home of their own within the chosen field of study. One may call this know-how phronesis. Drawing on Aristotle, Ben Flyvbjerg describes phronesis as practical wisdom. phronesis is responsible for our everyday negotiation with structures of power and knowledge.[1] Other kinds of knowledge also thrive in the making of disciplines. Aristotle refers to them as epistemé and techné. The former connotes abstract knowledge, and the latter specialist or technical vocabulary (Schram, 2012).

To summarize, in this chapter, I slip into cohort consciousness so as to gain autoethnographic insights concerning metanarratives of blindness. Practical wisdom or phronesis is a useful framework since it can show why special education assumes authority over blind people's everyday immersion into disciplines across life courses. To examine phronesis in operation in our cohort consciousness, I gather samples of biographical sketches, pedagogical interventions, and conversations on blind psychology that do not seem to rest.

Analytical discussion 1

Learnt suspicion of the social sciences

One special educational aspect of the metanarrative of blindness is a learnt suspicion about the social sciences that we were exposed to in our school, and with which some of us juggled later on. We the 'blind boys' were not encouraged to pursue social sciences. We were told that disciplines such as sociology were not our best bet. Dr Rambabu and Mr Anburajan not only went ahead with a career in social sciences but also pioneered newer ways of interpreting disciplinary anxieties concerning their formation. Their sense of phronesis reveals assumed authority by which the metanarrative of blindness operates across disciplinary ghettos.

In many ways, my biographical narrative of Rambabu is also a belated obituary for my dear friend. Rambabu passed away two years ago due to brain cancer. His special entry into sociology is a tribute to his discipline as much as our cohort consciousness. As a young undergraduate during the mid-1990s, Rambabu was concerned about his wholesome induction into (and future with) a discipline

---

1 Flyvbjerg coined the term *phronetic social science* in the year 2001 to describe a newly developing commitment among social scientists in favour of application-oriented knowledges (a move away from positivism, I must add). The latter is known to favour methods endemic to natural sciences so as to harness hypotheses that seem grand and universal.

about which he heard nothing favourable in his blind school. For one thing, he was required to deal with the incessant ideology of formation, and for another, he was required to redefine practicality so as to facilitate a trouble-free sociology pursuit. Because Rambabu inherited from his special school suspicion about pursuing the social sciences, something reaffirmed by local gatekeepers of sociology, he sort recourse to phronesis that works. This time, his phronesis involved a gradual release, of his peers and teachers alike, from a positivistic notion that sight is imperative for a sociology pursuit, especially in ethnographic work. Like Rambabu, a good many blind people harness phronesis so as to handle learnt suspicion concerning their suitability for a particular discipline, methodological intervention, career, membership in a professional association, and involvement in group projects. In this biographical sketch, I deal with Rambabu's phronesis in handling learnt suspicion concerning his location in sociology as a blind undergraduate. I gather his special story of phronesis with as much critical distance as I can muster.

Rambabu was a junior by one year in the school. We parted ways when I left St Louis so as to pursue 11th grade in a sighted school. Rambabu continued with 11th grade at St Louis. Rambabu and his classmates had a choice to stay back in the school for higher secondary school education. They could either choose a music major or a stream in advanced English. Rambabu chose the latter. All again, he was my immediate junior during an undergraduate programme at Loyola College, Madras. Rambabu chose to do sociology, while I went on to do English literature. To examine his fledgling immersion into sociology, I seek recourse to his research paper which he presented at the Center for the Study of Developing Societies (CSDS), where I organized a workshop on Disability Studies in 2012 (Rambabu, 2012).

Rambabu's research paper begins with his decision to opt for an undergraduate programme in sociology. Immediate resistance, so to speak, came from his parents. They always wanted him to study English literature, or something close to it, so that he could become a successful teacher in our blind school. This does not surprise me at all. 'I always wanted you to become a great teacher like Vincent sir in your school'. I am sure my mom said this recently as she might have a thousand times during my schooling. Such a confession seems so impressionable now as it was in those days. Like my mom, Rambabu's parents could not see any prospect in sociology. After all, no blind person they knew had opted for the field. When Rambabu actually chose sociology, he discovered that the discipline looked as much fortified as his school. The immediate gatekeepers such as his successful seniors, teachers, and the elderly pushed him towards a disciplinary ghetto that seemed suitable to the blind. For example, they used to ask, and I quote Rambabu: 'Would you be able to move around in new locations?' Maybe they were concerned about Rambabu's capacity to access disciplinary constituents such as primary materials and specialist vocabulary without sight. They could have had some concerns about the question of autonomy, not necessarily in Kagan's terms but by a persuasion that a person who depends on others for mobility cannot command individual judgement. Rambabu was damn sure that these questions were not meant for soliciting learnt responses. Instead, they were actually meant for shooing away seemingly unwanted intrusions. The gate-keepers who shooed him away this way often cited big names in the field such as Bronislaw Malinowski (1884–1942) and Marcel Mauss (1872–1950). Probably, the big names were invoked to validate what they were trying to claim about scopic inaccessibility. Further, irrespective of the relevance of such names to his entry into sociology, Rambabu heard the gatekeepers chant them as potential deterrents. To counter such deterrents, Rambabu was required to harness phro-nesis, which is where the assumed authority of special education kicks in from unexpected quarters.

As a first timer in the sociology business from our cohort, Rambabu was required to rely on phronesis, a basket of rhetorical strategies in favour of scopic survival as a blind undergraduate. Sociology included, most disciplines develop a way of saying no to blind people. To do so, they seek recourse to already thriv-ing disciplinary ghettos which are there in the first place to filter out seemingly unwanted intrusions. Disciplinary ghettos are hard to escape this way. Among other forms of filtering, disciplinary ghettos hold on to an old learnt suspicion that certain frameworks of knowledge are unsuitable for blind people. That good old idea emerges from special schools, and from nowhere else. In this way, special schools and disciplinary ghettos function as mirror images of each other. That is the point about the assumed authority of special education. As an undergraduate student, Rambabu could never resist such a nexus head on. Instead, he found himself doing visual stuff again and again. For example, whenever there was an opportunity to go for fieldwork, wholeheartedly he would opt for it, definitely not theoretical work. In the process, he gradually made everyone see the point about what Mia Mingus now calls access intimacy (Mingus, 2011). In Rambabu's scheme of things, access intimacy actually works like an antidote to ghettoiza-tion. Mia Mingus treats access intimacy as an affect experience that holds people together on account of accessibility. It is an intuitive bonding which disabled people and their companions build by way of personal chemistry. Most blind students get away from disciplinary ghettos via access intimacy. Typical examples include partnerships based on audio description, mobility requirements, youthful play, and other forms of cultural extravaganza. During moments of access inti-macy, the notion that certain frameworks are unsuitable for the blind undergoes irreversible dismantlement. Not surprisingly, Rambabu did everything visual in close tie with his friends so that a tendency for ghettoization gradually disap-peared. In that way, he was a pioneer among my cohort.

phronesis involving college life may also include some kind of strategic per-sonhood marketing. In Rambabu's case, he was required to play along with the idea that he possessed a rare gift for the art of listening and storytelling. Narrative turn in the social sciences was established long before the 1990s as a viable approach for fieldwork investigation. During the 1990s, it was not a taboo to go for fieldwork and come back with a bag of stories. But that did not favour

Rambabu in the least. It was one thing to gather stories with eyesight intact, and entirely different to do so without it. To break free from such a restriction, Rambabu was required to position himself as someone with a special knack for the art of listening. Of course, he did not create a mystical aura around his listening skills. Far from it, he was merely interested in drawing on the art of conversation which he so diligently mastered during his stay at St Louis.[2]

At this point it is useful to return briefly to Anburajan's sociology adventures. During our time, we all developed an unstated urge to opt for careers that have never been explored by our blind seniors (at least those of us who could afford it). Rambabu achieved this diligently, and so did Anburajan. 'The problem with choosing a career which is already well trodden by other blind people is that one can be ghettoised so irremediably'. 'This is why I chose to do a Masters in Social Work', says Anbu (Anburajan, 2020b). This does not mean a saying such as 'Unity is strength' is an anathema to our cohort consciousness. In fact, our cohort saw the maturing of a blind collective such as the College and Graduate Association of the Blind (CSGAB) founded in the year 1980 by Mr Kannan (Kannan, 1980). CSGAB was responsible for so many battles linked to the creation of employment opportunities for blind graduates from my city, and beyond. That said, like others, we too developed a strong inner urge to grow up as fuller individuals, and not as yet another member of an invisible ghetto. I guess this is natural given the fact that our protracted institutionalization ended when globalization was beginning to unfold in the neighbourhood.

In a nutshell, my cohort consciousness is shaped by learnt suspicion concerning the suitability of social sciences for the blind. As a consequence, we were specially attuned to detecting disciplinary ghettos like the ones we are used to in our special school. We remember Rambabu for his special role in this regard.

Analytical discussion 2

Learnt comfort with the humanities

The second aspect of the special educational metanarrative of blindness is a learnt comfort with the humanities. Not all of our cohort members have a reliable career, but those of us who do manage it by jumping on to the humanities bandwagon. We did not have much choice otherwise. All jobs earmarked for the blind by the state were primarily tied to the humanities arena. All the same, the state was never the source of the assumed authority over our long-standing affiliation with the humanities establishment. It emerged for the most part from our school. Our teachers at St Louis, for example, put into motion the aspect of the metanarrative of blindness that made us absolutely comfortable with certain

---

2 Rambabu does not make this point explicitly in his research paper. The insight is totally mine based on a vague memory of our school days together.

disciplines in the field of humanities, such as literary criticism. This learnt comfort is a total contrast to an affect such as learnt suspicion of the social sciences. That said, a deep sense of learnt comfort continued to push us into looking for a home within literary criticism, no matter what challenges we confronted by way of accessibility. To examine the dynamics of such a belief in humanities pursuit, I rely on dicta, idioms, sayings, propositions, proverbs, and stories that were in active circulation at the school during our time – not all of them, just a saying or two that offer an organic meaning to our cohort consciousness.

Our teachers at St Louis strongly believed in the importance of life of the mind for blind people, and how one can pursue the same via great literature. In fact, our sense of learnt comfort about a field such as literary criticism seemed to emerge from such a normative consideration. Great music, literature, and a corpus of cultural narratives possess their rare internal beauty. If we can have a hold on them, we can become equally handsome. So, we went ahead, relentlessly pursuing them while telling ourselves that it was completely worth the effort. Learnt comfort about humanities kept us going, always trying to suppress our concerns about mounting access issues. We learnt to laugh at misfortunes.

Our teachers also insisted that certain domains of knowledge, such as literature, could be mastered easily because of their internal beauty:

> They have rhythm, meter, form, prosody, and the rest. By sheer hard work and will, one can absorb all these literary constituents intracranially. This is how the great blind poets Andhagakavi Viraragavar from the Tamil world attained immortal glory.

Our Tamil sir was never tired of telling the story of the great poet[3] (Andhagakavi in Tamil means the poet of the interiors). 'Blind psychology is actually a blessing', Tamil sir proclaimed once:

Because you are not distracted by unwanted spectacles, you boys can easily meditate on the beauty of fine literature. Also, you can retain knowledge as much as Viraragavar who is supposed to have had a command over knowledge that was as immense as the great Himalayas.

Tamil sir's idea of internal beauty appealed to our sense of natural strength, which we all are supposed to possess as blind people – namely, blind psychology. Here I recall Cutsforth's verbalism. In that formulation, blind children can potentially mistake words for a thing. Our Tamil sir was not so sceptical. He encouraged us to relish diction for its own sake. Such a persuasion may eventually help us master literary knowledge, at least to the envy of the sighted out there. In Tamil sir's worldview, verbalism looked like a thing of dictional beauty and power. It was by no means a handicap. Again, Tamil sir's propositions were not out of place altogether. In the music circle, a good many people talk about blind people's

---

3 Viraragavar is a blind poet from the Saivite tradition.

special talent because of a freedom from distraction caused by eyesight. For example, during all of his concerts, K.J. Yesudas keeps his eyes shut so as to keep him distraction-free like the blind. I am sure my friend Karthik is drenched with this aspect of the metanarrative because he is a blind musician (Karthik, 2020).

I now turn back to Tamil sir's class. In due course, we were beginning to accept that blind psychology was some kind of intracranial capability and an embodied cognition. Intracranially, we were considered to be hosting a mind that was almost like a blob of sealing wax. The more one exercises the blob by way of cognitive moulding, the more impressionable it becomes. One may call this attitude rote learning. The metaphor of the mind as a sealing wax is not native to our Tamil class. All the same, thanks to our teacher's interventions, the metaphor became a synonym for affirmative blind psychology, particularly during our stay in the school. Broadly, we were culturally trained in the art of elocution, mimicry, *padam* (a Tamil word game involving film names), poetry recitation, and the art of creating musical rhythms on the classroom desk. At the risk of repeating myself, I must say that all these forms of training seemed like a modified form of verbalism. The modification involves the notion that word-mindedness is actually a distraction-free authority over the linguistic universe. Not all of us believe now that we are distraction-free. At the same time, we have not yet extricated ourselves from the idea that artefacts such as literature possess unique internal beauty, and it is not hard for blind people to carve out a professional connection with it.

So, we continue to echo Tamil sir's well-meaning advice concerning our special privilege in accessing the internal beauty of literature. This is not because of a slavish devotion to Tamil sir but due to a wide circulation of the notion concerning internal beauty of literature by the literati. For example, practical criticism was much popularized by IA Richards at Cambridge during the early part of the twentieth century (Bredin, 1986). Richards conducted literary experiments with his pupils. They were asked to interpret poems without any contextual information whatsoever. Later on, these experiments by Richards were modulated so as to include contextual information as well. Reader response criticism, for example, enabled a nuanced critique by including a judgement of the readers as indispensable means for analysis, evaluation, and interpretation (Abrams and Harpham, 2011). In the Indian subcontinent, literature teachers like me encourage our students to pay special attention to the mechanics and the craftsmanship of a literary text alongside contextual materials. My fellow cohorts, particularly teachers of English literature, find such a literary education somewhat in sync with Tamil sir's wisdom concerning the internal beauty of a work of art. Both seem to say the same thing: literature possesses a rare internal beauty; everybody, including blind readers, can absorb the same into their system by some effort:

> at the end of the day, we are better off doing literature. Unlike our visually challenged peers in disciplines such as sociology, we do not have to put up with inaccessible fieldwork environments.

For the literary kinds among us, the above statements appear existentially real, although we do not verbalize them that way. Perhaps such inner rumbles are our version of phronesis in brewing. As long as it works professionally in our favour, we do not see the point about challenging the view that we are ably guided by blind psychology in the appreciation of the internal beauty of literature. This renews the assumed authority of blind psychology at the behest of our professional dip into literary criticism.

Analytical discussion 3

Learnt withdrawal from the sciences

The third special educational aspect of the metanarrative of blindness in India is a learnt withdrawal from the sciences:

> 'Very good Jayachandran, you got a centum in science. You can become a computer scientist'.
>
> I am sure Jaya was pleased with my congratulatory note.
>
> 'Can blind people study science?'
>
> Durai sounded doubtful.
>
> 'Why not? Sir Isaac Newton's teacher Professor Nicholas Saunderson was in fact blind'.
>
> I felt really proud when I said this.
>
> We heard our science teacher Mr Raj (Name changed) walk into the room.
>
> 'I hear some debates about sciences?'
>
> 'Yes sir, Jaya wants to become a computer scientist'.
>
> 'How can he? God has given you some gifts. You should work on them rather than on those about which you cannot have any control. after all, you are not sighted'.
>
> 'Sir, a computer is just a machine. If I am trained well, I can work on it like the sighted'.
>
> We were frightened by such a comment from Jaya.
>
> 'What are you talking about? Can you see the blackboard? Can you drive a car? There are some things the blind can never do. You must get used to that idea. You will require some basic knowledge of science, and that's why we are training you in it until tenth class. Ok let us not get distracted anymore'.

This conversation is not designed to take revenge on Mr Raj. In fact, the conversation may not be real at all. However, I can testify that it is true in spirit. Such conversations did the rounds in our school. Despite their abundance, they were unanimous about one proclamation: keep away from sciences; they are not meant for the blind at all.

Staying away from sciences informed our phronesis as a cohort. In our systemic withdrawal from sciences, we also accepted the assumed authority of our special educators concerning the same. Their authoritative voices still echo in us. Naturally, I recount our collective withdrawal from sciences conversationally.

Concluding discussion

Special education is a culture-specific enterprise, and so are its reasons of being. In the Indian context, special education is shaped by approaches curated by Community-Based Rehabilitation (CBR). As a community-driven venture, Indian special education tends to recycle unresolved social anxieties concerning formation questions of people with disabilities. The metanarrative of blindness flows this way between special educational settings and communities at large. The unceasing flow of this metanarrative shapes the lives of disabled people, including their disciplinary choices. Such influences renew themselves constantly so as to sustain assumed authority over people with disability. It is time that disability studies take cognisance of such renewals in India. If not, the field may inadvertently miss out on formation questions, especially the ways and means by which they determine life chances of disabled people. Formation questions still make the staple of special education training. This is something worth examining with an open mind.

Locating myself within a cohort, I sketch how our special education influenced our journeys across disciplines. In doing so, I give due credence to phronesis (i.e. practical wisdom) that was influential all the way through. Somebody else may do it differently. The millennials, for example, may be influenced by phronesis of information economy, plus the power to share knowledge via an arrangement such as *Bookshare* and a spectrum of social media.

I am sorry, my cohort consciousness looks like a boys' club. Actually, it is not. Special schools in India, by and large, are monastic. They also put in place a strict gender segregation norm. That too is part of the metanarrative of blindness but beyond this chapter that I can only conclude by saying thanks to my cohort for a journey together.

References

Abrams, M. H. and Harpham, G. (2011) *A glossary of literary terms*, Boston: Cengage Learning.

Anburajan (2020a) Blind psychology, telephone conversation with author.

Anburajan (2020b) Career choice, telephone conversation with author.

Bolt, D. (2014) *The metanarrative of blindness: A re-reading of twentieth-century anglophone writing*, Ann Arbor: University of Michigan Press.

Bredin, H. (1986) IA Richards and the philosophy of practical criticism, *Philosophy and Literature* 10: 26–37.

Corning, A. and Schuman, H. (2015) *Generations and collective memory*, Chicago: University of Chicago Press.

Cutsforth, T. D. (1951) *The blind in school and society: A psychological study*, Arlington: American Foundation for the Blind.

Debord, G. (2012) *Society of the spectacle*, London: Bread and Circuses Publishing.

Kagan, J. (2009) *The three cultures: Natural sciences, social sciences, and the humanities in the 21st century*, Cambridge: Cambridge University Press.

Kannan, S. (1980) College students and graduates association of blind [Online]. Available: http://csgab.org/includes/aboutus.html [Accessed 26/08 2020].

Karthik. (2020) Blindness and music, telephone conversation with author.

Mingus, M. (2011) Access intimacy: The missing link [Online]. Available: https://leavingevidence.wordpress.com/2011/05/05/access-intimacy-the-missing-link/ [Accessed 30/8 2020].

Rambabu, A. 2012 Sociology and the study of disability: Disciplinary directions and personal reflections, *Workshop on the Emergence of Indian Disability Studies: Opportunities and Challenges*. (Unpublished).

Schram, S. (2012) Phronetic social science: An idea whose time has come, in, B. Flyvbjerg, T. Landman, and S. Schram (Eds.), *Real social science: Applied phronesis*, Cambridge: Cambridge University Press.

PART II

Beyond normative minds and bodies

4

THE METANARRATIVE OF MENTAL ILLNESS

A collaborative autoethnography

Katharine Martyn and Annette Thompson

Preliminary discussion

The critical context for this chapter is that the image of mental illness in cultural representations has changed little since biblical times, often with wild and emotive images of people possessed by evil or else having 'second site' with visitations by God (Millon et al., 2004; Watters, 1992). This mysterious and often frightening portrayal informs many headlines in the media and other stories (Carmichael et al., 2019), impacting on how society frames mental illness, and on how professionals and organizations support those who are struggling (Corrigan et al., 2012). The fictionalization of mental illness has been especially popular in medical, crime, and war dramas where the protagonist has a so-called problematic character; for example, addiction to drugs or alcohol (Greg House in the television show *House MD*), suicidal ideation (Aidan's exit storyline in *Coronation Street*), and a tendency to break the law or challenge professional boundaries (Jack Bauer in the television show *24*). Accordingly, media reporting of mental illness often uses familiar stigmatizing language and negative depiction. Individuals are groundlessly described as dangerous (e.g. homicidal and/or suicidal) when aligned with the metanarrative of mental illness.

That is not to deny that the twenty-first century has heralded a move towards a more inclusive society underpinned by legislation with policies to ensure that people with mental illnesses have equitable access to education, employment, and support. Both domestic and international disability legislation (e.g. Americans with Disabilities Act in 1990, Disability Discrimination Act in 1995) aimed to prevent all forms of discrimination. In the United Kingdom, for example, the Equality Act in 2010 identified mental illness as a protected characteristic. Nevertheless, such legislation has done little to change the metanarrative of mental illness and thus the stigma experienced by individuals who navigate and negotiate complex health systems, benefits, and employment opportunities (Temple et al., 2018). These are some of the lived realities we explore in this chapter.

Methodological discussion

This autobiographical journey as a living, dynamic narrative enables us to uncover meanings against a contemporary backdrop of social, political, and economic challenges. The personal narrative then transcends the individual as we explore how mental illness is perceived in lay and professional domains. As such, the autobiographical journey touches on themes familiar to many people.

Ethnography, the study of people in their natural surroundings, is concerned with understanding social meanings and activities. Hammersley (1990) argues that in ethnography the researcher seeks to study people's behaviour in everyday contexts. In contrast, autoethnography focuses on the narrative of an individual. This personal narrative is challenged through self-reflection to connect the autobiographical story to the broader cultural, political, and social meanings of the society within which it is situated. Nevertheless, Ellis and Bochner (2000) caution the reader to see autoethnography not as merely the retelling of stories but as a medium that allows readers to *feel* moral dilemmas; to think *with* the story, rather than *about* it. Indeed, Chang, Ngunjiri, and Hernandez, (2013) remind us that the autoethnographer, as any qualitative researcher, adheres to the rigours of research, including analytical approaches to interpretations of the individual narrative. We were certainly mindful of this point when ethical approval was considered, sought, and obtained for the research discussed in this chapter.

As a method, autoethnography incorporates cultural and personal aspects of individual narrative (Ellis and Bochner, 2000); it 'liberates a new generation of anthropologists to bring their personal stories to the centre stage of investigation' (Chang, 2008, 45). Collaborative autoethnography, involving two or more people, extends this concept further by still focusing on self-interrogation, but collectively, through shared personal narratives. It is in the sharing of our everyday experiences that the narratives and stories we tell – about how we live, why we live, and what is important to us – become shaped by our external and internal understandings of the world.

This collaborative autoethnography is written as a critical dialogue and draws on the dual lenses of the authors as we explore the experience of mental illness to disrupt the related metanarrative. We share our understanding of mental illness from very different perspectives. There is Annette's personal narrative about the lived experience of moving from adolescence to adulthood; from pre-diagnosis to diagnosis. There is Katharine's perspective as a nurse, academic, and researcher who works alongside students experiencing mental illness. This approach, as we move between individual and collaborative biography, allows an enriched understanding of the embedded, contextual character of mental illness, support, and care practices as they unfold amid education, employment, and so on.

Building research around the crafting of stories about our own experiences enables us to make sense of the complexities of a broader social world from the dual insider-outsider perspective. Stepping back from any particular disciplinary perspective (Ellis, 2007) and being challenged by the very process of collaboration, allows us to be critical, probing, and more analytical and self-conscious about our input (Chang, 2013, 32). Dual analysis sensitizes us to the individual nature of experiences and needs.

Analytical discussion 1

Voice and being heard

Voice is often critical to disruptions of the metanarrative of mental illness, as it is the main form of communication between the individual, the health care provider, and broader society. It communicates the individual's place within their mental health journey, their response to treatment, as well as the giving or withdrawing of consent. Voice illuminates how others respond to mental illness, with their acceptance or denial reflecting a societal position. This voice can be a combination of spoken words, non-visual and visual cues arising from an individual's actions, such as self-harm or a suicide attempt, and the persons' posture or lack of eye contact. Accordingly, the multifaceted concept of voice is relevant in many social interactions.

Voice and access to mental health services emerge as two of the recurring themes in our collaborative autoethnography. We begin with an exploration of the challenges in accessing mental health services within two cities in the United Kingdom and the concurrent changing social relationships. In understanding these relationships, Berne's theory of transactional analysis of phenomenological and social realities helps to describe how social behaviour can be relayed into a state of mind, formally known as ego states. In phenomenology, the ego state is 'a coherent system of feelings' (Berne, 1996, 154). However, in this chapter, Berne's definition of an ego state as a 'system of feelings which motivates a related set of behaviour patterns' is utilized (Berne, 1996, 154). Berne sets out three different types of ego states: the exteropyschic, neopsychic, and archaeopschic, also known as the parent, adult, and child. In our collaborative autoethnography, these states provide the framework for unpicking interactions with the health care system, as well as changing social relationships.

In one section of Annette's personal narrative a visit to the emergency department at the local hospital and an encounter with a nurse highlight how a shift between ego states changes the power dynamics. During this experience, an admission of heavy drinking prompts a conversation about alcohol and whether there is a drinking problem. The subsequent denial, followed by an explanation that it is the medication, implies guilt. At this familiar point of assumed authority, the dynamic shifts from two conversing adults to a parent and a child. Mills and Lefrançois (2018) suggest that this feeling of 'being a child' and the inference that one's behaviour is childlike is a common metaphor applied to the 'mad' to explain the apparent irrationality of behaviour and to enable others, such as health professionals, to assume authority in the encounter. The trouble is that, unable to respond differently, Annette is rendered shameful and guilty about being at the hospital, feelings of hopelessness and a lack of agency emerge.

In another section of Annette's personal narrative, the lack of agency is mirrored in a changing relationship at home. As adults sharing a flat, arguably the 'healthy' relationship is between neopsychics (i.e. adults). When sharing a home, each person assumes the expected roles of friend, colleague, flatmate; the relationship is mutually agreed upon and supportive. However, as with any relationship, it can deteriorate with one or more parties shifting roles. In this situation, the flatmates act as parents (i.e. exteropyschics), overseeing the running of the flat and creating a feeling of one-upmanship, that feels like a game, with one player as the child (i.e. archaeopsychic). Awareness of the changing relationships pre-empt deteriorating mental health and increasing despair that culminate in a suicide attempt:

> Annette. As things got worse in the flat, it all came to a crescendo one Friday evening, when I got a text message from one of them, insulting me. It was all about something insignificant. When I got to the flat, we had a blazing row, and I locked myself in my room. We were on the top floor of a small block of flats. I threw open the window as wide as it would go with the aim to jump. I wanted to end the pain that I felt, rather than wanting to die.

As adults, we always try to be reasoned in our interactions with others. We both recall times of emotional distress or despair when the ideal dialogue between fellow neopsychics was not maintained, and the destructive shift towards an exteropsychic and an archaeopsychic resulted in the latter 'storming off' and the former 'winning the game'. One such encounter was epitomized by the response of a general practitioner (GP) when I, Katharine, was seeking support for my daughter. The GP was unhelpful, and my cries for help were met by reassuring platitudes, telling me that 'she is playing up because you are divorced'. I can recall consciously relishing the slip into a childlike response as I sat on the floor of the surgery, refusing to move until someone listened to my daughter. Unlike Annette, my only label was that of a 'divorced mother', and once I had their attention, I resumed my adult stance. For Annette, the response of health care professionals and flatmates was clouded by the ever-present metanarrative of mental illness, every move accentuating an unwanted diagnosis, as well as the guilt and shame of the experience.

The feeling of shame that, as adults, we could not control the situation or behave in what we had perceived to be the correct way was ever-present in the encounters with health professionals and others. Shame is 'a cause for regret or disappointment' (Waite, 2012, 665). It is 'more than a mere mechanical reflection of ourselves but is also the imagined effect that this reflection has on others' (Cooley, 1922, 184–185), and far from simple when considered in Western culture (Scheff, 2003). It encapsulates some of the feelings experienced during mental illness (Walitza and Rossier, 2020; Riley et al., 2018; Mulfinger et al., 2018), and is made more tangible by the responses of others as they unconsciously reaffirm how behaviours or situations differ from those of peers. Shame and feelings of vulnerability can lead to increased awareness of perceived faults (Martens, 2005), leading to escapist or hiding behaviour, further increasing vulnerability as support becomes less secure. Feelings of shame can reflect how we perceive our health is understood by those who know us (Riley et al., 2018), including our family.

Feeling shameful, in accordance with the metanarrative of mental illness, sensitizes someone to the voice of health care professionals (Rivera-Segarra et al., 2019), as though *you* are the problem and *your* condition is a result of *your* actions. This is epitomized in Annette's personal narrative by a visit to the A/E department, involving a wait of 6 hours, only to be told to be kind to herself. For Annette, this influenced her view of the health service and, on reflection, her subsequent interactions when asking for help: 'I believed that health care providers had a subconscious scale of severity and that I needed to meet the threshold for further support'. Illustrating another aspect of the metanarrative, Vogel (2013) argues that the sense that one's mental illness is not legitimate is pervasive in society, often leading to disempowerment (Corrigan et al., 2020). In health services, particularly in settings that focus on physical health, the biomedical model of triaging individuals to treat appropriately is routine, yet often it fails to address the concerns of those with mental illness (Iserson and Moskop, 2007). As Beresford (2020) observes, despite the emergence of a new mental illness discourse, mental health continues to be defined by a biomedical framework. Carers and family members attending emergency departments reaffirm the biomedical stance. At the same time, those in a mental health crisis highlight a pattern of disempowerment and invisibility.

When considering the metanarrative of mental illness, changing relationships, be they with friends, family, or others, feature within several of our discussions. Some of these relationships become stronger, whereas others become damaged to the point of no repair. Friends and family can find it challenging to understand the internal anguish being experienced yet their response to individual distress is essential, often influencing the person's beliefs about their own mental health:

> Annette. I went home and met up with some friends from school. I cannot remember if I told them straight away (about my illness) or not. But these friends made me feel safe and normal, they have been with me through everything since, and I have a debt to them that I cannot pay. In contrast, when I returned to the flat, things were not always smooth, many arguments were had, and my mental health really deteriorated. I went from moderate to severe depression. This negativity was challenging and often fuelled the feelings of shame and inadequacy that led me to

self-harm. Despite my obvious distress, my flatmates accused me of faking my mental illness. In my head, this challenged my sense of self as simultaneously my medication had been switched from Citalopram to Fluoxetine (Prozac).

This form of assumed authority can be especially problematic, for Schomerus and Angermeyer (2018) describe how being accused of 'faking it' can add to the shame and stigma surrounding mental illness and can pre-empt maladaptive behaviour for coping that includes a cycle of pain relief, shame, and self-hate. That is to say, how health professionals respond to people experiencing a mental health crisis can trigger a cycle of events that further exacerbates the despair and loss of control:

> Annette. During one bank holiday weekend, I was very unwell and suicidal. I was referred by the local mental health rapid response service to be seen by a mental health nurse. The nurse that I saw was not compassionate, took no notes, just asked me questions. I knew that if I left without any help that I would try to take my life. But this did not sway her to get me help. Instead, I was told that I was not severe enough to be sectioned and that it would be better if I came back the next day to see a different nurse. Following this, I resorted to self-harm. Subconsciously, self-harm acted as a visual cue of my distress, when I felt that I was not being taken seriously. I believed that harming myself showed the severity of how I was feeling in my head and the pain that I was in.

Townsend (2019) stresses that self-harm needs to be taken seriously by frontline staff as it often begins when a young person feels patronized and not listened to. For many who self-harm, the relief experienced is short-lived, often replaced with feelings of guilt, shame, and worthlessness.

As we explore these interactions, difficulties in accessing mental health services emerge: the inequity of provision known as a 'postcode lottery'. MIND, United Kingdom (2019) identifies that local spending priorities influence the availability of mental health services. Gadamer's (2006) fusion of horizons provides a framework to explore the impact of difficulties in access to mental health services that, for Thompson (2011), allows for two contrasting opinions on the same experience to form a single, more rounded opinion. In London, then, access to psychological and psychiatric help was quick, with shorter waiting times for both the university services and the NHS from the time of referral. Furthermore, Annette felt believed and listened to, without resorting to desperate measures:

> At the time, I was also receiving Cognitive Behavioural Therapy (CBT) from the university health and wellbeing department. The hospital psychiatric assessment was pretty standard. What day was it? Who is the Prime Minister? Eventually, I was discharged and told to go home

with a letter from the doctor excusing me from the exam and a couple of Zopiclone and orders to take one and go to sleep.

In Brighton, however, the process was slow, with frequent referrals and reminders. It was only at the point of a mental health crisis that Annette believed she was heard:

> For many years, it was just me and my general practitioner (GP) battling against the mental health system in the Brighton area. I was seen by a psychiatrist in that time who confirmed that alongside depression and anxiety, I had Borderline Personality Disorder (BPD). But I did not receive proper help from the mental health services until my mum had lifesaving heart and lung surgery in 2015. After the operation, I was my mum's carer, and towards the end, I was breaking down again. My GP thought that I might have the start of Post-Traumatic Stress Disorder (PTSD). I was in crisis and was referred to the crisis team, who after discussing the least important aspects of my life and how I was feeling, referred me over to the Group Treatment Service (GTS) located in the local psychiatric hospital.

PTSD was first codified as a legitimate diagnosis in the *Diagnostic and Statistical Manual of Mental Disorders, Third Edition* (*DSM-III*) in 1980 and is said to arise from psychological trauma. In our collaborative autoethnography, the formal diagnosis allows access to mental health services previously denied. The diagnosis of PTSD provides gatekeepers with the reassurance they require that the individual is not a malingerer.

However, the acceptance of the diagnosis is challenged when, according to Hal and Hall (2006), the term *PTSD* has in recent times been applied to many different situations, most commonly for financial gain. The continued discord between formal diagnoses and whether an individual has a legitimate illness is evident in other conditions that sit uncomfortably with what society believes is normal:

> Katharine. For my daughter 'autistic spectrum disorder' (ASD) provided a label for the health professionals that they could refer to, it even excused their lack of understanding and frank disbelief. At that time, little was known about 'high functioning' autism, but her diagnosis was part of a research project and she was being seen by a well-known professor. This seemed to legitimise it for them. Before that, I was simply an over-anxious divorced mother.

Such doubt is a major factor in the metanarrative of mental illness. In the shadow of this disbelief, people are unable to access support, with several talking about having to be in a 'crisis' and many resorting to self-harm or verbalizing suicidal ideation as cues of distress. The feeling of not being ill enough is particularly resonant. The act of not being heard or being dismissed when attending acute services highlights a real fear held by those with a mental illness. The impact of being 'passed off' to someone else reinforces the belief that they are not worth the help and thus discourages them from asking for help when it is most needed.

The contrasting responses of the two cities illustrate how the experience of mental illness can vary. The lack of equity and underfunding of mental health services is not new and remains an issue for many health systems (Bartram, 2017; Ambikile and Iseselo, 2017; Jacobs et al., 2018). It highlights the 'postcode lottery' that impacts on health care provision, as indicated in the 2017/18 Care Quality Commission (CQC) review of the state of health and social care in England, United Kingdom (CQC, 2018). Together this indicates a service that needs to be designed better for people who struggle with accessing support.

Analytical discussion 2

Stigma

Given the ubiquity of the metanarrative, stigma is a phenomenon often experienced by people with mental illness. Stigma is 'a mark or sign of disgrace' (Waite, 2012, 716) which can be traced back to the ancient Greeks, where it showed something bad or unusual in the context of a person's mental status (Goffman, 2006). Goffman argues that stigma stems from blemishes on the social identity and character of the person, both personal (e.g. honesty) and structural (e.g. occupation), that are transformed into normative expectations. These include but are not exclusive to mental disorder, addiction, and alcoholism. Goffman further states that there is a belief that the stigma of the person makes them less human. Part of the metanarrative of mental illness, this pejorative discourse (Elraz, 2018) is often described by people who have direct experience – it remains prevalent in the twenty-first century (Turan et al., 2019). For example, the notion that mental illness equates with lacking competence or free choice was cited recently following a partial defence for a crime committed during the counter Black Lives Matter protests (Bowcott, 2020).

The attribution of stigma is a form of assumed authority that features in many aspects of life. Aspirations that a more inclusive society supported by legislation are positive, yet workplace discrimination by colleagues and laypeople, for those experiencing mental illness, remains evident (Elraz, 2018):

> Annette. I started to volunteer my time in a local charity shop. I was serving a woman who decided to comment on my scars – saying that I had ruined my life because of them. I tried to tell her a story that has worked in the past, that I got them from working in a sheet metal factory. But she did not believe me and kept on at me. Other people were queuing to be served and did nothing.

Corrigan et al., (2012) argue that it is incidents like this that chip away at a person's self-esteem, reinforcing the stigma that mental illness is a 'blemish' held by the individual and their families. The stigma associated with mental illness, and the self-stigma experienced by Annette as she struggles to own her identity as a person with a mental illness, leads her to consider a plausible explanation for her scars. This need to hide or excuse self-harm scars is not uncommon (Stirling, 2020), and it characterizes the individual's response to the unconscious bias associated with mental illness. Unconscious bias is a distortion of which the observer is unaware at the time, and is evident in issues of race, gender, and health (Fitzgerald and Hurst, 2017). It includes the attitudes and stereotypes that people unconsciously attribute to another person or group of people that affect how they understand and engage with a person or group.

Analytical discussion 3

Public identity and self-identity

Identity is 'the fact of being who or what a person or thing is' (Waite, 2012, 358). Identity can be divided into two sections: public identity and self-identity, also referred to as external and internal, respectively. A person's public identity can be defined by sociological constructs such as class, education, and job prospects. In contrast, self-identity is defined through a person's self-esteem and how they view themselves within society's norms. In Annette's personal narrative, there is a distinction between these two forms of identity, although often there is an overlap between the personal and public persona.

Goffman (1978) asserts that social interaction is akin to a theatre performance. In these terms, we play a role and only reveal certain aspects of the performance while shielding others, under what is known as impression management. This view is heavily criticized by Jenkins (2004), as being of cynical motivation. Goffman's framework illuminates three public identities that emerge in our collaborative autoethnography on mental illness: student, benefit claimant, and service user.

Being a student, at both sixth form college and university, is meant to be the 'time of your life'. However, students often experience pressure to succeed, and to exceed the expectations of peers and others, which negatively impacts on their mental health (Laidlaw et al., 2016). Nevertheless, public perceptions of student life are overshadowed by media articles and television shows such as *Skins* and *Fresh Meat*, where students are portrayed as lazy or intoxicated. These notions inform a metanarrative that is very different from the lived experience captured in Annette's personal narrative:

> In sixth form college I did manage to find some counselling, but I did not get on with the counsellor. As it seemed to me at the time that she just did not understand the pain I was in inside my head, and I could not find the words to explain it to her. I failed my first year of college. They wanted to

kick me out and not let me resit the year but let slip that they had noticed that I was not well and that they had done nothing. Teachers noted the deterioration of my mental health but, as it was not acted on, the time coincided with my experience of failure, adding to the mounting pressure in an already fragile person. This just adds to the perceived public identity that they (i.e. people with mental illness) are a failure and are not good for anything.

Seeking employment with an ongoing mental illness is also challenging, given the need to be seen as well and 'normal'. This often means not wanting to disclose a mental illness while simultaneously needing support:

> Annette. Eventually, I had to sign on at the jobcentre. There was one staff member who was so horrible that I would have a panic attack after each time I saw her. Then I snapped and told her exactly how she was making me feel and that I had a mental illness and that she was making it worse. I left the jobcentre crying. I had to have a medical under the Government's Work Capability test, and I was physically and mentally unwell. The medical was intense, and waiting for the assessment made me both physically and mentally ill, to the point where I was vomiting when they called my name.

Implicit in this abuse of authority is the fact that the external view of mental illness has not moved from being 'mad or bad' (Rüsch, 2012). In a time of professed equality and equity of opportunity, the ableist perspective of being 'normal' is challenged by the notion that someone can be struggling with a mental illness and attempting to work while needing help from the state (Young et al., 2019; Nario Redmond et al., 2019). To many people, including professionals such as the one in Annette's example, this non-normative dynamic is an alien concept.

The third branch of the public (i.e. external) image for this metanarrative of mental illness is that of a service user. In this context, the term *service user* refers to someone who is accessing (or has access to) mental health services. It is by no means a perfect system, and from Annette's personal narrative it has already been gathered that accessing the system can be dependent on where an individual resides. Even when in the system, the individual can experience stigma and other barriers that can prevent her, him, or them from getting treatment. This makes trusting the system in times of crisis exceptionally hard. Goicolea et al. (2018) identify the importance of trust, alongside other factors, as a determinant of a young person's utilization of mental health services. Moreover, a lack of trust can completely stop the person from attempting access when they are at their most vulnerable:

> Annette. The next day, it was the start of a new week, and I managed to get through to the doctor's surgery. I knew that the receptionist did not

believe me, so, I told her to check with the hospital and eventually I was told that the doctor would try and call me but not to hold my breath. The doctor did call me.

This extract from Annette's personal narrative provides a prime example of assumed authority and indeed the barriers faced when accessing the health care system: defensive gatekeeping to rationalize resource use and institutionalized gatekeeping through referral pathways (Aoki et al., 2018; McEvoy and Richards, 2007). Buchbindre (2017) recognizes the negative connotations but argues that, by redirecting, such gatekeepers are managing scarce resources. Wilson et al. (2013) conclude that this all reflects a system that requires urgent review.

The normative authority is complex, for being a service user often includes options for treatment that can only be received from a doctor's referral, including access to other services, such as a lead practitioner/community psychiatric nurse (CPN). This point is raised in Annette's personal narrative:

I had to leave GTS before my referral to the recovery centre was accepted and was handed over to the Assessment and Treatment Service (ATS) at the local polyclinic as well as to a mental health nurse who acted as my lead practitioner. It took me time to trust her, but she was good and helped me out when others could not.

Never is the normative authority of the metanarrative more complex than when it becomes internalized. The internal self-identity is the general or specific perspectives a person with a mental illness has towards themselves (Rise et al., 2010). Although self-identity can have a motivational root, in that, it is done for fear of rejection by others; it is also the lens through which people see themselves. Self-identity, as relevant to the metanarrative of mental illness, is formed by the assumptions made by others that often motivate an individual's actions, accentuating the internal struggle of the individual and making them unsure of who they are. These assumptions can influence both the treatment given and the treatment outcome as it affects the level of trust and faith that the individual has in the prescribed treatment:

Annette. I did put in a complaint about the first nurse that I saw, but this was swept under the carpet. It destroyed my trust in the rapid response service, and it was not regained until years later. The outcome of the complaint eradicated any trust that I had in the system and that they would not be able to keep me safe.

Finding the courage to speak up, only to be knocked back, can be very demoralizing; it encourages the person to suffer in silence. This can derail the personal narrative, in that it could stop it completely. The damage that can be done is on a par with social constraints and labels that are handed out by mental health professionals. Moreover, the person can start to believe the negative social perceptions about mental illness (Lally et al., 2013). In some cases, this can lead to a cycle of shame avoidance and further self-harm (Owens et al., 2018), a self-fulfilling prophecy, as the person will not expect help and does little to seek help thus making the prediction come true.

Concluding discussion

The metanarrative of mental illness can be viewed through many different lenses. In advancing a critical response, the emergent themes from this collaborative interpretation of experiences go some way to allow for the broad scope of mental illness to be explored. Capturing the real-world view via collaborative autoethnography allows for the exploration of the themes in more detail. Throughout this collaborative autoethnography, it becomes increasingly evident that the metanarrative of mental illness is defined by stigma and shame, against which the individual must work hard to ensure the more authentic personal narrative is voiced.

References

Ambikile, J. S. and Iseselo, M. K. (2017) Mental health care and delivery system at Temeke hospital in Dar es Salaam, Tanzania, *BMC Psychiatry* 17 (1): 109.

Aoki, T., Yamamoto, Y., Ikenoue, T., Kaneko, M., Kise, M., Fujinuma, Y. and Fukuhara, S. (2018) Effect of patient experience on bypassing a primary care gatekeeper: A multicenter prospective cohort study in Japan, *Journal of General Internal Medicine* 33 (5): 722–728.

Bartram, M. (2017) Making the most of the federal investment of $5 billion for mental health, *CMAJ: Canadian Medical Association Journal (CMAJ)* 189 (44): E1360–E1363.

Beresford, P. (2020) 'Mad': Mad studies and advancing inclusive resistance, *Disability and Society*, 35 (8): 1337–1342.

Berne, E. (1996) Principles of transactional analysis, *Indian Journal of Psychiatry* 38 (3): 154–158.

Bowcott, O. (2020) Man given 14-day jail term for urinating near PC Keith Palmer plaque, *The Guardian*, 15th June [Online] Available at: https://www.theguardian.com/uk-news/2020/jun/15/man-given-14-day-jail-sentence-for-urinating-near-pc-keith-palmer-plaque (Accessed: 22nd June 2020).

Buchbinder, M. (2017) Keeping out and getting in: Reframing emergency department gatekeeping as structural competence, *Sociology of Health and Illness* 39 (7): 1166–1179.

Carmichael, V., Adamson, G., Sitter, K. C. and Whitley, R. (2019) Media coverage of mental illness: A comparison of citizen journalism vs. professional journalism portrayals, *Journal of Mental Health* 28 (5): 520–526.

Chang, H. (2008) *Autoethnography as Method*. Walnut Creek: Left Coast Press.

Chang, H. (2013) Individual and collaborative autoethnography as method, in Jones, S., Adams, T., and Ellis, C. (Eds.), *Handbook of Autoethnography*. Walnut Creek: Left Cost Press.

Cooley, C. H. (1922) *Human Nature and the Social Order*, New York: Scribner's.

Corrigan, P. W., Morris, S. B., Michaels, P. J., Rafacz, J. D., and Rusch, €. N. (2012) Challenging the public stigma of mental illness: A metanalysis of outcome studies, *Psychiatric Services* 63 (10): 963–973.

CQC (2018) *The state of health care and adult social care in England*. Available at https://www.cqc.org.uk/sites/default/files/20171011_stateofcare1718_report.pdf [accessed 26 September 2020]

Ellis, C., Bochner, A. P. (2000) Autoethnography, personal narrative, reflexivity, in Denzin, N. K., Lincoln, Y. S. (Eds.), *Handbook of Qualitative Research* (2nd ed.). Thousand Oaks: Sage.

Ellis, C. (2007) Telling secrets, revealing lives: Relational ethics in research with intimate others. *Qualitative Inquiry* 13: 3–29.

Elraz, H. (2018) Identity, mental health and work: How employees with mental health conditions recount stigma and the pejorative discourse of mental illness, *Human Relations* 71 (5): 722–741.

FitzGerald, C. and Hurst, S. (2017) Implicit bias in healthcare professionals: A systematic review, *BMC Medical Ethics* 18 (1): 19.

Gadamer, G. H. (2006) *Truth and Method*, 2nd edition, London: Continuum.

Gadamer, H. G. (2006) Language and understanding (1970). *Theory, Culture & Society* 23 (1): 13–27.

Goffman, E. (1978) *The Presentation of Self in Everyday Life*. London: Penguin.

Goffman, E. (2006) Selections on stigma, in L. J. Davis (Ed.), *The Disability Studies Reader*, 2nd edition, London: Routledge.

Goicolea, I., Hultstrand Ahlin, C., Waenerlund, A. K. et al. (2018) Accessibility and factors associated with utilization of mental health services in youth health centers: A qualitative comparative analysis in northern Sweden. *International Journal of Mental Health Systems* 12 (1): 69.

Hall, R. C. W. (2006) Malingering of PTSD: Forensic and diagnostic considerations, characteristics of malingerers and clinical presentations. *General Hospital Psychiatry* 28 (6): 525–35.

Hammersley, M. (1990) *Reading Ethnographic Research: A Critical Guide*. London: Longman.

Iserson, K. V. and Moskop, J. C. (2007) Triage in medicine, part I: Concept, history, and types, *Annals of Emergency Medicine* 49 (3): 275–81.

Jacobs, R., Chalkley, M., Aragón, M. J., Böhnke, J. R., Clark, M. and Moran, V. (2018) Funding approaches for mental health services: Is there still a role for clustering?, *BJPsych Advances* 24 (6): 412–421.

Jenkins, R. (2004) *Social Identity*, 2nd edition, New York: Routledge.

Laidlaw, A., McLellan, J., and Ozakinci, G. (2016) Understanding undergraduate student perceptions of mental health, mental wellbeing and help seeking behaviour, *Studies in Higher Education* 41 (12): 2156–2168.

Lally, J., O Conghaile, A., Quigley, S., Bainbridge, E., and McDonald, C. (2013) Stigma of mental illness and help-seeking intention in university students, *The Psychiatrist* 37: 253–260.

Martens, W. (2005) A multicomponental model of shame, *Journal for the Theory of Social Behaviour* 35 (4): 399–411.

McEvoy, P. and Richards, D. (2007) Gatekeeping access to community mental health teams: A qualitative study, *International Journal of Nursing Studies* 44 (3): 387–395.

Mills, C. and Lefrançois, B. A. (2018) Child as metaphor: Colonialism, psy-governance, and epistemicide, *World Futures* 74 (7–8): 503–524.

Millon, T. (Ed.). (2004) *Masters of the Mind: Exploring the Story of Mental Illness from Ancient Times to the New Millennium*, Hoboken: John Wiley and Sons.

Nario-Redmond, M. R., Kemerling, A. A. and Silverman, A. (2019) Hostile, benevolent, and ambivalent ableism: Contemporary manifestations, *Journal of Social Issues* 75 (3): 726–756.

Owens, C., Hansford, L., Sharkey, S. and Ford, T. (2016; 2018) Needs and fears of young people presenting at accident and emergency department following an act of self-harm: Secondary analysis of qualitative data, *British Journal of Psychiatry* 208 (3): 286–291.

Riley, R., Spiers, J., Chew-Graham, C. A., Taylor, A. K., Thornton, G. A. and Buszewicz, M. (2018) 'Treading water but drowning slowly': What are GPs' experiences of living and working with mental illness and distress in England? A qualitative study, *BMJ Open* 8 (5): e018620.

Rise, J., Sheeran, P., and Hukkelberg, S. (2010) The role of self-identity in the theory of planned behavior: a meta-analysis, *Journal of Applied Social Psychology* 40 (5): 1085–1105.

Rivera-Segarra, E., Varas-Díaz, N. and Santos-Figueroa, A. (2019) 'That's all fake': Health professionals' stigma and physical healthcare of people living with serious mental illness, *PloS one* 14 (12): E0226401.

Rüsch, N., Evans-Lacko, S. and Thornicroft, G. (2012) What is a mental illness? Public views and their effects on attitudes and disclosure, *Australian and New Zealand Journal of Psychiatry* 46 (7): 641–650.

Scheff, T. J. (2003) Shame in self and society, *Symbolic Interaction* 26 (2): 239–262.

Schomerus, G., and Angermeyer, M. C. (2008) Stigma and its impact on help-seeking for mental disorders: what do we know? *Epidemiologia e Psichiatria Sociale* 17 (1): 31–37.

Stirling, F. J. (2020) Journeying to visibility: An autoethnography of self-harm scars in the therapy room, *Psychotherapy and Politics International* 18 (2): 1–14.

Temple, J. B., Kelaher, M. and Williams, R. (2018) Discrimination and avoidance due to disability in Australia: Evidence from a National Cross-Sectional Survey, *BMC Public Health* 18(1): 1347.

Thompson, A. (2011) H.L.A. hart and hermeneutic philosophy, assignment for *LA3900, LLB (Hons) Law*, University of East London: Unpublished.

Townsend, E. (2019) Time to take self-harm in young people seriously, *The Lancet Psychiatry* 6 (4): 279–280.

Turan, J. M., Elafros, M. A., Logie, C. H., Banik, S., Turan, B., Crockett, K. B., Pescosolido, B. and Murray, S. M. (2019) Challenges and opportunities in examining and addressing intersectional stigma and health, *BMC Medicine* 17 (1): 7–15.

Vogel, D. L., Bitman, R. L., Hammer, J. H. and Wade, N. G. (2013) Is stigma internalised? The longitudinal impact of public stigma on self-stigma, *Journal of Counseling Psychology* 60 (2): 311–316.

Waite, M. (Ed.). (2012) *Paperback Oxford English Dictionary*, 7th edition, Oxford: Oxford University Press.

Watters, W. W. (1992) *Deadly Doctrine: Health, Illness and Christian God-Talk*, Buffalo: Prometheus Books.

Wilson, A. B., Barrenger, S., Bohrman, C. and Draine, J. (2013) Balancing accessibility and selectivity in 21st century public mental health services: Implications for hard to engage clients, *Journal of Behavioral Health Services and Research* 40 (2): 191–206.

Young, R. E., Goldberg, J. O., Struthers, C. W., McCann, D. and Phills, C. E. (2019) The subtle side of stigma: Understanding and reducing mental illness stigma from a contemporary prejudice perspective, *Journal of Social Issues* 75 (3): 943–971.

5

THE METANARRATIVE OF OCD

Deconstructing positive stereotypes in media and popular nomenclature

Angela J. Kim

Preliminary discussion

Obsessive Compulsive Disorder (OCD) is a mental disability characterized by involuntary, recurrent, obsessive thoughts that cause distress and anxiety. These obsessions are often quelled by compulsive behaviors in order to ease anxiety and suppress intrusive thoughts. These behaviors can manifest as visible actions, while others are internal and mental. Common obsessions include germ contamination, sexually explicit or violent images, the need for symmetry, or the fear of harming others. Common compulsions involve excessive re-checking, rearranging items, counting, and hoarding. There is not always a logical connection between obsessions and compulsions, so people with OCD recognize that their behaviors can be irrational. However, they still feel an immense urge to perform various repetitive behaviors throughout the day to ease their mental distress and to prevent something 'bad' from happening. The OCD cycle is vicious and unrelenting. It begins with an obsessive thought, which creates anxiety. To quell the anxiety, one performs a compulsive behavior, which provides temporary relief. This cycle is repeated multiple times a day. OCD is oftentimes chronic and can severely interfere with a person's daily routine of work, school, family, or social activities.

The metanarrative of Obsessive Compulsive Disorder is one bound by appropriations which are disseminated yet often stand in direct opposition to the actual lived experiences of personal narratives. It is a mental disability routinely trivialized in media, commodified by callous modes of production, misapplied to unrelated personal narratives, and largely misunderstood by a misinformed public. A brief cultural survey would yield the immensity of misconceptions about OCD, punctuated by a recurring tone of levity and two key themes: cleanliness and organization. One recalls characterizations of OCD in film and television, such as Howard Hughes in *The Aviator* (2004), Melvin Udall in *As Good as It Gets* (1997), Monica in *Friends* (1994–2004), and Sheldon Cooper in *The Big Bang Theory* (2007–2019). Buzzfeed quizzes that inquire 'Just How OCD Are You?' or articles that claim 'These Pictures will Trigger the Hell out of Your OCD' give the impression that the disability is up for grabs while undermining its severity and pushing a metanarrative of frivolity. Furthermore, festive shirts displaying 'Obsessive Christmas Disorder' or 'Obsessive Cat Disorder' bypass the complexities of the disability and bastardize the phrase in the name of humor.

When society exclusively associates humor with OCD, the unintended consequence is that our experiences are downgraded from a serious mental disability to funny habits that warrant laughter instead of care and understanding. In this chapter, I connect this association of humor to positive stereotyping, as, in the metanarrative of OCD, it has become synonymous with 'good' qualities such as cleanliness and order. While society may view this as a positive effect, it erases the reality of OCD as a debilitating mental disability that affects 1 in 40 adults and 1 in 100 children in the United States (CDC, 2020).

Ultimately, the most visible, well-known, and widely circulated strands of the narratives of OCD are those of white men and women whose OCD categorically predicates a prickly, unsavory, virtually misanthropic behavioral subset. These false narratives embed these uncouth personality traits within the disability itself, for indeed, an individual predisposed to anxiety about the order of the world around them cannot fit seamlessly into the social fabric. I argue that the 'socially acceptable' form of OCD, therefore, is characterized by cleanliness and order – a characterization that is endlessly reproduced in popular culture.

OCD, as reduced to germaphobia and organization, is easily digestible to the greater public. The determination of 'goodness' in both of these qualities have long-standing sociocultural precedents in Western civilization. Practices like washing hands or coughing into the sleeve to avoid the spread of germs are ingrained into us from childhood. Our institutions condition us, therefore, to fear the spread of germs. This is in our best interest, after all, since a sick person is a nonproductive person. Education systems also condition us to be organized – to follow strict, predetermined schedules, to keep our finances, employment, relationships, and so on, all in order, lest we suffer the consequences. When these deep-seated sociocultural mandates interact with predominant, narrow, and exclusionary narratives of OCD, the impact is the production of favorable perception. In other words, it must be good to have it since it forces one to be organized, clean, and productive. Needless to say, the perception of OCD as a 'good' mental disability is demonstrably harmful.

Methodological discussion

In Western culture, disabled people have been portrayed as monsters, markers of evil, freaks, and test subjects. We have been labeled as useless burdens on society, unproductive and worthless. We are deemed excessive, undisciplined, incapable.

Our disabilities have been appropriated to depict tales of tragedy, despair, and caution. The proliferation of much of this language may have subsided in recent times, but the inherent sentiments are still deeply ingrained into the Western social fabric. Even in the present day, people who presumably share an enlightened mode of thinking still respond to disability in ways that hark back to unexamined sentiments of the past (Quayson, 2007, 56). With various metanarratives of disability in culture, these misrepresentations come to set the terms for how disabled people are treated and how we view ourselves. Misconceptions around disability can be further explained by Rosemarie Garland-Thomson's concept of the 'normate': the imagined everyman whose individualism, self-determination, and logical thinking abilities allow Western capitalism and democracy to flourish. The normate is built from the idea that disability is the object of a negative comparison to what is constituted as corporeal normality; the cripple, the invalid, the mad come to represent everything that the normate is not and should not be.

Disability studies can offer a critical perspective to explore why OCD evokes mixed responses of laughter and fear from nondisabled people. Paul K. Longmore explains that people harbor unspoken anxieties about the possibility of disablement of ourselves or our loved ones. Popular entertainment offers disabled caricatures to reify what people shun, stigmatize, and fear most about disability. Additionally, popular culture addresses these fears in an oblique or fragmentary manner, as a means to reassure nondisabled people of themselves (Longmore, 2003, 32). Furthermore, representations of OCD in popular culture evoke comparisons to Garland-Thomson's writing on freak shows. She explains that in Victorian America, the exhibition of freaks proliferated into a public ritual that bonded a 'sundering polity together' in the collective act of looking (Garland-Thomson, 1997, 2). Crowds gathered at these freak shows to gaze intently at the ineffable other. For these onlookers, the spectacle of the extraordinary body stimulated curiosity and ignited speculation, while provoking disgust and horror. The visual exchange between the 'freak' and the audience rendered the audience comfortably common and safely standard. Thus, disabled bodies threaten the post-Emersonian ideal of a regulated, disciplined body, as they fit outside the normative principles of 'self-government, self-determination, autonomy, and progress' (Garland-Thomson, 1997, 42).

Both Longmore and Garland-Thomson concur on the situation of the disabled bodymind as Other, and representations of OCD in film and television reflect this recurring 'square peg, round hole' dynamic, often exploiting the perceived abnormalities of OCD for comedy. The most prominent depictions of OCD fall into that genre category (*As Good as It Gets*, *Friends*, *The Big Bang Theory*). Two things are true at once: as the behaviors of OCD seem to reflect an overexaggerated version of capitalist exceptionalism – the safe, productive, orderly laborer – OCD subverts the threat to the well-governed able bodymind that disability traditionally poses. However, OCD is still a disability – a label that designates the individual as Other – and therefore a threat to the capitalist world order. Additionally, OCD demands that the individual try to control facets of their world to eschew impending doom, and this amount of control can never be relinquished by institutional forces built on the direct, uncomplicated extraction of labor.

While conducting research on the metanarrative of OCD, it is important to consider how media and visual analysis can be useful for exploring disability via various objects of popular culture and entertainment. Media and visual analysis offer disability studies the opportunity to investigate multiple forces, such as discursive constructions or symbolic meanings, that impact disability representations (Fraser, 2018, 74). Similarly, Mitchell and Snyder posit that narrative analyses in disability studies is crucial, as it involves the production of stories that shape our lives and allows a greater understanding of how narrative plays a crucial role in how we imagine social worlds (Mitchell and Snyder, 2005). Breaking down misconceptions and metanarratives will allow us to de-essentialize constructions of normative disability, disrupt preconceived perspectives on disability, and help determine possibilities for a crip futurity. Through rigorous media, visual, and discourse analysis, perhaps we can begin to understand the extent to which media and cinematic portrayals of OCD suggest that people with OCD can be utilized as punch lines, as stereotypes of OCD are often constructed as humorous quirks.

This chapter centers on three analytical discussions with overlapping facets. The first is a critique of the positive perceptions assigned to Obsessive Compulsive Disorder, with a specific focus on commonly circulated, reductive qualities and their relationship to productivity and capitalism. The second supplements this critique with analyses of representations of OCD in advertising, social media, and popular culture, and how these representations shape and perpetuate harmful behaviors and mindsets. In the third discussion, I take an ontological approach to dissecting the particular language those with OCD use and do not use when relating their experiences to others, especially with respect to oversimplified and overdone narratives. I strive to include a crip politics of bodymind (Clare, 2017) by incorporating autoethnographic reflections and foregrounding vulnerability in this chapter, in the hope of bridging the intersection between the academic and the crip. This serves to bring in more representations of 'madness', specifically mental disability, into the academic realm, as Margaret Price and other disability studies scholars do (Price, 2011). Autoethnography and cripistemology separate us from the perspective of the normate, and through these methods, disabled scholars are greater able to articulate their own deeply felt sense of existence in an ableist world. This is especially important since the academic institution as a system produces human oppression and oftentimes exacerbates disabilities. For this reason, I begin with a personal narrative of my OCD and my various experiences with this chronic disability.

Tracing my experience with OCD, I recall a formative adherence and near evangelical belief in the immutable laws of superstition. At the age of 11, a friend and I were perusing the internet when we found a list of superstitions and their antidotes. Afterward, my fascinated, impressionable young mind dove deep into research, but at some point along the way, curiosity gave way to study, then memorization. Soon, I shaped my life around them: avoid walking under ladders, do not break mirrors, throw spilled salt over the left shoulder, and so on. If I bit my tongue, it meant that someone was talking negatively about me somewhere, and I needed to bite my sleeve to stop it. If I saw a face-up penny on the ground, I could carry it around in my right shoe for continued good luck. I purchased four-leaf clovers on eBay as well, desperate to fend off the looming threat of misfortune.

In 8th grade, I was informally diagnosed by a pediatrician, but a lack of understanding both on my and my parents' part meant it went unaddressed. The symptoms, however, became worse as new habits and compulsions arose – arbitrary gestures or affectations to the outside observer, but ones I needed to do to ward off my anxiety and intrusive thoughts. The habits became debilitating, my energy routinely drained from performing rituals, and it began to interfere with my schoolwork. It was not until 11th grade that I underwent Cognitive Behavioral Treatment Therapy (CBT) and tried medication. The former quickly proved more effective at curbing my symptoms, as Zoloft left me excessively fatigued and Prozac produced excruciating migraines. I stopped CBT after four months, noticeably more adept at coping with my symptoms.

Confronting the social misconceptions was an entirely different animal. I first became aware of access barriers in high school when the College Board rejected my petition for extra time accommodations during the SAT. This was suddenly an obstacle whose burden I was chosen to shoulder. The narrow discourse on OCD I critique in this chapter became another obstacle; researching OCD online yielded merely a bevy of the typical characteristics associated with it. I learned plenty, but only in relation to germaphobia and cleanliness. Nothing I read addressed my religion-related habits, for example, borne from my Catholic upbringing. Catholicism leans heavily into daily tradition, ceremony, and ritual as mandates for cleansing oneself of sin and avoiding a cursed fate – a rearticulation of the superstition I feared. One habit, for example, dictated that I say exactly one 'Our Father' and two 'Hail Mary' prayers every single night before bed for six years. I could never throw away my withered old rosary or charms with pictures of Catholic saints and figures, lest I bear the consequences. I became a hoarder, but without resources evident in the research I explored as a child to help articulate my behaviors, I lived largely unaware of the problem.

Even during and after CBT, it was difficult to talk openly with people about my OCD. The common perception of OCD as a quirk of cleanliness made it seem trivial and, at best, a good thing. For years, when referring to it to others, I exclusively referred to it by its full name, 'Obsessive Compulsive Disorder', in an attempt to tap into the legitimacy that the elongated, medical terminology inherently carries. Using 'I have OCD', alternatively, was met with misplaced expressions of sympathy: 'Me too – I love to clean!' or 'I'm so OCD, too – my closet is all color-coordinated!' References to OCD in the everyday typically appropriate the disorder to explain a preference, such as the specific arrangement items on the table, following a particular routine, and, most commonly, a preference for cleanliness. Therefore, those who erroneously use the term OCD to explain their preference for a certain aesthetic arrangement of things perpetuate a false metanarrative which, in turn, tends to promote and circulate misinformation, thereby imbuing the average consumer with assumed authority. For, in other words, if aesthetic preferences, which are infinitely more commonplace than anxiety disorders, can be explained by OCD, then it virtually becomes a reflex to adopt it. This assumed authority accredits the misinformed merely for having heard of OCD and privileges the nondisabled person's perspective and understanding over the disabled person's perspective. Effectively, in this social context, my ability to articulate my mental disability, as well as others' ability to understand it, was and still is severely impaired by the pervading cultural misconceptions of OCD.

There is no aspect of my life that OCD does not touch, and writing this chapter has borne its own set of personal complications. As someone with OCD, I do not have the luxury of a detached analysis; conducting autoethnography, researching the narratives of others, and critiquing misconceptions in popular culture have exacerbated the worst of my disability. Since I live with it every second of my life, it oftentimes fades into the background. Writing about it, however, brings it right to the fore, and consequently, I am unwillingly reminded to keep performing my habits and compulsions. Researching it, too, while empowering, provides new habits and obsessions to adopt or reinforces the necessity of ones I already have (to be clear, adopting the habits of others is not a conscious choice, but when my mind is presented with the possibility that doing something will prevent misfortune, it makes the performance of that action a necessary precaution). Unsurprisingly, the simultaneous COVID-19 pandemic has induced major complications, stemming both from the existential threat of merely going outside and the inevitable dip in productivity. All of these factors contribute to my anxiety, which hyper-activates my OCD. As I write this, the number '4' and letter 'n' on my keyboard are hidden by stickers, since physically interacting with either of those symbols, by mistake or not, predicates misfortune. That is the true nature of OCD.

Analytical discussion 1

Capitalism and discipline

Germaphobia, the pathological fear of germs, microbes, or contamination, is linked to disease prevention practices such as handwashing or bathing. In fact, one could argue, germaphobia is disease prevention taken to the extreme, stoked by anxieties around the spread of infection and compromised health. Disease prevention, in turn, has long been established as a vital principle to the efficacy of capitalism. Disease and illness are well-established threats to the machinery of industry, to worker productivity, and to economies that revolve around the direct exploitation of the laborer's body. In the United States, for example, signs instructing employees to wash their hands before returning to work are posted in the bathrooms of virtually every business. Additionally, mandatory health inspections ensure accountability and safety in food service. These codified practices and procedures serve a socially valuable purpose: It is a net good to reduce disease in society, for it inflicts undue harm and increases mortality. However, disease prevention within capitalist structures exists more so to ensure productivity and profit, not for the general well-being of the populace.

This is because diseased and disabled people are regarded as, at best, useless and, at worst, detriments to a given economy. Disability and capitalism have served as contradistinctive systems as disabilities, diseases, and defects have been considered threats to national economic prosperity and growth. The essentialist thought that the possession of a disability directly affects the individual's potential for productivity has been fully integrated into our social fabric. Notions of 'worth' and 'value' are borne directly from capitalism, which rearticulates a person's value as the potential for meaningful economic impact. Therefore, disabled people jeopardize a nation's economic sanctity because they threaten the principle that the industrial worker should be interchangeable (White, 2012, 112). Grouped with the disabilities that impede economic efficacy are anxiety disorders, for anxiety can often be debilitating and render the individual unproductive.

The preeminent characteristic of Obsessive Compulsive Disorder, propagated by popular culture, emphatically entails germaphobia. When this disability interacts with ingrained notions of economic virtue – the demand to be productive, clean, and interchangeable – suddenly, the desire for cleanliness is deemed an asset. With this perception, anxiety over contamination instead appears as constructive caution; in other words, OCD is deemed an asset, too, by association. While in some ways OCD can be beneficial (within these parameters), assigning OCD a positive value diminishes the realities those with the disability confront.

The portrayal of infectious diseases has historically been linked to inherent racial deficiencies and savagery. Nayan Shah pinpoints how health authorities in San Francisco's Chinatown depicted Chinese immigrants as filthy and a diseased race, who were responsible for spreading smallpox, syphilis, and bubonic plague to white Americans (Shah, 2001). Similarly, Neel Ahuja points to the ways in which native Hawaiians with Hansen's disease were photographed and depicted as monstrous, often blurring the boundaries between the human and nonhuman, the living and the dead (Ahuja, 2016, 47). Even today, President Donald Trump has repeatedly labeled COVID-19 as the 'China virus' or 'Kung-flu virus', intentionally grouping illness with the racialized Other. Germ-related fears are attributed to geographies of risk, and these looming fears are quelled through disease prevention techniques such as vaccinations, medicine, and the narrative of humanitarian technology. Racial fears of contagion produce a public dependency on the usage of pharmaceuticals, medical experimentation, military intervention, and quarantine to regulate the immune capacities of the body.

Given that efficiency of labor is defined as productivity across 'man-hours' (time), Western medicine and capitalist structures traditionally frame disability with regard to temporality. For example, disability-related terms such as 'chronic', 'intermittent', 'recovered', or 'cured', as Alison Kafer argues, place disability on the time line of normative progress (Kafer, 2013, 25). Curative time, in which medical professionals cannot imagine anything other than intervention and cure, oftentimes violently forces the disabled person to arrive at the nondisabled state and molds the disabled individual to fit into a constricting kind of normative future (Kafer, 2013; Kim, 2017). Living within an ableist neoliberal regime partly means living in prognosis, self-managing between processes of living and dying by monitoring indicators of how and why some live for longer or shorter periods of time, live healthier or sicker, or are nondisabled or disabled.

These principles inform the treatment of disability within capitalist structures as well. 'Sick days' were designed to grant the worker a specially designated period of recovery should they temporarily lose their productivity (as hiring and training a replacement would be far too expensive of an investment). Yet, chronically ill and disabled people find themselves at constant war with this construction. With the intention geared toward a curative model of disability, the expenditure of time necessary for a chronically ill individual is too great a risk for a company to incur. Disabled people, therefore, lose their value within the system.

The other prevalent attributes associated with OCD – orderliness, organization, and perfectionism – are similarly valued highly in the workplace and industrial spaces. Rob Imrie explains that space is defined intrinsically to human existence, and the human body is emplaced, and its placement is conditioned. Therefore, the disabled body is 'constructed as not normal, unsightly, and 'out of place' in everyday environments' (Imrie, 2015, 170). This notion of space is taken to the extreme in considering the history of disabled people confined in prisons, mental or psychiatric institutions, or asylums. The space in which disabled people often existed is one of discipline, regulation, and management. The disorderly, disabled body contrasts the orderly space in which their bodies will be changed into a disability-free, orderly, docile, and disciplined subject, in line with Foucault's theorizations on the panoptic regime. This evokes Foucault's work on discipline and regulatory controls that govern the anatomopolitics of the individual and govern the species-being or the overall population (Foucault, 1977). The disciplining of bodies has developed an entire economy and politics for bodies and new techniques by which the body's operations can be controlled. Discipline is enforced by coercing and rearranging the disabled person's movements and their experience of space and time. Therefore, the concepts of 'perfectionism', 'orderliness', and 'organization' engender positive connotations.

Orderliness and organization are key to sustaining the principle of the worker's interchangeability, since those characteristics, in theory, make it easier to conform bodyminds to measurements and practices predetermined to maximize productivity. In other words, it does not require extraneous effort to train the orderly individual to accept and adopt the rhythms of labor; the orderly individual will exhibit punctuality, adhere to rules and regulations, and more readily abide by hierarchies that subjugate them. The workspace can be trusted to stay clean and the habits of repetitive labor will be followed since deviation from them bears significant repercussions. Therefore, as the perception dictates, the individual with OCD should easily slip into these spaces. Indeed, since someone with OCD tends to alter their behaviors based on anxieties that stem from individually or socially determined subsets of consequences, they can become more susceptible to systems of reward and punishment within capitalism.

However, orderliness and organization for the individual with OCD does not necessarily predicate alignment with the order and organization of capitalist structures. At its core, individuals with OCD reflexively assign meaning to specific things, actions, events, or thoughts that others might not deem symbolic. Frequently, these manifest in behaviors targeted toward avoiding 'bad' or 'unlucky' meanings (for example, the number '13' is often associated with bad luck, but the anxiety that interaction with the number generates can be worse in the individual with OCD than others). Therefore, individuals with OCD alter their behaviors in an attempt to organize their life and stave off anxiety. This organization does not necessarily correlate to behaviors or attitudes that will improve job performance or help an individual achieve success. What good could possibly come of avoiding the number 13, for example?

Analytical discussion 2

OCD on camera

Stereotypes of OCD prevalent in media are often constructed as humorous and quirky. For example, in the romantic comedy *As Good as It Gets* (1997), the protagonist, the deeply misanthropic Melvin Udall (played by Jack Nicholson), exhibits the stereotypical symptoms of OCD: revulsion of human contact, excessive handwashing, and extreme cleanliness. The film deserves a modicum of credit for depicting a range of obsessions and compulsions, such as re-locking doors and turning on and off lights a certain number of times, following a meticulously structured routine, and avoiding signifiers of bad luck, such as stepping on cracks in pavements.

Problems arise, however, when these habits are juxtaposed and intermingled with Udall's abrasive personality. Udall's arc is one of redemption and transformation; the dramatic questions the film asks and answers are (1) Will Udall 'get the girl' in the end? and (2) Can Udall shed his unfeeling persona and become a generous soul in order to do so? The events of the film all serve to challenge Udall's reliance on other people and force him to overcome his wanton misgivings about forming intimate relationships to achieve his goal. However, the film seems to posit that his compulsion to avoid physical contact with pedestrians is emblematic not just of his surly nature but also of his mental disability. The implication here is that individuals with OCD want an unattainable social order around them, and the demand for such is necessarily an act of malice. Often, Udall's compulsions are played for comedy, frequently in awkward, confrontational scenarios, which further perpetuate the notion that OCD (and, by extension, all disability) exists in a constant state of conflict with society.

As Paul K. Longmore emphasizes, representations of disabled characters in media often share tropes of 'the evil cripple', where the disability, often framed as a burden on the character, motivates malevolence. For these characters, in other words, their disability makes them hate the world (as with Melvin Udall) and usually creates a desire to enact revenge (like Raoul Silva in *Skyfall* (2012) or Captain Hook in *Peter Pan* (1953)). While this trope is usually associated with the villain, *As Good as It Gets* inverts the arc for its protagonist; Udall starts the film volatile, hostile to the innocuous passersby whose minuscule interactions he perceives as sleights. Udall reflexively insults those who interfere in his carefully cultivated lifestyle, or impede the performance of his habits. These moments, again, are played for comedic effect. He begins the film, in other words, in a state of compulsive revenge and is tasked with overcoming it. In the finale, Udall conquers his disdain for other people and forms a relationship with put-upon single mother Carol (played by Helen Hunt). However, the film offers an implicit marriage between Udall's antagonistic disposition and his OCD, cemented when in the film's conclusion, after uniting with Carol, Udall steps on a brick walkway (earlier, desperately avoided) and shrugs it off. With this final image, we are given the resolution to the arc, and Udall is finally 'cured' of his OCD.

The motif of 'cure' is all-consuming in films depicting disability. In a medium (especially commercial cinema) where character arcs are prioritized, nondisabled creators tell the stories of disability as they perceive it – from a lens of burden. Disability, in these stories, is framed as the roadblock to a character's goal. For example, King George VI in *The King's Speech* (2011) must overcome a speech impediment, and only once he has done so can he reclaim his self-worth. Frequently these narratives station self-worth, or objective worth, as antithetical to life with a disability; they either necessitate conquest of the disability (*As Good as It Gets*, *The King's Speech* (2011), *Regarding Henry* (1991)) or escape through suicide (*Me Before You* (2016), *Million Dollar Baby* (2004), *The Elephant Man* (1980)). Furthermore, the former narrative can facilitate the 'supercrip' trope, such as in *Daredevil* (2003) or recent Nike advertisements featuring disabled athletes. With these stories, disabled characters must prove their worth by overcoming disability – an endgame that positions the ultimate goal as becoming or embodying 'normal' (i.e. nondisabled).

This normative-nonnormative dichotomy is amplified when OCD is played for comedy in media representations. Monica Geller from *FRIENDS* (1994–2004), for example, whose OCD manifests in excessive and intrusive cleaning habits, often yields canned laughter. The same can be found in *The Big Bang*

Theory (2007–2019), the most-watched primetime network sitcom by the time it had ended. Sheldon Cooper, one of the main characters, has OCD, which the writers meld with his very meticulous and abrasive personality. His compulsions – mostly germaphobia and organization-related – often provoke ire from his contemporaries and, inevitably, laughter from a laugh track. The effect of these depictions is threefold: they turn OCD into a punch line, situate the mental disability as inextricable from irascibility, and perpetuate the reductive stereotype that OCD is germaphobia. The lived experiences of those with OCD are often overshadowed by the narrative of OCD associated with the spectacle of entertainment.

Interestingly, the conduits through which mainstream depictions of OCD are presented are uniformly white characters: Melvin Udall, Monica Geller, and Sheldon Cooper. In film and television, the representations of characters of color with mental disabilities are nowhere near parity with white characters with mental disabilities. The hegemonic forces of media designate what is not just socially acceptable but also visible. Therefore, at the intersection of race and disability, the potential disruption that narratives of mental disability pose seem routinely mitigated by packaging those narratives within whiteness.

In recent years, Howie Mandel has extensively detailed his experiences with OCD in television interviews and in his memoir *Here's the Deal: Don't Touch Me* (2009). While Mandel is a real person and not a fictional character, his high profile and media presence inform a reading of his story as an object of popular culture. Mandel's metanarrative mostly focuses on his debilitating germaphobia, and in his memoir, he recounts experiences where others have intentionally stoked his anxieties for their amusement. While it is admirable that Mandel has taken up this mantle, and he emphasizes the severity and complexity that the resulting anxiety causes, the circulation of his metanarrative broadly enforces widely held misconceptions about the nature of OCD. Furthermore, in viewing these interviews and scrutinizing his accounts, one cannot shake the feeling that the public has turned his mental disability into a spectacle, further reinforcing Garland-Thomson's theories on the gaze of the 'normate'. In an interview with Ellen DeGeneres (2013), Mandel could not take his seat to begin the interview. On camera, he explained that his overwhelming anxieties about remaining sedentary and its negative health effects stem from his OCD, and compel him to walk around the studio. The explanation is met by jeers and chuckles from the audience, despite Mandel's visible discomfort. One wonders if this reaction would have happened in a reality without the canned laughter at Monica Geller or Sheldon Cooper.

Media representations, as Patricia Friedrich explains, have the potential to 'un-other and de-stigmatize people living with mental difference', yet oftentimes end up ultimately downplaying the challenges that the same people face (Friedrich, 2015, 69). The crux of the problem with most representations of OCD that revolve around obsessions and compulsions with cleanliness is that it completely disregards all the other aspects of OCD and reduces the disability to one compulsion. Living with OCD does not solely equate to compulsive hand-washing because OCD is not simply about contamination concerns. More commonly, OCD flies under the radar, often making those diagnosed feel extremely isolated and misunderstood.

Analytical discussion 3

OCD in the everyday

OCD is frequently a target for comedy and insensitive parody. Amazon, Target, Redbubble, and Etsy have all been under fire for selling merchandise with offensive slogans involving OCD. Currently, on Etsy, there are over 300 results tagged with 'Obsessive Christmas Disorder' and over 200 results tagged with 'Obsessive Coffee Disorder'. The first result of the key term 'Obsessive Compulsive Disorder', on the other hand, is a t-shirt labeled 'I suffer from O.C.S.D. Obsessive Compulsive Sushi Disorder'. The successive two mugs are labeled 'Obsessive Compulsive Gardening Disorder' and 'Obsessive Coffee Disorder'. By contrast, a quick search of key terms such as 'depression', 'anorexia', or 'schizophrenia' results in a deluge of affirming artwork, therapy journals, Urgent Medical Notice emergency cards, ribbon awareness shirts and pins, and therapeutic essential oils. The signal is clear: Cracking wise about cancer, Down Syndrome, acquired brain injuries, or quadriplegia is absent from the mainstream, yet puns about OCD are not just permissible but common. Buzzfeed quizzes that ask, 'What percent OCD are you?' treat OCD as a benign trend. Within these parameters, OCD can seem almost trivial, and the reproduction of these punch lines can continue ad infinitum.

These OCD slogans are offensive toward people whose lives have been consumed and debilitated by OCD. OCD is vastly complex and multidimensional. While the perception of OCD is influenced by media representations, it does not encompass the entire macrocosm of OCD. Although there are overlaps and spillovers, to understand the metanarrative of OCD, one must also delve into the microcosmic – the small interactions of everyday life and the language we use to talk about it.

Unfortunately, in the minds of many, OCD has been transmogrified into a trivialized version of itself, and I, personally, am often obliged to employ carefully cultivated language to reclaim OCD as a legitimate mental disability. First, it bears mentioning that social stigma around mental disabilities implicitly suppresses free discussion in the general sense. However, even past that barrier, the associations attached to OCD in the minds of the general public directly obstruct my ability to relate my experience to others. Since prevalent misconceptions of OCD hyper-exaggerate germaphobia and the fear of contamination, I am often placed in the position of having to explain and elaborate the many complexities of my specific obsessions and compulsions – in other words, justifying and legitimating it.

Furthermore, the same popular narratives prime the nondisabled individual to view OCD in a humorous light, and as such, I inevitably fear that I will not be taken seriously. For years, to either circumvent or confront this misconception, I have entirely avoided saying simply, 'I have OCD'. Instead, I make sure to say, 'I am *diagnosed* with OCD', in order to lend it an air of credibility – of seriousness – and reclaim the narrative. Additionally, the sentence 'I have OCD' is syntactically and phonetically so similar to the erroneous 'I *am* OCD' that it leaves room to vindicate the latter phrase. While using the aforementioned specific medical diction usually does the trick, it also entails that I privilege medical diagnoses as most valid and thus feed into the medical industrial complex which has historically been rooted in violent and curative practices.

Interestingly, those without OCD (who nevertheless co-opt the phrase to describe a personality quirk) will frequently say, 'I *am* (rather than have) OCD'. Disabilities, however, are not adjectives; we might think how ridiculous it would be to announce 'I am depression' or 'I am bipolar disorder'. When people say, 'I am so OCD', they are literally saying 'I am Obsessive Compulsive Disorder', which signals precisely how removed some are from the meaning of the phrase. In bastardizing the initialism *OCD* and turning it into a protean label, we have removed not merely its potency but its identity as a mental disability; it is no longer a noun, but an adjective, a modifier, to be flung around and attached to anything we see fit. Instead of sustaining its own subjectivity, it becomes the descriptor, and without that identity, suddenly we are uninterested in describing it, defining it, and, therefore, understanding it.

Concluding discussion

A central principle of disability justice is to practice and embody an anti-capitalist politic, as the nature of our bodyminds resists conformity to capitalist expectations (Berne, 2015). Capitalism places sole value on productivity and labor capacity, and it directly perpetuates disability oppression by enforcing a standard of normalcy that all people should strive to maintain or obtain. However, the disabled community does not evaluate our purpose within the framework of capitalist productivity, and our personhood, our value, and our purpose are not predicated upon the amount of labor our bodies produce. This principle links directly to another of disability justice: recognizing wholeness. This principle encourages us to recognize the value of people for who they are, not how they could be, and understanding that people are worthy outside of commodity relations (Berne, 2015). After all, the most anti-capitalist protest, as Johanna Hedva asserts, is simply to care for another and care for ourselves by taking on the historically feminized and invisibilized practice of nurturing and caring (Hedva, 2015). Thus, I hope for others to recognize the wholeness of people living with Obsessive Compulsive Disorder, to produce nuanced and complex representations of OCD.

The year of writing, 2020, is a particularly salient time to think through the misrepresentations of OCD in contemporary culture, as erroneous narratives of

OCD as a positive preventative measure to combat COVID-19 reemerge and gain footing. There are no lives, it seems, untouched by the virus, either in direct form or a natural hyperawareness – it has consumed our everyday. With that has come a global scrutiny and revision of potentially disease-spreading behavior. As the world struggles to put language to a deadly virus in the hopes of attenuating vacillating social conditions, stubborn misguided conceptions of OCD reappear, rehashed for this new era of global precaution.

The fear of contamination (the most common associated symptom of OCD) has globalized, and, understandably, people from all echelons of society are frightened of contagion from this invisible airborne virus. To cope, institutional leaders have implemented, among other things, rigorous handwashing, sanitizing, and cleaning practices. Recently, movie theaters, gyms, shopping centers, and restaurants have attempted to bring Americans back to a semblance of normalcy by boasting innovative sanitization technology, such as UV lighting in HVAC systems, electrostatic disinfectants, vacuums with HEPA filters, and medical-grade sanitizers. The World Health Organization and Center for Disease Control recently published step-by-step handwashing tutorials to encourage the public to wash their hands frequently and for at least 20 seconds with water and soap, as well as sanitizing clothes, groceries, cardboard delivery boxes, cloth masks, shoes, and just about every other household item that may be touched by others in the course of everyday life. Individuals without contamination OCD are likely to follow protocol and move on with limited to no anxiety. With these new guidelines, those considering contamination OCD from the outside may view this mental disability as an overall boon – a safety net, of sorts.

However, while those with OCD are, generally speaking, more cautious and aware of contact with bacteria, to equate it with safety would be a disastrous misrepresentation. The individual with contamination OCD does not feel safe. In fact, the disability is characterized by debilitating anxiety, the antithesis of feeling safe, and, if anything, they suffer the more so because of it. Furthermore, many individuals with contamination OCD have been through Exposure and Response Therapy to unlearn harmful compulsions – often a lifelong undertaking. The heightened prioritization of hygienic practices, while crucial to slow COVID-19 and end the pandemic, problematize the relationship that those with contamination OCD have to cleanliness and germs.

In summary, in the time of COVID-19, one might be tempted to view those with OCD as responsible, clean, and safe, and place other value-judgments upon them due to the positive stereotypes of OCD as hygienic, organized, and tidy. However, what happens when you have been living with Obsessive Compulsive Disorder for years and your obsession with germs leads to excessive handwashing and cleaning? What happens when your fear of germs and contagion has been exacerbated by COVID-19, particularly while living with people and under government regimes who refuse to take the pandemic seriously? Too often, the discourse concerning the post-pandemic 'return to normalcy' ignores the complexities it entails for people with contamination OCD. Today, we must consider with renewed consciousness the harmful impact of asserting OCD as a 'cure' for the disease.

References

Ahuja, N. (2016) *Bioinsecurities: Disease Intervention, Empire, and the Government of Species*, Durham: Duke University Press.

As Good as it Gets (1997) Film. Directed by James L. Brooks, Culver City: TriStar Pictures; Gracie Films.

Berne, P. (2015) Disability Justice – A Working Draft by Patty Berne. Available from: https://www.sinsinvalid.org/blog/disability-justice-a-working-draft-by-patty-berne#:~:text=The%20first%2C%20a%20primary%20principle%20of%20Disability%20Justice%2C%20is%20Intersectionality.&text=Like%20the%20above%20principles%2C%20Disability,Commitment%20to%20Cross%20Movement%20Organizing. [Last Accessed 3 August 2020].

Center for Disease Control and Prevention (n.d.) Obsessive-Compulsive Disorder in Children. Available from: https://www.cdc.gov/childrensmentalhealth/ocd.html [Last Accessed 1 August 2020].

Clare, E. (2017) *Brilliant Imperfection, Grappling with Cure*, Durham: Duke University Press.

Foucault, M. (1977) *Discipline and Punish: The Birth of the Prison*, New York: Pantheon Books.

Fraser, B. (2018) *Cognitive Disability Aesthetics: Visual Culture, Disability Representations, and the (In)Visibility of Cognitive Difference*, Toronto: University of Toronto Press.

Friedrich, M. (2015) *The Literary and Linguistic Construction of Obsessive-Compulsive Disorder: No Ordinary Doubt*, London: Palgrave Macmillan.

Friends (1994–2004) TV Series, Burbank: Warner Bros Television.

Garland-Thomson, R. (1997) *Extraordinary Bodies: Figuring Physical Disability in American Culture and Literature*, New York: Columbia University Press.

Hedva, J. (2015) Sick Woman Theory, *Mask: The Not Again Issue*. Available from: http://www.maskmagazine.com/not-again/struggle/sick-woman-theory [Last Accessed 4 August 2020].

Howie Mandel Won't Sit Down (2013) *The Ellen Show*. Available from: https://www.youtube.com/watch?v=R4acRnB2v9M [Last Accessed 29 June 2020].

Imrie, R. (2015) Space, in Adams, R., Reiss, B., and Serlin, D. (Eds.), *Keywords in Disability Studies*, New York: New York University Press.

Kafer, A. (2013) *Feminist, Queer, Crip*, Bloomington: Indiana University Press.

Kim, E. (2017) *Curative Violence: Rehabilitating Disability, Gender, and Sexuality in Modern Korea*, Durham: Duke University Press.

Longmore, P. (2003) *Why I Burned My Book and Other Essays on Disability*, Philadelphia: Temple University Press.

Mandel, H. and Young, J. (2009) *Here's the Deal: Don't Touch Me*, New York: Bantam.

Mitchell, D. T. and Snyder, S. L. (2005) *Narrative Prosthesis: Disability and the Dependencies of Discourse*, Ann Arbor: University of Michigan Press.

Price, M. (2011) *Mad at School: Rhetorics of Mental Disability and Academic Life*, Ann Arbor: University of Michigan Press.

Quayson, A. (2007) *Aesthetic Nervousness: Disability and the Crisis of Representation*, New York: Columbia University Press.

Shah, N. (2001) *Contagious Divides: Epidemics and Race in San Francisco's Chinatown*, Berkeley: University of California Press.

The Aviator (2004) Film. Directed by Martin Scorsese, Los Angeles: Forward Pass; West Hollywood: Appian Way; IMF; Santa Monica: Initial Entertainment Group.

The Big Bang Theory (2007–2019) TV Series. CBS, Burbank: Warner Bros Television, 24 September.

White, S. (2012) Crippling the Archives: Negotiating the Notions of Disability in Appraisal and Arrangement of Description, *The American Archivist* 75(1), 109–124.

6

THE METANARRATIVE OF LEARNING DISABILITY

Vulnerability, unworthiness, and requiring control

Owen Barden and Steven J. Walden

Preliminary discussion

A metanarrative is a cloud of a story that displaces personal narratives and knowledges with overarching ones derived from dominant, etic discourses (Bolt, 2014, 2020). It is a globalizing or totalizing cultural narrative schema which orders and explains knowledge and experience (Stephen and McCallum, 1998). In this chapter, we explore the cultural evolution of the metanarrative – specific tropes and stereotypes – associated with what are now frequently termed learning disabilities. Conceptualizations of, and responses to, learning disabilities have varied dramatically between cultures and across eras. It has been suggested, for example, that the Mexican Olmec tribe considered people with Down Syndrome to be the offspring of humans and the main Olmec totem, the jaguar, and so revered them as godlike (Gonzalo and Milton, 1974; Slorach, 2016). Currently, attitudes are much more prejudicial. Contemporary Western culture tends to characterize learning-disabled people as vulnerable, unworthy, and requiring control. We trace the roots of these conceptualizations as far back as the mid-nineteenth century, although, of course, they go back much further (Barnes, 1997). This was the first period of institutionalization and medicalization, occurring against a backdrop of urbanization and population control, social Darwinism, scientism, capitalism, colonialism, and imperialism. These conditions helped establish and sustain a dehumanizing metanarrative of deficiency and deviance. This metanarrative, in turn, paved the way for the strategic eugenic targeting of people with learning disabilities, from antilocution to attempted extermination (Allport, 1954) – most overtly under the genocidal Nazi Aktion T4 programme yet continuing today through genetic screening and editing technologies. Definitions, descriptions, and ascriptions of learning disability may be historically contingent, and yet there is one point of continuity: society remains anxious of the outgroup it creates through its shifting conceptualizations of learning disability, because the group appears to challenge the essence of what it means to be human. It is this 'inclusion phobia' that is the genuine cross-historical phenomenon (Goodey, 2015, 2017). Whether worshipped as gods or dismissed as disposable, the metanarrative of learning disability bolsters the normate subject position (Garland-Thomson, 1997): learning-disabled people are always Other, never Us. They are what ordinary people are not.

In this chapter, we adopt historicism as a critical analytical paradigm. Historicism recasts epistemological questioning of historical knowledge as onto-logical questioning, acknowledging contemporaneous sociocultural tensions to maintain a logic of enquiry when being utilized to interpret the ascription of meaning in context (Iggers, 1995). Historicism assumes that every expressive act is embedded in a network of material practices and that no discourse within that network gives access to unchanging truths or expresses inalterable human nature (Veeser, 1989). The metanarrative of learning disability, encompassing ascriptions of meaning, as well as perceptual and attitudinal shifts, and the lived experiences of people with learning disabilities can be argued to both express and influence cultural historiography, if this is read as a network of changeable material practices from within which these tropes ultimately arise. The intention here is to analyze the tropes inductively as reflective of the liminal spatial dialectic between culture and the shifting dynamics of its underpinning psychosocial milieu, refracted through the historiographic lens. Rearticulating the historicist discourse pertaining to sociocultural shifts in terms of concomitant cultural anxieties within this framework thus examines the psychosocial evolution of this metanarrative over the last two centuries. People who are physically, psychologically, or cognitively different have always been marginalized (Meininger, 2010). This notion of 'the other' as a construction opposing 'the self' at its most simplistic, or perhaps reductionist, pervades the literature and indeed philosophical inquiry (Brons, 2015; Jensen, 2011). Brons enquires further: framing the Hegelian dialectic of self-other self-identification and distanciation to conceptualize othering as a more fluid and complex dichotomy that could be perceived as a spectrum conceptualization. This dichotomy comprises crude othering constructed through self-other distanciation, concurring with the commonly held notion of othering that perpetuates marginalization, and sophisticated othering predicated on an element of self-identification, whereby one perceives aspects of the self within the other, engendering empathy rather than prejudice, if not unconditional acceptance. Meininger (2010) posits a paradox that in all periods and all cultures people who are perceived as different have also been presented as symbolic of what it is to be human. This paradox can be argued to be resolved by Brons's (2015) dichotomous spectrum construct of othering if we align Meininger's juxtaposition with its opposing loci extremis and accepting the liminality between. The traversing of this liminal space by people with learning disabilities from the marginalization and prejudices encompassed by crude othering to the empathy of sophisticated othering, to hopes of eventually transcending othering entirely, can arguably be charted via the historicist perspective, framing their metanarrative and its inherent tropes as a discourse with and punctuated by concomitant historic shifts in contemporaneous sociocultural dynamics over time.

Methodological discussion

Although contributing to autocritical disability studies, we cannot claim to be learning disabled. My (i.e. Owen) first job in education was as a support worker for disabled students at my local community college (Barden, Youl, and Youl, 2016); my doctoral research investigated literacy practices and social media use among a small group of sixth form students labelled with dyslexia (Barden, 2014a, 2014b); and more recently, my research has focused on the cultural history of learning disabilities (Barden, 2020a, 2020b). I (i.e. Steve) have had an eclectic career path, initially studying human biology and medical genetics before training to become an actor and working in theatre and television, then training as a producer, all the while working as a healthcare support worker for people with learning disabilities, and latterly qualifying as a certified forensic anthropologist (Walden et al., 2017, 2018, 2020). I continue to work on my research interests in these disparate fields, but it is my role as a registered learning disabilities nurse and lecturer with an ongoing research interest in the social history and cultural anthropology of people with learning disabilities that is foregrounded here.

We recognize that although disability studies emerge from and seek to speak to the lives of disabled people, research in disability studies written by and for the academy can be perceived as distant from the lives and experiences of the people it hopes to serve. We also recognize that applying the historiographic method directly to the research outlined below would produce a series of metaphoric still life images of given moments that could be construed as both overtly subjective and arbitrary. We intend to counter this potential criticism by taking an objective view of the lived experiences of people with learning disabilities ranging in age from their early 20s to their early 70s, and facilitating comparative discussions framed around the documented experiences of their historical counterpart, Antonia Grandoni. Our methodology has sought to address these concerns. We cannot claim the experiential knowledge that learning-disabled people have of the metanarrative they inhabit. However, we can bring our scholarly expertise to bear on helping to elicit and illuminate this metanarrative. Our recent joint, participatory project with learning-disabled researchers helped to do just that. *Inside the History of Learning Disability* used a bespoke two-step methodology. Traditional methods and academic expertise in archival research and textual analysis were combined with a series of workshops designed to enable a group of learning-disabled co-researchers and their advocates to access, interpret, respond creatively to, and report on the archive material. In the first step, the academic researchers accessed and selected archive material about people with learning disabilities from the UK Medical Heritage Library (UKMHL). The UKMHL is an online archive of 66,000 digitized nineteenth-century European history-of-medicine texts. In the second step, the academic and learning-disabled researchers worked together to explore, analyze, question, and respond creatively to the archive material. During these workshops we use analytical prompts and questions alongside less orthodox techniques, sometimes facilitated by graphic illustrators, to elicit insider knowledge about so-called learning disabilities. This knowledge was then expressed in a range of ways: spoken, written, and artistic. The varied sets of knowledge and expertise each contributor brought to the project were interdependent and illuminating in developing a rich and emotive appreciation of both the history of learning disabilities and the lived experience of learning disabilities today.

Learning-disabled people today encounter systems of oppression, segregation, and discrimination. *Inside the History of Learning Disability* examined the origins of these systems in nineteenth-century Europe. To do so, it focused on narratives surrounding and precipitated by one person. Exploring, analyzing, and discussing the narrative presented in the UKMHL archive brought a number of other narratives out into the open; both individual narratives relating to experiences of learning disability and their relationship to the metanarrative of learning disability. The person in question was called Antonia Grandoni. She lived in Milan in the mid-nineteenth century. According to Croce et al. (2017, 81):

> At this time in Italy, the first institution for the education of people with intellectual disabilities opened in Aosta in 1848 for the cure of cretinism, followed in the 1884 by a structure in Rome specifically for 'idiots and imbeciles'. The positive reasons for these institutions rapidly diminished, and it was not long before they turned into places of segregation. By the end of the century, there was a recognizable change in society's view of disability, and in the way people with disabilities were served.

This ascriptive shift was underpinned by a contemporaneous ideology of institutionalization and moral treatment that not only pervaded Grandoni's Italy, but also the UK and the post-colonial new world of the mid-nineteenth century, under the burgeoning sociocultural influence of Edouard Seguin and his contemporaries (Wright, 2000; Chouinard, 2009; Webmeyer et al., 2017; Barden, 2020a). This ideology was characterized by its inherent dichotomy. It was on the one hand couched in the biomedical positivist drive towards a cure and the patriarchal religious moral imperative to care for those perceived as unfortunate, juxtaposed with the equally patriarchal desire to control and segregate those perceived as different on the other. After her death, and during her life, Antonia was perceived less as a person with all the inherent ascription of self that comes with that perception, and more as a reductionist conglomerate of diagnoses, analyses, and accounts of presentation. Her voice, her choice, and her human identity were absent from the historical record. To return to Brons (2015), we might say she was, for the most part, crudely othered. Antonia lived in an era characterized by marginalization, othering, and ultimately physical and cultural segregation for people with learning disabilities, rendering the parallels encountered within the discourse with her present-day contemporaries all the more stark.

Antonia features prominently as a case history in Dr William Ireland's book *On Idiocy and Imbecility* (Ireland, 1877). Ireland presents a translation of the accounts of Professor Cardoni, who seems to have taken an interest in Antonia while she was alive, and the report of five Italian doctors who examined her after her death. At the time, Ireland was considered an authority on the nature and treatment of idiocy and imbecility (these were clinical diagnoses then, rather than the naked pejoratives of today). Ireland's 13-page account of Antonia was chosen because it contains some details of her life before she was institutionalized, some description of her character and behaviour while she was institutionalized, two pencil portraits (a rare find), as well as tables and descriptions of anatomical measurements and comparisons with other 'microcephalic idiots'. Our intent was to work with learning-disabled researchers and look beyond the documented judgements and assumptions of Ireland's medical colleagues, glean inklings of who Antonia Grandoni was as opposed to an impression of the disability she lived with, refracted through the lens of her modern-day contemporaries' own parallel and divergent personal experiences. Three distinct metanarrative tropes emerged from this process.

It would be useful at this juncture to look at some of the sociocultural origins of the segregation that Antonia experienced before drawing contemporary comparisons. The rambling gothic institutions of Europe built to 'other' and contain people with learning disabilities grew from the backyards of similar institutions that marginalized people living with mental health disorders (Parmenter, 2001). Antonia Grandoni's life may well have been touched by Seguin, who had a radical and transformative impact on the perceived educability of 'idiots', from the 1850s onwards, predicated upon his use of intensive sensory-motor activities in this context. Seguin adopted an unreservedly biomedical stance, taking more interest in the conditioned neuromuscular responses of his patients than in his patients themselves (Parmenter, 2001; Kraft, 1961). Parmenter goes on to posit that the influence of the medico-psychologists of the nineteenth century, including Seguin, extended throughout much of the then Western world and continued into the early twentieth century. It was only towards the end of the nineteenth century in Italy that a more benevolent, if still patriarchal and certainly clinically positivist, attitudinal shift became apparent, as illustrated again by Croce et al. (2017):

> Sancte de Sanctis, one of the fathers of neuropsychiatry in Italy, was the founder of the first kindergarten and school for children with intellectual disabilities. In his career, he introduced the first ambulatories for neurodevelopmental psychiatry (1899) and introduced the clinical practice of maintaining a file containing biographical information for each person.
>
> *(Cimino, 2004)*

Antonia, unfortunately, did not live to see this tropic shift of nascent humanist recognition of the individuality and personhood, if not citizenship as conceptualized today, of people with learning disabilities. In fairness to Ireland, he did alight upon some of her reported strengths – an empathetic consideration on his part and those of Antonia's reporting physicians more in tune with Brons' (2015) concept of sophisticated othering whereby the other is allowed to share some of the qualities ascribed to the self. This apparent benevolence was far from universal, however, and must also be weighed against broader cultural shifts in attitudes across much of Europe as well as the United States and Australia, which identified people with learning disabilities as menacing and degenerate rather than pitiable (Barden, 2020a, 2020b).

To segue to the present day, the current postmodern neoliberal milieu that pervades Western democracy continues to foreground risk as an overarching principle informing social responses to people with learning disabilities, seated in a paradoxical dialectic with marketized dependency that argues to promote choice while in many ways negating it (Dowse, 2009). People with learning disabilities, if independent of their families, often live in supported living arrangements with other people with learning disabilities and are subjected to sets of rules that wider society may not be. The overt segregation that Antonia was subjected to is thus sublimated by a more nebulous, covert segregation for her modern-day counterparts predicated on disability as a commodity (Brown, James and Hatton, 2017; King et al., 2017).

Analytical discussion 1

Vulnerable

A very significant component of the metanarrative of learning disability is vulnerability. People with learning disabilities are cast as vulnerable: needing protection from the hazards of the physical world, from exploitation by unscrupulous others, and from harming themselves. However, people who nowadays carry the label of learning disabled are not necessarily inherently vulnerable – in our pre-industrial agrarian society they would not have been thought of as so, and they could perhaps have functioned and participated perfectly well (Barnes, 1997; Goodey, 2015; Slorach, 2016). Rather, they are trapped in a regime of truth, established during Antonia's lifetime, which depicts them as vulnerable (Barden, 2020a; Simpson, 2014). This is a powerful representation of learning disability because it circulates and so is constantly reinforced in medical discourse, popular culture, mass media, and people's everyday speech; indeed, it is such a powerful and all-encompassing hegemonic as to be almost inescapable (Smith and Smith, in press). Vulnerability is then used as a justification for segregation. During Antonia's lifetime, notions of vulnerability and justifications for segregation and discrimination were established and reified in part through diagnostic criteria and biomedical definitions. These definitions positioned their subjects as vulnerable both to common physical dangers (Clive, in press) and to being out-competed by their fellows. As such, they had a distinctly Darwinian feel, and so it is perhaps no surprise this metanarrative helped feed the pseudoscience of eugenics, which sought to eliminate people deemed 'unfit' – another Darwinian term – from the population. In Antonia's case, the concern over her perceived vulnerability is evident in a biographical sketch, which precedes the more extensive anatomical evaluation:

> She was not much later than usual in beginning to walk and speak, but her intelligence was inferior to children of her age. She, however, learned in time to do easy work in the house, and to go out of doors to buy provisions. She was fond of learning amorous poetry, and showed erotic tendencies. On getting older she took to wandering about, and might be seen dancing with grotesque movements to her own singing.
>
> For many years she led a wandering life, an object of curiosity, of pity, or of ridicule to all. At last she was removed to the hospital where she died. [...] I have little doubt that, by a well-planned education in childhood, her mental powers could have been considerably increased, and her wandering and erotic tendencies repressed. Apparently she was a poor neglected creature.
>
> *(Ireland, 1877, 106–107)*

This narrative tells us that Antonia was seemingly abandoned, or at least not cared for, by her family – perhaps her brothers and sisters, mentioned earlier in the story, out-competed her for her parents' affections – and that she led 'a wandering life' for 'many years' before being institutionalized. The justification given for this course of action is that she was both neglected at home and not safe by herself in the outside world because of her exposure to ridicule. This is apparently sufficient to warrant a decision to separate her from her family and incarcerate her, condemning her to a lonely existence for the rest of her days. Moreover, her supposed 'erotic tendencies' are probably an even greater concern than her wanderlust, given Ireland's stated desire to suppress them. Again, this relates to broader eugenic concerns about promiscuity and degeneracy as well as the potential for Antonia to be taken advantage of or do things of which she does not understand the consequences. The idea that people with learning disabilities should not have sexual relationships or become parents is one that is still prevalent today, still part of the metanarrative of learning disability.

Our learning-disabled researchers recognized this narrative of vulnerability and drew parallels with contemporary experiences. Their relationship to this aspect of the learning disability metanarrative was complex. On the one hand, they appreciated the potential for exploitation, for example, through sensational-ist daytime television shows[1]:

---

1 The transcript excerpts use initials to preserve anonymity.

Sa. Well I think that – well I know it's been axed now but – the Jeremy Kyle Show would be quite often young women, nobody knew who the father was, this kind of thing. Very vulnerable people, you could just tell, very vulnerable people. So it's a big cause for concern that, I suppose, as well.

L. We've got other ways of exploiting people...

A. But nowadays there's also that kind of idea of fandom, sensationalism and fetishism, so I think nowadays it'd be like, would she be like on Tinder or whatever, and getting like 100 likes. I don't use Tinder. [laughter, hubbub] I've got a coffee date tomorrow, that's all!

H. I think when Jeremy Kyle first started I think I saw it once and I thought 'Well, how sad. You bring people on for basically Joe Public to watch and laugh at'. Because it's cheap TV to get people who have problems and are vulnerable, get them on so Joe Bloggs can have a cheap laugh.

Sa. It's what they did in the old asylums, isn't it? People would come and view them.

A. Chuck tomatoes at them and stuff.

H. I saw it [Jeremy Kyle] once and I thought 'That is just sick'.

This exchange touches on a number of aspects of vulnerability and exploitation: media manipulation, sexual fetishism, freak shows and exhibitions, verbal and physical abuse; and how these can be traced to asylums of the kind where Antonia was held. Vulnerability to abuse and exploitation was thus clearly a concern for the co-researchers. These concerns are borne out of the lived experience of learning disability and can be read as a perpetuation of the metanarrative. However, other aspects of the co-researchers' insights can be read as challenges to the metanarrative. Several times the co-researchers expressed a wish to take Antonia for a night on the town; Ireland's account tells us she was 'a good and agile dancer' as well as being 'gay and sociable' and 'fond of attracting the attention of the opposite sex':

Sa. we talked about her lifestyle as well, that she liked to dance provocatively, and ...

Cr. And she smiles.

Sa. ... and we talked about her sexuality and stuff, and we just joked, you know, think of describing any girl out on a Saturday night in Liverpool city centre you know [laughter] but she obviously seemed different to other people around her, and her behaviour, she was more open, more kind of, bohemian I suppose, in her own way.

[...]

Ja. Somebody mentioned that you could do the Twitter from a cell, but I'd have thought she wouldn't be in a cell today, these days. I hope she'd be out in the community. She liked dancing – maybe she'd be looking forward to Glastonbury or something! I don't know.

Part of the motivation for wanting a night out with Antonia we all began to think of her as 'one of us', belonging to our groups and being part of our lives, doing the things we do. But part of it also stemmed from wanting to resist the characterization of learning-disabled people as vulnerable. There was a recognition that a good life is one that balances challenges and risks – that protecting from risk also means protecting from success and inner growth (French and Jones, in press). And wanting a good life for Antonia was part of the broader project of rehumanizing her, an objective established to counter the dehumanizing narrative of Ireland's account and characteristic of the metanarrative of learning disability.

Analytical discussion 2

Unworthy

The second aspect of the dehumanizing metanarrative of learning disability we explore in this chapter is that such lives are barely human – that people with learning disabilities are not really people at all. As medicalization took hold, animalization became a well-established tactic of patriarchal disability and oppression, aligned to a belief that because animals lack certain traits and abilities, they exist outside our compass of moral responsibility, and are therefore fair game for domination and abuse (Taylor, 2011). This tendency to equate learning disability with non-human status is evident in Ireland's book. Here he relays Cardoni's opinion of Carlo Guiseppe Cioccio, an Italian man who lived at the same time as Antonia and also received a diagnosis of microcephalic idiocy:

> But, observes Cardona, 'the smallness of the brain of Cioccio induced stupidity, idiocy, deaf muteness – in short, simply animal life; the poverty of the brain of our Grandoni in that small size accorded to it by nature, could admit of a sensibility, an intelligence, and an education, which has not fallen much short of the average of her countrywomen'.
>
> *(Ireland, 1877, 105)*

In this second excerpt, he quotes Dr Adriani, one of the five Italian physicians who examined Antonia after her death:

> An examination of the brain strengthens the conclusion that microcephales do not represent a degeneration in the sense of retrogression to the organic type of certain apes, but rather an arrest of development without aberration from the typical laws of organic formation through a pathological cause.
>
> *(Ireland, 1877, 105)*

In both cases, the doctors liken their subjects to animals: Cardona in the most general and therefore perhaps dismissive terms; and although Adriani seeks to maintain a distinction between microcephalic idiots and apes, the very fact that the comparison is reported is telling. Our co-researchers were highly alert to this tendency. Their analysis of and responses to Ireland's narrative highlighted his tendency to objectify Antonia in this way, as well as how she continued to be neglected once institutionalized, even though familial neglect was part of the original justification for removing her to hospital:

Cl. Yeah, she was just judged by appearances, is what we came up with, and we picked up on one thing that it said on attachment that, you know, she attached to people who were kind to her and we thought that the very wording made us think, you know, had she been in contact with people who were unkind to her and how would she respond to them, and she would respond very differently, she was quite happy to smile at people when they smiled at her. We went along the lines of you know being on the autistic spectrum kind of thing. We thought it sounded as though she was not, had not been given many opportunities in her life and was judged by appearances, that's pretty well what we talked about.

OB. Okay, super, thank you very much. So, there's a handy little bit of summary from one group there, who would like to go next?

Sa. Can I just say that reading just that, I wouldn't surmise that she had any kind of learning disability … ?

St. Exactly.

Sa. … if you haven't told us beforehand, she just sounds, she sounds a bit like a lab rat, really, you know, here's her measurements …

St. Exactly.

Sa.… she sleeps, she does this, that's what I … that's kind of, that's how she's treated, she's treated like a subject rather than a human being. But just reading that from the paragraph, I wouldn't just think oh, this person has a learning disability at all.

As well as in these discussions, the 'lab rat' metaphor and Antonia's degrading treatment were featured in the artworks the groups produced as creative responses to the narrative presented.

The idea that a person with a learning disability is unworthy of education, opportunities, even of life itself has persisted, through the Nazi characterization of 'useless eaters', used to justify the genocidal Aktion T4 programme, to post-war characterizations of some children being ineducable, to a catalogue of abuse and neglect in so-called care homes like Winterbourne View, Whorlton Hall, Yew Trees, and Muckamore Abbey; and on into learning-disabled people receiving inferior healthcare, dying prematurely in disproportionate numbers (LeDer, 2018), and being regarded, along with other disabled people, as disposable during the ongoing Coronavirus pandemic (Wong, 2020). Again, our co-researchers had experiences which resonated with the way Antonia was apparently regarded and treated:

V. I was called a spastic.

Os. I was walking home, eating my lunch, and somebody shouted you're eating like a spastic.

Y. That was recent, wasn't it?

SW. That's another term that was used and we've got two people now who've had experience of that label and been called spastic.

V. Another one I was called was Mongol.

Y. That used to be the medical name though, when I was growing up, that's what my sister's diagnosis was; it wasn't Down syndrome, it took people a while to get used to that. Then people started using it to be mean to people and as an insult. Down syndrome was chosen because Dr Down first described it.

SW. As an insult, it's racist as well as being disablist.

[...]

W. R, has anybody ever called you any names that you didn't like?

Hi. I might've been called spastic once or twice.

W. ... and how did that make you feel?

Hi. Annoyed.

Os. W, when I was in school, I was called dick-head. The boys were doing the action. I'm not going to do what they did, and they said to my friend I was a freak.

W. That's terrible.

V. They called me a donkey.

Y. When I was little my sister punched another girl on the nose for calling her a Mongol. She didn't like that label being put on her.

In this exchange, we see the tendency towards animalization persist, as V is called a 'donkey'. A number of other insults are reported, all of which imply that the target is unworthy of respect or basic human decency. Moves to label people in this derogatory way are of course moves to subjugate them: to exert control. This brings us to our third and final trope.

Analytical discussion 3

Requiring control

So far we have argued that people labelled with learning disabilities are often conceived of as vulnerable, and also as not fully human. During Antonia's lifetime there was a shift in the impact of these conceptualizations; the pity and sympathy which initially motivated the creation of asylums were replaced by hostility and fear, because 'idiots', 'imbeciles', the 'feebleminded', and 'moral defectives' came to be seen as threats to the health of nations. This was an overriding concern for capitalist, empire-building governments, who wanted populations who were fit to work and fight. Herein lie the origins of eugenics – which we must remember was a mainstream politico-scientific movement in the late nineteenth and early twentieth centuries, with support from, for example, UK and US governments, before it fell out of favour following the abhorrent Nazi Aktion T4 extermination programme. T4 remains the ultimate expression of our third trope: that people with learning disabilities need to be controlled. Whether because they are seen to need protecting from risk, to a degree most other people are not, or because they represent a threat to other people, the metanarrative demands that people labelled with learning disabilities must be controlled. We can map these moves to control against Allport's (1954) scale of prejudice. Antilocution is evident in the diagnostic criteria and definitions formulated in Antonia's lifetime, and continues both in biomedical terminology – as embodied in the ever-expanding Diagnostic and Statistical Manual of Mental Disorders – and in the kind of insults our researchers reported above. Indeed, the unfortunate fact is that many diagnostic terms evolve into insults. Avoidance and discrimination are evident in moves to segregate learning-disabled people from the rest of the population in the 'archipelago of confinement': penal, medical, and educational settings, including asylums, madhouses, special schools, colonies, hospitals, and more recently prisons, immigration, and detention centres and care homes (Adams and Erevelles, 2017; Drinkwater, 2015; Foucault, 1977; Spivakosky, 2017). Many such places create marketized dependency: privatized supported living supposedly promotes choice while paradoxically maintaining segregation and imposing myriad restrictions. Residents find themselves living lives in the workplace of others, subjugated to available resources and 'Human Resources' logistics predicated on maximizing profit. Physical attacks are common, both outside such settings and as a means to control residents within them, as the continuing litany of horrendous cases like Winterbourne, Whorlton, Yew Trees, and Muckamore demonstrates. The will to exterminate persists through genetic modification and screening programmes, as well as forced sterilizations.

Antonia was subject to a good deal of control, and our co-researchers reported many ways in which their lives were controlled to a far greater extent than most other people's. The very fact that Antonia was removed from her family, to prevent her 'wandering existence', tells us that the authorities felt the need to control her life, as do the attempts to suppress her 'erotic tendencies' and make her attend Church and abide by the moral code of the day, even though she was deemed ineducable:

> She had the sentiment of good and evil, and made sensible remarks upon the conduct of her companions. She was religious through imitation and habit, and behaved well in church. Every attempt to instruct her was without success.
>
> *(Ireland, 1877, 107)*

Similarly, our co-researchers talked about ways in which their conduct, relationships, and choices were controlled – from the food they ate, to what time they went to bed or were allowed to shower, the clothes they wore, whether they were allowed boyfriends or girlfriends, to being administered medicines they knew didn't work and even electro-convulsive 'therapy'(ECT) against their will. We present a series of transcript excerpts which help illuminate the influence of the 'controlling professions' (Mitchell and Snyder, 2006). In the first, researchers in Steve's group discuss daily routines in supported accommodation:

Os. The staff say we can't have a nap in the afternoon.
SW. You can't have a nap in the afternoon?
Os. We're only allowed to have granny naps if we're ill.
Y. Oh really? She has just said that where she works the doors are locked at 11 o'clock and everyone's got to be in bed.
W. This is not an unusual thing for people with learning disabilities.
Os. In the mornings they are knocking us up.
SW. In the mornings, Sh is saying that everyone has to get up between 7 and 10, have had breakfast and have showered in that time, everyone who lives there.
W. So, what happened to 'this is my home'?
E. It's not their home.

In the next excerpt, one researcher from Steve's group describes moves to control what people wear in their own home, something that would never happen to most people:

Os. I had a Christmas top on one morning, and the staff said what are you doing wearing a Christmas top, go and change it.
SW. Was that the staff at your school or the staff at your house?
Os. The staff at the house. They say we're not to keep our Christmas top on. They'll tell R.
W. What?!
D. You don't always get a choice in what you wear then?
Os. I get a choice, but if wear a Christmas top when it's nowhere near Christmas then I have to change it.

The researchers also discussed repeatedly and at length controls over their friendships and romantic relationships, of which we can only present a tiny fragment here:

W. Is that the same for you Nicole? You still live at home, do your family encourage you to have relationships? Would they be OK with you taking somebody home with you?
I. Yeah, I've already got a boyfriend.
M. If you didn't have a boyfriend, would they be happy with you taking someone home?
I. No, I don't think so.
W. So it's OK for you to take your boyfriend home, but not some randomer you picked up in a pub?

I. No. But I've already found a boy!

    [...]

D. My parents wouldn't allow that either.

W. ... and L you're saying there was no way your parents would ever have allowed any of it?

E. No.

D. My parents would never let that happen.

W. Young people these days, they go out, there's no strings attached ... we're talking about relationships, yeah?

D. My mother would probably lock me up for years if I brought a random person home.

The final excerpt is harrowing as one researcher describes being subjected to ECT:

St. I, one day I suffer from what's that called that you get when you're on, oh, oh ... dzh dzh dzh dzh [making buzzing noise] ... Yeah, yeah, I suffered from 1, 2, 3, 4, 5, 6, 7, 8, oh god, it was horrifying. I didn't know whether I'd be right again. I didn't believe it, well dzzzzzzz oh god, so, oh, crying duh duh duh.

Ja. This is in recent times Stella, this isn't so long ago.

An. ECT, ECT.

Jn. ECT'll do it yeah.

H. They were gonna do it on me but didn't.

St. Yeah. I got this when I was younger, 18–19, really, really go on, in my head. I lost conscious of the oh, and then a month time, it was for me to go again, I dreaded that, dreaded, I cried, really, and don't get me wrong, it is abomination of that to happen, I spoke out about that, but every day, oh I felt frightened because only for the 8 and finish, oh my god der der der der der duh. I got energy back in myself, I got the, you know what I mean, I got, I was elated to not have this treatment.

The transcripts and the account of Antonia's life amply demonstrate both the degree and the various ways in which people labelled with learning disabilities are subject to control, stemming from their persistent conceptualization as an outgroup.

Concluding discussion

From the meta-analytic vantage point of the historicist perspective then, we see a shift in the meaning ascribed to what it was to be a person with learning disabilities in Antonia's time, concomitant with an associated attitudinal shift on the part of Western society responsible for their othering. The atavistic and irredeemable 'idiot that must be segregated' trope had been superseded by a more benevolent, if patriarchal and overwhelmingly positivist 'idiot that must be conditioned to resemble the perceived norm while remaining segregated' trope that circulated among at least some of the medical profession, at the same time as eugenics was gaining ground as a mainstream politico-scientific movement. It was this shift from crude to sophisticated othering, to draw once more upon Brons (2015), that may have prompted the recognition and documentation of some of Antonia's personal strengths, if not going so far as to document Antonia's actual personhood. Antonia was not entirely rejected by the society in which she lived, but she was never entirely accepted either, a perception of the world that, as outlined in this chapter, is still all too familiar to people with learning disabilities today. As our analysis demonstrates, the tropes of vulnerability, unworthiness, and requiring control are still very much in operation. The metanarrative may at times seem inescapable, and yet there are grounds for cautious optimism. It may indeed be possible to transcend narrative othering through embracing and appreciating the insider knowledge and perspectives that people living with learning disabilities bring, and continued advocacy work. Our co-researchers spoke, for example, of generational shifts in parental attitudes towards relationships, with younger people in our groups reporting more choice and freedoms than their older counterparts. However, our teams also recognized that learning disability communities can often be quite insular – and this is, of course, itself a manifestation of the metanarrative. The real challenge is to shift attitudes outside learning disability circles and networks, not just in disability-related communities, but in culture more broadly.

References

Adams, D. L. & Erevelles, N. (2017) Unexpected spaces of confinement: Aversive technologies, intellectual disability, and "bare life.", *Punishment & Society* 19 (3): 348–365.

Allport, G. W. (1954) *The Nature of Prejudice*, London: Addison-Wesley.

Barden, O. (2014a) Facebook levels the playing field: Dyslexic students learning through digital literacies, *Research in Learning Technology* 22 (18535). http://www.researchinlearningtechnology.net/index.php/rlt/article/view/18535#alm

Barden, O. (2014b) Winking at Facebook: Capturing digitally-mediated classroom learning, *E-Learning and Digital Media* 11 (6). http://www.wwwords.co.uk/rss/abstract.asp?j=elea&aid=6117&doi=1

Barden, O. (2020a) A cultural history of learning difficulties in the modern age, in D. T. Mitchell, and S. L. Snyder (eds) *A Cultural History of Disability in the Modern Age*, London: Bloomsbury.

Barden, O. (2020b) Demanding money with menaces: Fear and loathing in the archipelago of confinement, *Journal of Literary and Cultural Disability Studies* 14 (1): 91–108.

Barden, O., Youl, W., and Youl, E. J. (2016) Including adult learners from diverse cultural backgrounds, in Fehring, H. and Rodrigues, S. (eds) *Teaching, Coaching and Mentoring Adult Learners: Lessons for Professionalism and Partnership*, Abingdon: Routledge.

Barnes, C. (1997) A legacy of oppression: A history of disability in western culture, in Barton, L. and Oliver, M. (eds) *Disability Studies: Past Present and Future*, Leeds: Disability Press.

Bolt, D. (2014) *The Metanarrative of Blindness: A Re-Reading of Twentieth-Century Anglophone Writing*, Ann Arbor: University of Michigan Press.

Bolt, D. (2020) The metanarrative of disability: Social encounters, cultural representation and critical avoidance, in N. Watson and S. Vehmas (eds) *Routledge Handbook of Disability Studies*, 2nd edition, Abingdon: Routledge.

Brons, L. (2015) Othering, an analysis, *Transcience. A Journal of Global Studies* 6 (1): 69–90.

Brown, M., James, E., and Hatton, C. (2017) A trade in people: The inpatient healthcare economy for people with learning disabilities and/or autism spectrum disorder. University of Lancaster: CeDR Briefing Paper. 2017:1. Available from: http://wp.lancs.ac.uk/cedr/files/2017/06/A-Trade-in-People-CeDR-2017-1.pdf [Accessed 27.6.17].

Chouinard, V. (2009) Impairment and disability, in T. Brown, S. McLafferty, and G. Moon (eds) *A Companion to Health and Medical Geography*, New Jersey: Wiley-Blackwell.

Cimino, G. P. L. (2004) *Sante de Sanctis tra psicologia generale e psicologia applicata*, Milano: Franco Angeli.

Clive, R. (2021) Panarchy 3: River of the sea, *Journal of Literary and Cultural Disability Studies*, fin press.

Croce, L., Di Cosimo, F., and Lombardi, M. (2017) A short history of disability in Italy, in R., Hanes, I., Brown, and, N., E., Hansen (eds) *The Routledge History of Disability*, Abingdon, Oxon: Routledge.

Dowse, L. (2009) 'Some people are never going to be able to do that'. Challenges for people with intellectual disability in the 21st century, *Disability and Society* 24 (5): 571–584.

Drinkwater, C. (2015) Supported Living and the Production of Individuals, in S. Tremain (Ed.), *Foucault and the Government of Disability*. Ann Arbor: University of Michigan Press.

Foucault, M. (1977) *Discipline and Punish: The Birth of the Prison*. New York: Vintage.

French, J., and Jones, L. (2021) Recipe for a good life. A self-advocate's perspective on curating the 'good life' to explore happiness and living well, *Journal of Literary and Cultural Disability Studies*, in press.

Garland-Thomson, R. (1997) *Extraordinary Bodies: Figuring Physical Disability in American Culture and Literature*, New York: Columbia University Press.

Gonzalo, R., and Milton, G., 1974. Jaguar Cult-Down's Syndrome-Were-Jaguar, *Expedition* 16 (4):33.

Goodey, C. F. (2015) Why study the history of learning disability?, *Tizard Learning Disability Review* 20 (1): 3–10.

Iggers, G. G. (1995) Historicism: The history and meaning of the term, *Journal of the History of Ideas* 56 (1): 129–152.

Ireland, W. W. (1877) *On Idiocy and Imbecility*, London: J. & A. Churchill.

Jensen, S. Q. (2011) Othering, identity formation and agency, *Qualitative Studies* 2 (2): 63–78.

King, E., Okodogbe, T., Burke, E., McCarron, M., McCallion, P., and O'Donovan, M. A. (2017) Activities of daily living and transition to community living for adults with intellectual disabilities, *Scandinavian Journal of Occupational Therapy* 24 (5): 357–365.

Kraft, I. (1961) Edouard Seguin and 19th century moral treatment of idiots, *Bulletin of the History of Medicine* 35: 393.

LeDer Annual Report 2018 (2019) University of Bristol Norah Fry Centre for Disability Studies, Healthcare Quality Improvement Partnership. Available here: https://www.bristol.ac.uk/media-library/sites/sps/leder/LeDeR_Annual_Report_2018%20published%20May%202019.pdf [Accessed 6.2.20]

Meininger, H. P. (2010) Connecting stories: A narrative approach of social inclusion of persons with intellectual disability, *Alter* 4 (3): 190–202.

Mitchell, D. T., and Snyder, S. L. (2006) Regulated bodies: Disability studies and the controlling professions, in D. Turner and K. Stagg (eds) *Social Histories of Disability and Deformity: Bodies, Images, and Experience, 1650–2000*, London: Routledge.

Parmenter, T. R. (2001) Intellectual disabilities-quo vadis, in Albrecht, G. L., Seelman, K., and Bury, M. (eds) *Handbook of Disability Studies*, Thousand Oaks: SAGE Publications.

Simpson, M. K. (2014) *Modernity and the Appearance of Idiocy: Intellectual Disability as a Regime of Truth*, New York: Edwin Mellen Press.

Slorach, R. (2016) *A Very Capitalist Condition: A History and Politics of Disability*, London: Bookmarks Publications.

Smith, S., and Smith, K. (2021) Down syndrome as pure simulacrum, *Journal of Literary and Cultural Disability Studies*, in press.

Spivakovsky, C. (2017) Governing freedom through risk: Locating the group home in the archipelago of confinement and control. *Punishment & Society* 19 (3): 366–383.

Stephens, J. and McCallum, R. (2013) *Retelling Stories, Framing Culture: Traditional Story and Metanarratives in Children's Literature*. Abingdon: Routledge.

Taylor, S. (2011) Beasts of burden: Disability studies and animal rights, *Qui Parle* 19 (2): 191–222.

Veeser, H. (ed) (1989) *The New Historicism*. Abingdon: Routledge.

Walden, S. J., Evans, S. L., and Mulville, J. (2017) Changes in vickers hardness during the decomposition of bone: Possibilities for forensic anthropology, *Journal of the Mechanical Behavior of Biomedical Materials* 65: 672–678.

Walden, S. J., Mulville, J., Rowlands, J. P., and Evans, S. L. (2018) An analysis of systematic elemental changes in decomposing bone, *Journal of Forensic Sciences* 63(1): 207–213.

Walden, S. J., Evans, S. L., Mulville, J., Wilson, K., and Board, S. (2020) Progressive dehydration in decomposing bone: A potential tool for forensic anthropology. *Journal of Thermal Analysis and Calorimetry* 8: 1–8.

Wehmeyer, M. L., Shogren, K. A., Singh, N. N., and Uyanik, H. (2017) Strengths-based approaches to intellectual and developmental disabilities, in K. A. Shogren, M. L. Wehmeyer, and N. N. Singh (eds) *Handbook of Positive Psychology in Intellectual and Developmental Disabilities*, Berlin: Springer.

Wong, A. (2020) I'm disabled and need a ventilator to live. Am I expendable during this pandemic? *Vox*, April 4th. Available here: https://www.vox.com/first-person/2020/4/4/21204261/coronavirus-covid-19-disabled-people-disabilities-triage [Accessed 22.7.20].

Wright, D. (2000) Learning disability and the new poor law in England, 1834–1867, *Disability and Society* 15 (5): 731–745.

7

THE METANARRATIVE OF AUTISM

Eternal childhood and the failure of cure

Sonya Freeman Loftis

Preliminary discussion

Neurotypical (non-autistic) people have suggested to me in a variety of contexts and on diverse social occasions that my autistic traits could be decreased if I just exercised more and ate more yogurt. Having eaten a lot of yogurt in my life, I can say with complete confidence that, while yogurt is delicious, it does not cure autism (exercise does not work either). However, one of the governing aspects of the metanarrative of autism is the notion of eternal childhood. Western culture persists in the erroneous belief that all autistic people are children or child-like (McGrath, 2017; McGuire, 2016). This naturally leads to a second, equally dangerous assumption: Autistic adults have failed to be properly 'cured' of their autism. Unfortunately, for many people, such an imagined failure of cure seems to suggest an implied moral failing on the part of the autistic adult. This chapter traces the cultural origins of such metanarratives while interrogating the problematic assumptions they reinforce – particularly the way in which conceiving of autism as a 'child-like' condition lends a fake credibility to the assumed authority that neurotypical adults frequently claim over their autistic counterparts. In analyzing cultural examples of these metanarratives, I look at three recent cultural texts that offer depictions of autistic characters: ABC's popular drama *The Good Doctor* (2017–), Netflix's dramedy series *Atypical* (2017–), and *The Umbrella Academy* (2019–), a Netflix adaptation of a popular graphic novel. All of these television shows infantilize autistic characters, depict autistic characters as passive pawns in neurotypical affairs, and/or draw attention to failed attempts to cure autism. In analyzing these cultural texts, I employ what is introduced elsewhere in this volume as autocritical discourse analysis and what disability studies scholars have described as 'Cripistemology' – using my own lived experience as an autistic person to form part of my approach to analyzing cultural texts about autism (Price, 2009; Johnson and McRuer, 2014, 247).

Methodological discussion

Psychologists describe autism as a 'spectrum', which means that autistic people demonstrate extremely diverse impairments. In general, autism is diagnosed when individuals exhibit difficulty with language and communication, difficulty with social interaction, restrictive routines and repetitive behaviour (often referred to as 'self-stimulatory behaviour' or 'stimming', for short), and sensory sensitivities (hyper- or hypo-sensitivity to sound, touch, etc.) (Atwood, 2007). Autism is, according to medical definitions, a developmental disability: This means that autism is fundamentally defined by perceived deviations from what is considered 'normal' childhood development. Although autism is usually diagnosed in early childhood, it is a condition that is life-long. While mainstream modern medicine currently acknowledges that there is no cure for autism, this has not stopped some people from seeking a cure. This search for a cure is controversial, since many autistic adults do not want to be cured and recognize being autistic as a fundamental part of self-identity (Loftis, 2015). Others believe that the search for an impossible cure may implicitly encourage violence against autistic people, since the desire to eliminate a disability that cannot be cured may eventually be transformed into a desire to eliminate the *people* who cannot be cured (Loftis, 2015; McGuire, 2016). Nevertheless, popular culture beliefs that autism might be cured in some way, or that autistic people might be made more neurotypical through therapy, contribute to cultural attitudes that implicitly blame autistic adults for the failure to be cured.

Although the infantilization of adults with various disabilities is an all-too-common phenomenon, there is an especially strong association in the popular imagination between autism and childhood. Disability studies scholars have frequently noted and critiqued stereotypes that infantilize adults with disabilities: 'The West has a long history of infantilizing the disabled subject … the image of the disabled child is central to the ideological and economic success of charity and advocacy work' (McGuire, 2016, n.p). However, when it comes to representations of autism in the mainstream media, this trend is extreme – a cultural focus on the autistic child nearly effaces any notice of autistic adults whatsoever. According to one study,

> Parents portrayed the face of autism to be that of a child 95% of the time on the homepages of regional and local support organizations. Nine of the top 12 charitable organizations restricted descriptions of autism to child-referential discourse. Characters depicted as autistic were children in 90% of fictional books and 68% of narrative films and television programs. The news industry featured autistic children four times as often as they featured autistic adults in contemporary news articles … Adults with disabilities in general, and those with developmental disabilities in particular, have long been treated as childlike entities, deserving fewer rights and incurring greater condescension than adults without disabilities. The stereotype of the 'eternal child' has burned a disturbing path through history and continues

to wreak havoc in arenas ranging from employment discrimination to forced sterilization.

(Stephenson, Harp, and Gernsbacher, 2011, n.p)

Indeed, McGuire describes adult autism as a 'culturally incoherent subjectivity' and points out that focus on the autistic child often 'paints a utopic picture of a non-autistic future' (2016, n.p). Thus, the very term *autistic adult* is coded as failure – the existence of autistic adults disproves the fantasy of cure.

The narrative of autism as childhood also excludes autistic adults from narratives about autism in potentially dangerous ways. Focusing exclusively on autistic children results in a lack of support services for autistic adults. For example, the widespread cultural assumption that autistic people will not become parents means that there are no resources in place to support autistic parents. As Annie McGuire explains, 'the dominance of cultural representations framing autism as a condition linked with childhood structure dangerous material exclusions for disabled/autistic adults' (2016, n.p.). As I discovered when I became pregnant, lack of adequate pre-natal care can definitely be a 'dangerous material exclusion'. James McGrath points out that

> Online searches for information regarding autism and pregnancy almost overwhelmingly bring up speculative theories and counter-theories around what causes autism. There is contrastingly little public recognition that the experience of pregnancy ... may present particular sensory (and other) adjustments for women with autism.
>
> *(McGrath, 2017, 69)*

When I was pregnant, my neurotypical husband and I had an extremely difficult time finding a physician who was willing to work with an autistic mother – let alone one who had any training that would prepare him or her to do so. Indeed, our difficult encounters with various doctors and nurses in our attempts to find a suitable physician or midwife to deliver our child ranged from embarrassing to traumatic. Neither of us was surprised by this difficulty: In our encounters with medical professionals over the years, it had become clear that, at least in the world of modern medicine, I am thought of as a child rather than as an adult. Such encounters routinely display a sense of assumed authority on the part of medical professionals: There is an assumption that neurotypical people understand what it means to be autistic – and that assumption usually includes the belief that I am child-like. For example, after discovering that I would need a support person in the recovery room after surgery, one nurse argued with my husband about whether I should be classified as a 'child' or an 'adult' on my hospital paperwork. I was 33 years old at the time. When a friend of the family expressed concern about the hospital's readiness to perform surgery on an autistic adult, another nurse told her not to worry: 'We did this same surgery on a kid with Down's Syndrome last week'. It did not seem to occur to the hospital staff that the needs of a child with Down Syndrome and the needs of an autistic adult might be different. Another nurse asked my husband whether I was able to sign my own paperwork. 'She can read', he said with quiet exhaustion: 'she has a PhD'.

Thus, when I became pregnant, my husband and I were already well aware of the challenges we would face, having become accustomed to ableist discrimination in our previous attempts to access medical care. A few private practices told us up-front that they would not or could not work with a pregnant autistic woman. Others bungled through attempts to give pre-natal 'care' (I cannot resist the scare quotes) in offensive ways. At one office, the nurse read questions aloud from a form, directing each inquiry at my husband. When she got to 'And does she work?', her tone clearly implied that she already knew the answer. She was writing 'not applicable' on the form, in medias res of her ableist assumptions, when my husband explained patiently that 'She's a professor of Shakespeare'. At yet another office, a nurse pulled my husband out into the hallway to inform him that 'your wife's therapy didn't work'. He explained that 'This is just the way she is. She's not going to be "cured" by therapy'. We were having such a hard time finding someone to deliver the baby that my husband began to joke (with increasing levels of seriousness) about delivering the child himself, perhaps on the floor of our kitchen. The governing assumptions in my encounters with hospital personnel seemed to be that an autistic person should not be having a child – *because an autistic person is a child*. Even worse, an autistic adult is automatically seen as an adult who has failed in some important but unspoken way. If therapy had not cured me of autism, by the age of 34, I had obviously done something terribly wrong.

Analytical discussion 1

The Good Doctor

ABC's *The Good Doctor* is a drama that builds on a number of common autism stereotypes – however, infantilization and the failure of cure are both themes that underpin the show's narrative in subtle ways. *The Good Doctor* follows the story of an autistic doctor, Shaun Murphy (played by Freddie Highmore), who is completing a surgical residency at a large hospital. One might argue that the show's pilot episode offers a progressive depiction of autism. In the pilot's climatic scene, the hospital's president, Dr. Glassman (played by Richard Schiff), makes a compelling boardroom speech in favour of hiring an autistic surgeon. The speech clearly argues that social discrimination (and not impairment) is the primary barrier faced by many autistic people, a perspective rarely voiced in the mainstream media. Although Dr. Glassman's speech (falsely) equates disability with gender and race to make its point, the speech is clear in its intent to ask viewers to focus on social discrimination rather than on perceived impairment.[1] Glassman gives a variety of reasons to hire Shaun:

We should hire him because he is qualified and because he is different. How long ago was it that we wouldn't hire Black doctors in this hospital? How long ago was it that we wouldn't hire female doctors at this hospital? … Aren't we judged by how we treat people? … especially those who don't have the same advantages that we have. We hire Shaun, and we give hope to those people with limitations that those limitations are not what they think they are – that they do have a shot.

('Burnt food')

In this opening episode, the show seems to acknowledge neurodiversity, a paradigm that views mental disability as a form of diversity. Glassman asks his listeners to acknowledge neurotypical privilege (someone with a mental disability does not have the same 'advantages' that many neurotypical people have). On the other hand, this potentially progressive statement is undercut by a number of other factors. Shaun (like most autistic characters on television) is played by a neurotypical actor who is 'cripping up' (i.e. pretending to have a mental disability): The makers of the show did not choose to cast an autistic actor in the role. Furthermore, Shaun, like most fictional autistic characters, is presented as a savant – and such seemingly 'magical' savant superpowers are not a realistic representation of the majority of autistic people, who are not savants (Loftis 2015; Murray, 2008).

In addition, later episodes turn back on the potentially progressive message of the pilot in a variety of ways, as the topic of curing autism becomes a recurring theme throughout the show. The first episode emphasizes that autistic people are discriminated against in the workplace, depicting autistic people as a marginalized minority group and emphasizing the social model of disability. However, later episodes revert to the medical model in which autism is depicted not as a source of identity but as a pathological disorder that needs to be cured. Indeed, *The Good Doctor* structures itself around a series of characters who serve as foils for Shaun, as various patients with different disabilities, injuries, and/or illnesses come into contact with the surgical team. For example, in one episode, Shaun tells a man who is experiencing hallucinations that he can be 'cured' by having a brain tumour removed: He convinces the patient to undergo surgery by comparing a brain tumour to autism and pointing out that autism (unlike the tumour) cannot be removed. In giving this speech, Shaun seems to imply that if a cure were available for autism, he would be happy to take it. This episode seems to undercut the ostensible message of the pilot regarding neurodiversity: now autism is presented not as a natural form of diversity but rather as pathology that needs to be cured. In this scene, the audience is encouraged to pity Shaun, who cannot be cured, and to be glad that the patient decides to have his tumour removed in response to Shaun's speech.

In another episode, Shaun works with a patient whose condition physically prevents her from smiling or displaying any kind of facial expression ('Smile'). The surgery that would 'cure' this condition is said to be risky. Shaun, who rarely smiles himself, does not understand why the patient and her family are willing to risk her life in order for her to have 'normative' facial expressions. In the third season, Shaun convinces the parents of a boy who cannot speak to do a dangerous surgery in order to create an artificial voice box for the boy ('Unsaid'). The boy communicates using American Sign Language (ASL), but Shaun devalues ASL in favour of spoken language, displaying an auralist prejudice against deaf people and other people who sign to communicate. At the end of the episode, Shaun gives a speech in which his own struggles with communication, social interaction, and making friends serve as the evidence for why this dangerous surgery is 'needed'.

In yet another episode, Shaun has a patient who is unable to be touched by other people ('Heartfelt'). Specifically, the teenage girl expresses a desire to hug her family and friends. Because of his sensory issues, Shaun does not like to be hugged or touched, and he does not see any need for the procedure that will 'correct' this 'problem' for the patient. The episode ends by showing Shaun standing alone in the hallway watching as the (now 'cured') girl is able to hug her friends. This scene juxtaposes Shaun (who remains uncured and isolated out in the hallway) with the vivid and joyful social engagement of the now 'cured' patient. The moment is made even more symbolically evocative by the fact that Shaun is about to attend a fundraising gala at the hospital – a crowded party scene at which he feels socially excluded. In season three, Shaun encounters a young woman with a condition that physically prevents her from having intercourse with her partner. Scenes of Shaun interacting with this patient are intercut with scenes in which Shaun struggles, because of his autistic sensory issues, to be physically intimate with his girlfriend. All of these episodes have nearly identical plots. In each, Shaun encounters a patient with a condition that is meant to mirror some aspect of autism (mental difference, flat affect, differences in communication, and hypersensitivity to touch). In each, the audience is invited to compare the situation of Shaun with the situation of the patient – and possibly to pity Shaun because autism cannot be cured.

Not only does the larger narrative arc of the show focus on the concept of cure but the show also infantilizes Shaun in subtle ways – in doing so, *The Good Doctor* reinforces the larger metanarrative of autism in which autism is associated with childhood, and thus, neurotypical society implicitly blames the autistic adult for the failure to 'grow up' and be cured. In the show, Shaun is figuratively haunted by the ghost of his younger brother, who died when they were children. Although the character often appears in childhood flashbacks, he also appears to counsel Shaun in moments of anxiety and stress. The memory of his dead brother giving him advice, a ghostly image that manifests on the screen as a child who is now many years younger than the adult Shaun, seems to return Shaun to a child-like status: He needs and craves the advice of his nine-year-old brother. Moreover, in the first season, Shaun carries a toy scalpel around with him in his pocket wherever he goes. Although this treasured object is part family memento (his brother gave it to him), part symbol (representing his dreams of becoming a surgeon), and partly for stimming (Shaun pulls the scalpel out and rubs it with his thumb in moments of stress), it is also a child's toy. Overall, *The Good Doctor* not only infantilizes Shaun in subtle ways, but it also loops back to the subject of cure in many episodes.

Analytical discussion 2

Atypical

Although Netflix's dramedy *Atypical* avoids the savant stereotype employed by *The Good Doctor* and seems disinterested in the subject of cure, it still finds ways to infantilize its autistic protagonist. In fact, the main character, an autistic teenager named Sam Gardner (played by the neurotypical actor Keir Gilchrist), may not even be the show's main character. Sam's neurotypical family gets more screen time than the ostensible main character does, and the show often focuses on the 'problems' Sam causes (or is perceived to cause) for his neurotypical family. In the first season, Sam is a high school senior interested in dating; in the second, he begins college. His mother Elsa (played by Jennifer Jason Leigh) has such a difficult time with Sam's increasing independence that she copes with the stress by having an affair. Like Mark Haddon's popular novel, *The Curious Incident of the Dog in the Night-Time*, the show implicitly blames the autistic son for the irresponsible behaviour of his mother, falsely depicting autism as a force that disrupts marriages and families (Loftis, 2015; Murray, 2008). According to some sources, 'studies show that raising a child with autism is more stressful than raising a child with any other disability' (Autism Ontario, 2009 qtd in McGuire, 2016). The belief that neurotypical parents encounter unusual stress in raising autistic children has resulted in a frequent trope in literature and film: the neurotypical mother who has an affair as a 'result' of the stress of raising an autistic child. The show's strong emphasis on Sam's parents and their ailing marriage emphasizes Sam's role as a child even though he is 18 years old when the series begins. *Atypical*'s narrative places the mother of the autistic son (not the autistic son himself) in the centre of the show's narrative arc.

Part of the reason that Sam's mother Elsa has such a hard time letting Sam gain more independence is that she continually infantilizes her son. Elsa is definitely over-involved in Sam's life, and she is uncomfortable with the fact that her son wants to start dating. In fact, she has a conversation with Sam's psychiatrist in which she tries to convince the therapist that her son is not mature enough to handle potential 'heartbreak' (pilot). Sam's sister Casey (played by Brigette Lundy-Paine) is also over-protective of her older brother and becomes involved in his dating life, going so far as to tell him whom he should and should not date. When Sam begins dating a neurotypical classmate, Paige (played by Jenna Boyd), Casey confronts her brother's new girlfriend and tells her to break-up with Sam:

Paige. I think maybe he's avoiding me because we were talking yesterday, and I don't know … maybe I just upset him because he kind of disappeared after that. I don't know. Maybe it's nothing

Casey. Well, it's not nothing. Because of you he didn't eat lunch yesterday, which I know is an annoying thing to have to think about when you are dating an 18-year-old dude, but that's what you get with Sam.

Paige. Do you have any advice?

Casey. Yeah, stop seeing my brother. Why are you with him? What's in it for you? Are you desperate or do you think you're going to get extra credit for dating the weird kid?

Paige. No, no. Casey, I really like Sam a lot. He's honest, and he's so cute. And have you seen his notebook thing? It's amazing. The way his brain works is so interesting.

Casey. Interesting? My brother is not a science experiment … what happens when he starts to rely on you? And then you leave … because then he'll need you. And that shit can really mess him up. ('That's my sweatshirt')

Casey implies that no one would want to be with Sam if they didn't have ulterior motives ('what's in it for you?') as well as expressing an ableist notion that being with an autistic person is a kind of sacrifice ('do you think you're going to get extra credit?'). She implies that choosing a partner with a disability is a sign of being 'desperate' for companionship. Finally, she ends by accusing Paige of seeing an autistic boyfriend as exotic and of objectifying Sam: 'my brother is not a science experiment'. Both Elsa and Casey infantilize Sam by trying to prevent him from dating and attempting to control whom he dates.

The Good Doctor features a nearly identical scene in which the nosy and bossy Morgan (played by Fiona Gublemann) confronts and interrogates Shaun's girlfriend Carley (played by Jasika Nicole). Like the scene from *Atypical*, this encounter between the two women shows how the neurotypical characters infantilize Shaun, and specifically, how they feel that they have a right to comment on his dating choices. Such attitudes are informed by the metanarrative of autism, which dictates that autism is an inherently child-like state. Autistic adults are imagined as too immature for romantic relationships, and they are seen as needing the advice and guidance of the neurotypical adults around them in all matters:

Morgan. I like Shaun and I love that he's dating. But I can't help thinking that the kind of person who would go out with Shaun might be seeing him more as a project than a person. And I'd rather not see him get his heart broken …

Carley. I am not going out with Shaun because I have a martyr complex. I'm going out with him because he's a great guy who treats me well. And the condescending notion that someone needs an ulterior motive to be interested in him means you are the one who isn't seeing him as a person. ('Incomplete')

Like Casey, Morgan accuses a neurotypical woman of having ulterior motives for dating an autistic man. Like Elsa, Morgan claims that she is worried about whether an autistic adult can handle heartbreak. Just as Casey feels that she has the right to interrogate her brother's girlfriend, Morgan feels that she has the right to interrogate her co-worker's girlfriend. But unlike the teenaged girl-friend in *Atypical*, Carley points out the ableist assumptions underpinning such inappropriate interrogations: 'you are the one who isn't seeing him as a person' ('Incomplete'). Clearly, *The Good Doctor* and *Atypical* have some important simi-larities: a key one is that both infantilize their autistic adult characters.

Analytical section 3

The Umbrella Academy

Unlike *The Good Doctor* and *Atypical*, *The Umbrella Academy* does not feature a main character on the autism spectrum: rather, it has a minor autistic character who appears in only a few episodes. However, the show's depiction of autism emphasizes the perceived passivity of its autistic child character as well as bringing a 'desperate' search for a cure into its narrative.

Based on a graphic novel, *The Umbrella Academy* follows the adventures of seven time-travelling siblings with superpowers who attempt to prevent the apocalypse. In the show, Vanya Hargreeves (played by Ellen Page) is the most non-descript of the seven super siblings, and she encounters an autistic child named Harlan when she time travels from 2019 to the 1960s. Although Vanya's superpower is extremely destructive and uncontrollable (she inadvertently causes the apocalypse twice – in two different timelines), she was raised to believe that she is 'normal' and passed for most of her life as a non-superhero. Harlan, the son of Vanya's lover Sissy (Marin Ireland) in the show's second season, is a non-verbal child who has frequent meltdowns and engages in self-harm. Like most representations of autistic people in the media, Harlan (played by Justin Paul Kelly) is a child. And like most representations of autism in the mainstream media, the word *autism* is never spoken in *The Umbrella Academy*. Harlan's character is an example of a literary character type Robert Rozema would describe as 'coded autistic' and James McGrath refers to as 'implicitly autistic' (Rozema, 2020, 20; McGrath 2017); such characters clearly display autistic traits, although they are never explicitly labelled as being on the spec-trum. Like many cultural representations of autism (*The Curious Incident of the Dog in the Night-Time, Atypical*), *The Umbrella Academy* gives a great deal of focus to the autistic character's neurotypical mother. And like Hadden's novel and Netflix's dramedy, the show also depicts the parents of the autistic child as having a failing marriage and implies that the stress of raising an autistic child leads the neurotypical mother to have an affair. Sissy tells Vanya about how lonely she feels:

> Do you know what it's like when you have a man that can't see you? A son who won't talk to you? Your life gets small – a little smaller every day. And

you don't even notice the box that you're in until somebody comes along
and lets you out.

('The majestic 12')

This revelation is followed by Vanya and Sissy's first kiss, inaugurating an affair
in which Sissy cheats on her cold and indifferent husband.

It seems symbolically significant that this affair takes place in the 1960s, an
era in which mothers were often blamed for their children's autism. This was a
time period in which the mothers of autistic children were famously described
as 'refrigerator mothers', and their 'cold' mothering was thought to cause the
condition (McGuire, 2016; McGrath, 2017). As McGuire explains,

> psychoanalysis takes up the role of the mother as a crucial arbiter in the
> psychosocial development of the child. In the 1950s and 1960s, various
> foundational precepts of psychoanalysis became popular – particularly
> in white, middle-class households – in relation to maternal practices of
> child-rearing. While the mother was understood to be uniquely and even
> 'naturally' positioned as the rearer of children and as the prime nurturer
> of their psychosocial development, she was nonetheless always (and
> differentially, with respect to, say, the mother's social class, race, disability
> identification) framed to be at risk of mothering wrong and so always (and
> differentially) positioned as at risk of catalyzing 'poor' child development
> outcomes. (McGuire)

When Sissy's husband, Carl, learns of her affair with Vanya, he defends himself as
a 'good' husband, saying to his wife, 'I never blamed you for the boy' ('743'). In
Carl's mind, the fact that he has not blamed his wife for their autistic child is in
itself a sign of his inherent goodness as a spouse and father. However, now that he
knows of the affair, he threatens the two women by threatening Harlan. He claims
that their lesbian relationship sets a bad example for the child and threatens to put
Harlan in an institution 'for his own good'. In this way, *The Umbrella Academy*
allows its historical setting to imbue the ableist and homophobic attitudes of
Sissy's husband, who perceives 'the disorder of the child' as 'a reflection of the
disorder of the mother and her home' (McGuire).

Like many of the non-verbal autistic children who are represented on
television, Harlan is depicted as magical or mystical, and there is a narrative
emphasis on trying to cure his autism. Mark Osteen has noted the prevalence
of the trope in which autistic children are represented as magical (2008, 31).
Another dangerous cultural stereotype of autism depicts non-verbal autistic
people as lacking in subjectivity (Loftis, 2015). In *The Umbrella Academy*, Harlan
takes on both of these stereotypes: He is represented as a passive or empty
receptacle that can contain Vanya's superpower. In one scene, Harlan suddenly
elopes, running away from his mother. The terrified women search for him, and
Vanya is horrified to find the boy drowned at the nearby lake. However, she is

able to use her superpowers to resurrect the child – who magically absorbs some of her power when he is brought back to life. The cultural perception of non-verbal autistic people as lacking in subjectivity clearly informs this depiction, since Harlan is presented as though he were an empty vessel that can absorb Vanya's abilities. When he is resurrected, Harlan seems to be exactly the same character – except that he has absorbed some of Vanya's power. In the climax of the second season, Harlan inadvertently unleashes this destructive force. Because Harlan has frequent meltdowns, Vanya's uncontrollable and explosive power is conflated in this scene with an autistic meltdown, as though the two symbolically stand in for each other. Furthermore, the heroes of the Umbrella Academy are not only called upon in this episode to save the world but also to save an autistic child. The innocence of this disabled victim stands in (as children so often symbolically do) for the future of the world. Only saving Harlan will prevent an apocalypse. After Vanya manages to re-absorb her power, thus resolving the meltdown/explosion that threatens to end the world, she begs Sissy to return to 2019 with her. In a conversation with her brother, Vanya makes the argument that Sissy should travel to the future for Harlan's sake: 'There's a name for what he has! We can get him the help that he needs' ('Oga for Oga'). A potential cure for autism, the right therapy that would 'help', Vanya claims, would be worth time-travelling in order to find.

Concluding discussion

There are many other examples I could give of cultural discourses that perpetuate the notion of autism as childhood, that depict autistic adults being infantilized, or that represent autistic children as passive beings who merely symbolize the tribulations of their mothers. There are many other cultural stories about autism in which the search or desire for cure is a reoccurring motif. There are plenty of cultural discourses in which autistic adults are blamed (sometimes implicitly, sometimes overtly) for not partaking of a cure which does not exist and was never offered to us in the first place. The popular television shows I have analyzed here, *The Good Doctor*, *Atypical*, and *The Umbrella Academy*, are merely three recent examples of ways in which popular culture manifests autism's metanarrative of eternal childhood. It is a metanarrative that has real implications in the lives of autistic adults and that impacts their lived experience of disability. As an autistic adult, I grow weary of being treated as a child and spoken to like a child. I am tired of being told that my 'therapy did not work'. As McGrath argues,

> To society (including psychiatry), adult autistic identities – and responses to them – remain a point of much uncertainty. There is not yet a cultural or medical space in which to acknowledge adult autism as an entity or identity in its own right. In its own way, infantilization of autistic adults is a form of normalization: to liken us to children is to expect our subservience.
>
> *(McGrath, 2017, 75)*

The metanarrative of autism as eternal childhood contributes to the perception of autistic people as passive characters in neurotypical stories. It prioritizes the perspectives of neurotypical parents over the perspectives of autistic people. It contributes to a lack of services and supports being provided for autistic adults. Ultimately, it can both drive the search for a cure and also lead to the blaming of those of us (all of us) autistics who fail to find it.

Note

1 For more on the problems that arise when people compare disability with race and gender, see Samuels (2017).

References

Atypical (2017–2020) Created by Robia Rashid, Netflix.

Atwood, T. (2007) *The Complete Guide to Asperger's Syndrome*, London: Jessica Kingsley.

Johnson, M. L. and McRuer, R. (2014) Introduction: Cripistemologies and the masturbating girl, *Journal of Literary and Cultural Disability Studies* 8 (3): 245–256.

Loftis, S. F. (2015) *Imagining Autism: Fiction and Stereotypes on the Spectrum*, Bloomington: Indiana University Press.

McGrath, J. (2017) *Naming Adult Autism: Culture, Science, Identity*, London: Rowman and Littlefield.

McGuire, A. (2016) *War on Autism: On the Cultural Logic of Normative Violence*, Ann Arbor: University of Michigan Press.

Murray, S. (2008) *Representing Autism: Culture, Narrative, Fascination*, Liverpool: Liverpool University Press.

Osteen, M. (2008) *Autism and Representation*, New York: Routledge.

Price, M. (2009) 'Her pronouns wax and wane': Psychosocial disability, autobiography, and counter-diagnosis, *Journal of Literary and Cultural Disability Studies* 3 (1): 11–33.

Rozema, R. (2020) Waiting for autistic superman: On autistic representation in superhero comics, *Ought: The Journal of Autistic Culture* 1 (2): 26–41.

Samuels, E. (2017) My body, my closet: Invisible disabilities and the limits of coming out, in L. J. Davis (ed.) *The Disability Studies Reader*, 5th edition, New York: Routledge.

Stephenson, J., Harp, B. and Gernsbacher, M. A. (2011) Infantilizing autism, *Disability Studies Quarterly* 31 (3), n.p.

The Umbrella Academy (2019–2020) Created by Steve Blackman and Jeremy Slater. Netflix.

The Good Doctor (2017–2020). Created by David Shore. *ABC*.

8

THE METANARRATIVE OF DOWN SYNDROME

Proximity to animality

Helen Davies

Preliminary discussion

In 2018, the Canadian Down Syndrome Association launched a campaign under the banner 'Endangered Syndrome', featuring a short video of actors with Down syndrome costumed as various endangered animal species, including a polar bear, lion, panda, rhinoceros, and sea turtle. Sharing the lines, the actors state, 'like some animals [...] people with Down syndrome are endangered. That's why we're applying to be the first people on the endangered list'. Further details can be found on the campaign's website, where visitors are encouraged to sign a petition to be sent to the International Union for Conversation of Nature. A letter addressed to the IUCN indicates that the global Down syndrome community is 'shrinking' (although not explicitly stated, this implicitly refers to prenatal screening and subsequent termination), and highlights the barriers that people with Down syndrome experience in relation to access to education, housing, employment, and quality of living (2018, 1). Although the goals of the campaign – improving all aspects of the lives of people with Down syndrome, and awareness raising – are certainly laudable, the connection being made between animals and people with Down syndrome proved problematic for some commentators. There was a social media backlash,[1] and David M. Perry, whose son has Down syndrome, remarked: 'Cute, well-intentioned depictions of people with Down syndrome as charismatic megafauna [...] literally dehumanize them' (Perry, 2018). Francie Munoz, a woman with Down syndrome, was interviewed by CBC Toronto, and she explained: 'It doesn't matter who you are ... I don't like people comparing me as an animal, it's not fair [...] Love us for who we

---

1 See Barr (2018) and Wanshel (2018) for a summary of social media responses to the campaign.

are, not a character, not an animal' (Brown, 2018). In contrast, however, Dylan Harman, one of the actors with Down syndrome who starred in the video, perceived the comparison as relevant: 'This campaign is about our existence in life [...] everyone has a purpose' (Stechyson, 2018).

This chapter seeks to explore the ways in which a particular aspect of the metanarrative of Down syndrome – a comparison to animals, the implication that people with Down syndrome are less than human – has come to be established and perpetuated in cultural discourse. The discomfort over the 'Endangered Syndrome' campaign from some members of the Down syndrome community is unsurprising when understanding that nineteenth-century medical discourse around 'idiocy' repeatedly made comparisons between intellectual disability and animality, mired in colonial, racist, and ableist stereotypes. As this chapter shows, such ideologies cast a long shadow into the twentieth century, and also find resonance in the championing of animal rights by philosophers such as Peter Singer. My reading of Doris Lessing's *The Fifth Child* (1988) demonstrates the way in which such comparisons can be reiterated in literary representations of Down syndrome. I argue that Lessing depicts Amy, a child with Down syndrome, as having a *proximity* to animality; the novel does not go as far as to articulate that people with Down syndrome are animals, but it does replicate constructions of Down syndrome as a sort of mid-point in a hierarchical chain of human and non-human animals, which has a troubling resonance with nineteenth-century ideologies. However, I also offer a reading of Sarah Kanake's *Sing Fox to Me* (2016) as a counterpoint to this metanarrative. Kanake's inclusion of a central character with Down syndrome, against the backdrop of postcolonial Tasmania, has a keen eye on the discourse of 'extinction' when it comes to subjugated human and non-human animals. I argue that Kanake's novel, contextualized via critical animal and disability studies, offers alternative, more productive points of connection and affiliation between human and non-human animals.

Methodological discussion

This chapter is a text-based study,[2] but metanarratives of Down syndrome are of significant personal interest to me; my older sister Elizabeth, who died in 1998, had Down syndrome and my childhood and teenage years were spent as part of local and national Down syndrome/disability communities. This gives me no special claim to speak on behalf of people with Down syndrome, of course, and I do not intend to do so: My concern here is to interrogate a metanarrative – a normative social order which has constructed and perpetuates a medically approved

2 My research towards this chapter is part of a larger project, *Reading Down Syndrome: Fictions of Intellectual Disability*. As part of this project, I am working with the Down's Syndrome Association in the United Kingdom to set up book groups for people with Down syndrome and their families and friends to discuss literary representations of Down syndrome.

story about Down syndrome as being a perpetual deficiency, lack, abnormal, less than *human*. My choice of the term *story* in relation to the metanarrative of Down syndrome is pointed, for some of the finest times of my childhood were spent listening to Elizabeth's stories. We would sit in our bedroom, and she would spin elaborate, hilarious yarns featuring a girl named Georgina, her excellent companion Super-Dog, and the pranks they played upon their arch-nemesis, Mr Gorbachev (in our mitigation, it was the late 1980s, and his real-life counterpart was often on television). But what of the stories that other people told about Elizabeth? I do not mean stories told by family and friends, by people who knew *her*. I am referring to the metanarrative that was routinely imposed upon her and us in relation to what having an additional copy of chromosome 21 meant for her personality, her identity, her agency, her capabilities, her life.

Some of the less-than-fine times of my childhood were spent listening to other people's stories about Elizabeth, the assumptions they felt they could make about her based on what the social order dictates people with Down syndrome are or can be. A pertinent example for the focus of this chapter came in a secondary school biology lesson in the 1990s. The class was asked to copy some notes about chromosomes from a textbook, and on turning to the required section there was an illustration of a child with Down syndrome but also a photograph of an orangutan on the adjacent page. In retrospect, this could have been coincidence, but I hesitated, considering what might be being implied by this *proximity* between a representation of Down syndrome and animality. Eventually, the teacher came to see why I was not following her instructions. I did not have the words then to articulate my unease, and angrily waved my hand in the direction of the book, saying 'This ... this. ... Did you know that my sister has Down syndrome?' The last remark was articulated as defiantly as I dared, and the meaning I intended to convey was that there was something offensive about this positioning of representations. However, her manner changed, and she sat down next to me, cooing with sympathy about what a 'shame' this was for my family but that 'it must be a great comfort that people with Down syndrome are so happy and affectionate'. This was truly extraordinary to me at the time, not least because Elizabeth was just as cynical and reserved as myself and the rest of my immediate family. But as the years have passed, the mysterious reasons for why she would make such an assumption have become all too clear. Down syndrome has so often been represented in both medical and cultural discourse as a 'tragedy' to befall a family (Kanake, 2019, 62), and people with Down syndrome have routinely been presented as 'happy idiots' (Smith, 2011, 53).

There is another point to be made here about locations of social power in relation to who constructs and controls the metanarratives of Down syndrome. The medicalized discourse in a school textbook intersects with the assumed authority of the science teacher, who is in a position to impose her cultural metanarrative of Down syndrome onto a teenaged student and, more importantly, the teenager's disabled sister. Julie Avril Minich, naming critical disability studies as a methodological approach, is attuned to these relationships of power when it comes to epistemology; who produces knowledge, and to what ends: '[critical disability studies] scrutiny of normative ideologies should occur [...] with the *goal of producing knowledge in support of justice* for people with stigmatized bodies and minds' (Minich, 2016). In this chapter, therefore, my aim is to weave some aspects of my experiential knowledge of Down syndrome with a critical disability studies approach to expose the ableist – and speciesist – ideologies of cultural representations that construct both humans with intellectual disabilities and non-human animals as deviant and inferior.

Analytical discussion 1

Racist science, ableism, and speciesism

What of those two images, the child with Down syndrome and the orangutan? As critics such as Patrick McDonagh (2008) and Licia Carlson have identified (2010), there is a long history of associating intellectual disability with animality, but it is during the course of the nineteenth century that a pernicious matrix of associations between 'idiots', colonial subjects, and non-human animals becomes entrenched in scientific and medical discourse. This is exemplified by Charles Darwin's analysis in *The Descent of Man* (1871), remarking on traits such as 'imitation' being found in 'monkeys, in microcephalous idiots and in the barbarous races of mankind' (Darwin, 1871, 16).[3] The Victorian zeal for taxonomization ensured that the umbrella term of 'idiocy' begins to give way to various gradations for intellectual disability on both sides of the Atlantic,[4] and John Langdon Down's publication of his brief article 'Observations on the Ethnic Classification of Idiots' in 1866 coins the classification of the 'Mongolian' type of idiocy (Langdon Down, 1866, 259). This designation persisted, in various forms, until a collective of scientists in the early 1960s petitioned for the name of the condition, now understood as chromosomal, to be changed.[5] Langdon Down's seminal publication is making a transparent connection between intellectual disability and racialized categorization, borrowing from Blumenbach's use of 'Mongolian' as a generalized term to refer to people of northeastern Asian heritage and loaded with implications of racial inferiority to white, Western, non-disabled subjects (Keevak, 2011, 62). Langdon Down does invoke the concept of degeneration in his initial studies (Down, 1866, 262), and in his later work offers a long description of the "congenital class" of idiot, concluding that

3 See Gelb (2008), for a fuller discussion of Darwin's use of intellectual disability in *The Descent of Man*.
4 See Snyder and Mitchell's concept of the 'Eugenic Atlantic' as a way of articulating the exchange of ideas about intellectual disability and race during the nineteenth and early twentieth century (2006, 100–132).
5 See Wright (2011, 115–118) for further discussion of the process and politics of the introduction of the term Down['s] syndrome.

'so far as instinct is concerned, the young animal is on a higher platform than an idiot baby' (1887, 116–117).

The continuum of animals, idiocy, and non-white Western people became more pronounced as the century progressed: Sunaura Taylor, among others, has highlighted the ways in which eugenic principles applied to human populations (especially disabled and colonial subjects) originated in selective animal breeding practices (Taylor, 2017, 215). Although there were some contemporaries of Langdon Down, such as William W. Ireland, who ultimately discounted direct comparisons between people with intellectual disability and animals (namely monkeys), Ireland spends a great deal of time trying to find such connections by detailing skull and palate shape (Ireland, 1877, 50) and comparing the relative intelligence of animals and 'idiots' (Ireland, 1877, 271–272). By the early twentieth century, a routine conclusion of studies of idiocy – which always made reference to Mongolian idiots or imbeciles, 'primitive' people, and animals of some sort or other – would be that separation from the general population (e.g. institutionalization) was necessary to ensure 'racial progress' (Tredgold, 1920, 501–502; Shuttleworth and Potts, 1910, 208–209). F.G. Crookshank's *The Mongol in Our Midst* (first published in 1924, with a third expanded edition being published in 1931) represents a nadir for the conflation of Down syndrome with those deemed racially 'other', and animals. Crookshank's thesis was actually a revival of nineteenth-century anthropological/pseudo-scientific theories of reversion which had largely been discounted by this point in the twentieth century – ironically, therefore, something of a throwback – and his suggested connection between 'imbecile mongoloids' and orangutans is ultimately based on copious, spurious remarks about supposed visual similarities between the two. But such a comparison did not wholly expire even with the discovery of the chromosomal origin of Down syndrome; Thomas A. Merton's *Mankind in the Unmaking: The Anthropology of Mongolism*, published in 1968, encourages the reader to: 'Try this test! Take a full face photograph (a) of a Caucasian with Down's syndrome, (b) of an orangutan', concluding that the shape of the respective eyes proves interchangeable (Merton, 1968, 24). Merton's slim volume is illustrated with numerous photographic comparisons of children with Down syndrome, monkeys, and apes. Lest we reassure ourselves that Merton was an exception, another throwback to an earlier time, the chapter on 'Down's Syndrome' in L. Crome and J Stern's *Pathology of Mental Retardation* (1972, second edition) features a photograph of a 'young chimpanzee showing some facial feature of Down's syndrome' (Crome and Stern, 1972, 205).

To return to my anecdote about the school science lesson, I can note that my teenage sense of discomfort about what might be signified by the proximity of an image of Down syndrome and the face of an orangutan seems well-founded based on the above historical overview. Furthermore, such ideologies have had material, terrifying consequences for the lives of people with Down syndrome and other intellectual disabilities: institutionalization and enforced sterilization in the name of eugenics; extermination in the Third Reich's T4 programme; and, as indicated by the 'Endangered Syndrome' campaign, increased rates of selective abortion when foetuses with Down syndrome are detected.[6] Donna Haraway, borrowing Bruno Latour's concept of the 'Great Divides, the principal Others to Man' lists 'gods, machines, animals, monsters, creepy crawlies, women, servants and slaves, and noncitizens in general' at various points standing in for the non-human, those who are located '[o]utside the security checkpoint of bright reason' (Haraway, 2008, 9–10). People with intellectual disabilities should definitely be added to this litany. But there is a detail in Elizabeth Davies's stories – rather than the metanarratives of the normative social order – which bears further consideration: the role of Super-Dog. For Elizabeth's imagining of Super-Dog had much in common with Haraway's progressive vision of what can happen 'when species meet'; Elizabeth's fictional creation was most definitely a dog, but worked and played alongside Georgina, in his own, canine way. They had their obvious differences, but their lives, interests, and emotions were inextricably entwined. Their relationship was not hierarchical; Georgina might issue instructions to Super-Dog, but he was just as likely to modify and challenge Georgina's decision making. They shared mutual respect, appreciation, and understanding. Elizabeth never specified if Georgina had Down syndrome, but I suspect that this was the case. I also suspect that Peter Singer probably would not have had a great deal of time for Georgina, and would have preferred Super-Dog.

Peter Singer's position as a trailblazer for philosophical theorizations of animal rights – and the pitfalls of speciesism – is rivalled only by his reputation as the bête noire of disability rights. His argument in *Animal Liberation*, first published in 1975, that the oppression of animals should be considered in the same vein as racism and sexism is provocative. However, his use of intellectual disability as a test case for exploring the respective ethics of killing humans and non-human animals is deeply problematic:

> Adult chimpanzees, dogs, pigs, and members of many other species far surpass the brain-damaged infant in their ability to relate to others, act independently, be self-aware, and any other capacity that could reasonably be said to give value to life. With the most intensive care possible, some severely retarded infants can never achieve the intelligence level of a dog [...] The only thing that distinguishes the infant from the animal [...] is that it is, biologically, a member of the species Homo sapiens.
>
> *(Singer, 2015, 18)*

Although Down syndrome is not mentioned in *Animal Liberation*, he devoted a co-authored book to exploring issues around the euthanasia of infants with

---

6 See Snyder and Mitchell for a discussion of the history of institutionalization, and the T4 programme from a disability studies perspective (2006, 121–125); see Kaposy (2018) on Down syndrome and the ethics of prenatal technologies.

Down syndrome and other disabilities, concluding that such killing might well be in the best interests of families and society more broadly in some cases (Kuhse and Singer, 1985). Such views are reiterated in his later work as well (Singer, 1994; Singer, 2010, 331–344). There have been some excellent interrogations of Singer's ableist assumptions about what counts as a valuable human life from critics such as Harriet McBryde Johnson (2003), Eva Feder Kittay (2010, 393–413), Michael Bérubé (2010, 97–110), and Licia Carlson (2010), among others. For my purposes, Sunaura Taylor's identification of the ways in which Singer's remarks are, ironically enough, speciesist are invaluable: 'Singer's arguments reinforce not only a hierarchy of ability but also a hierarchy of species' (Taylor, 2017, 146). In the above quotation from Singer, the value of non-human animals is still linked to a normative, medicalized construction of intelligence (hence my suggestion that Singer might have appreciated Super-Dog more than Georgina or, indeed, Elizabeth).

Taylor's work considers comparable sites of oppression between humans with disabilities and non-human animals, including 'ableist paradigms of language and cognitive capacity' (Taylor, 2017, 53), which have led to the use and abuse of both groups in a myriad of ways. She also offers the radical possibility of *identification* between disabled human and non-human animals; while always sensitive to the dangers of such connections, given the 'histories of animalization and pathologization' of disability (Taylor, 2017, 20), she explores the value in 'claiming animal' from the perspective of her own physical disabilities. Understandably, her commentary about the ways in which people with intellectual disabilities might claim animality is tentative, acknowledging that '[s]peciesism doesn't necessarily keep people from wanting to identify as animal; dehumanization does' (Taylor, 2017, 110). This is amply demonstrated by the criticisms of the 'Endangered Syndrome' campaign discussed in this chapter's preliminary discussion. Furthermore, I am certainly not the person to make any case for people with Down syndrome 'claiming animal', though it is interesting to note that the actors in the CDSA video are doing this. Instead, I turn now to two fictional depictions of Down syndrome to explore how the metanarrative of Down syndrome as proximity to animality has been engaged with in literary representation. Although Doris Lessing's *The Fifth Child* replicates the Victorian discourse of degeneration and animality in relation to Down syndrome (and intellectual disability more broadly), Sarah Kanake's *Sing Fox to Me* imagines the anti-ableist and anti-speciesist potential of representing interconnectedness between people with Down syndrome and animals.

Analytical discussion 2

Degeneration, dogs, and Down syndrome

Doris Lessing's novel *The Fifth Child* (1988) tells the story of a couple who have had a number of children in close succession, much to the annoyance of family members who believe that their actions are selfish. Nevertheless, the first four pregnancies run smoothly, and the children are a source of happiness and pride for Harriet and David. On the other hand, Harriet's sister, Sarah, gives birth to Amy, a baby with Down syndrome. Harriet labels Amy as 'the mongol child':

> yes, yes, of course she knew one shouldn't call them mongol. But the little girl did look a bit like Genghis Khan, didn't she? A baby Genghis Khan with her squashed little face and her slitty eyes?
>
> *(Lessing, 1988, 22)*

Harriet evidently invokes the assumed authority of the Victorian medical, racialized discourse of 'Mongolian idiocy' here, and the reference to Genghis Khan also exposes the racist anxieties that construct the stereotypical traits of 'Mongols'; in Michael Keevak's analysis, by the nineteenth century, these were firmly solidified to connote the 'exotic, and threatening', 'a common symbol of monstrosity', and a 'reputation as inhuman invaders' (Keevak, 2011, 4; 76; 73). Amy is thus introduced into the narrative as a symbolic menace, and the 'mongol' baby carries associations of savagery, monstrosity, and the non-human.

Nevertheless, the perceived threat that Amy poses to the extended family is supplanted by the arrival of Ben, the eponymous fifth child. Harriet experiences a nightmarish pregnancy due to the unborn child's size and vigorous movements: the foetus is imagined as a 'savage thing' (Lessing, 1988, 41); 'the creature' (1988, 49); '*monster*' (1988, 47). On his birth, Harriet labels him 'Neanderthal baby' due to his size, strength, and unusual appearance (Lessing, 1988, 53) and throughout the narrative, Ben is repeatedly represented as an atavistic, bestial throwback (Lessing, 1988, 106). Significantly, Bridget – a cousin of David who has come to visit Ben – asks: "'What is wrong with him? Is he a mongol?", to which Harriet responds: "Down's syndrome [...] no one calls it mongol now. But no, he's not'" (Lessing, 1988, 61). Bridget's assumption that the 'changeling' child has Down syndrome is telling (Lessing, 1988, 59); the 'mongol' label becomes a catch-all expression for any child deemed abnormal or degenerate. Harriet's correction of Bridget's terminology is ironic given her own prior invocation of such language, and could be interpreted as a progression of Harriet's attitudes towards disability. However, she returns to referring to Amy as the 'mongol child' shortly afterwards (Lessing, 1988, 66).

Although Ben is routinely represented in animalized, bestial terms, Amy's proximity to animality is reasserted via the children's dealings with family pets. A visitor's dog and neighbour's cat are found dead in mysterious circumstances and Harriet suspects Ben (Lessing, 1988, 62). Sarah becomes more tentative in her visits, asking 'if it would be "all right" to bring Amy. This meant that she had heard – everyone had – about the dog, and the cat' (Lessing, 1988, 66). Harriet confirms that '[i]t'll be alright if we are careful never to leave Amy alone with Ben', and she reiterates to her older children: 'Please look after Amy. Never leave her alone with Ben' (Lessing, 1988, 66). The implication is that Amy is more vulnerable to Ben's violence than the 'normal' children, and her position of being closer to the state of the household pets is reiterated when the day of their visit arrives:

> Amy, who expected everyone to love her, would go to Ben [...] this afflicted infant, who was radiant with affection, suddenly became silent; her face was woeful, and she backed away, staring at him. Just like Mr. McGregor, the poor cat.
>
> *(Lessing, 1988, 67)*

The characterization of Amy thus references the aforementioned metanarrative strand of the happy and affectionate 'nature' of people with Down syndrome, and she is also figured as possessing some sort of animal instincts as to Ben's deviance. Seemingly, both animals and children with Down syndrome are to be pitied in some way, evidenced by the vocabulary of tragedy – 'afflicted', 'poor' – that is being applied to their respective positions in relation to Ben.

Sometime later we learn that Sarah has bought a 'cheerful [...] mongrel', who by the time they come to visit Harriet's family again, is firmly established as Amy's companion:

> [Harriet] watched how the big dog seemed to know that Amy, the loving child in the big ugly body, needed gentleness: he moderated his exuberance for her [...] Sarah said this dog was like a nursemaid to Amy.
>
> *(Lessing, 1988, 71)*

The relationship between Amy and the unnamed dog could be interpreted as a profound cross-species connection, but Amy's otherness – the 'ugliness' of her body – is reiterated; the dog is cast as having an almost superior emotional intelligence to the child with Down syndrome. This said, it is difficult not to note the resonance between mongrel/mongol, and both are defined by their happiness. Predictably, the dog is not keen on Ben, and one morning Harriet catches Ben creeping up on the sleeping canine and intervenes just in time. The very same day the assembled family pressure Harriet into putting Ben in an institution, and the description of this place is filled with abject, bestial, Gothicized imagery: 'In the cots were – monsters [...] every bed or cot held an infant or small child in whom the human template had been wrenched out of pattern' (Lessing, 1988, 81). Harriet ultimately rescues Ben from the institution and he stays in the family. As he grows older, he is frequently couched in canine terms: 'as if Ben were [...] a puppy that needed training' (Lessing, 1988, 91); 'like a frightened dog' (Lessing, 1988, 107); 'he bared his teeth and snarled' (Lessing, 1988, 109). The novel concludes with Harriet's imaginings of what might become of her son in his adulthood, and the final image of the text is of Ben 'searching the faces in the crowd for another of his own kind' (Lessing, 1988, 133).

The Fifth Child constructs a hierarchy of inhabitants of the household, a microcosm of the normative order of society more broadly. Children who are non-normative – Ben, Amy, the unnamed inhabitants of the institution – are repeatedly figured as being non-human and closer to the state of animals. Interestingly, Amy stays in the bosom of the family, while Ben is placed, temporarily, in the institution, but she is placed on a continuum with the children who are 'wrenched out of pattern', for the quotations provided above repeatedly focus on the difference – and abnormality – of her physicality and cognition. Ben is framed via the discourse of degeneration and atavism, but Amy's Down syndrome is historically rooted in the same nineteenth-century ideological othering of disability, people of colour, and animals. Her perceived vulnerability to Ben's aggression renders her closer to the state of household pets in the novel's rendering of a chain of beings: the metanarrative of Down syndrome's proximity to animality persists.

Analytical discussion 3

Claiming animal

Sarah Kanake's *Sing Fox to Me* (2016) follows the fates of the Fox family: Samson and Jonah Fox, twin brothers, travel with their father, David, from Australia's mainland to the island of Tasmania. David grew up with his mother, Essie, his sister, River, and his father, Clancy, on the mountain, living near to George and his son, Murray, who is Aboriginal. However, Essie dies of cancer during their teenage years, shortly after which River experiences mental health problems and goes missing in the bush. David appears to have separated from his wife, and his fractious relationship with his father and their complicated history mean that he struggles to return to the family home, leaving the twins in Clancy's care. Tasmania was the home of the thylacine – otherwise known as the Tasmanian Tiger, a marsupial predator that was hunted to extinction after the island became a colony of the British empire in the nineteenth century. By the early twentieth century, the Tasmanian Tiger was rare in the wild, and the last thylacine in captivity died in a Hobart zoo in 1936. Although sightings were regularly reported through the decades and even into the twenty-first century, the thylacine was declared extinct by the IUCN in 1982, and by the Tasmanian government in 1986, the year in which *Sing Fox to Me* is set. River became obsessed with the continued existence of the Tiger on their mountain, and by the time the twins arrive, Clancy is also tortured by the possibility of the thylacine's – and River's – endurance in the wilderness surrounding his home.

In contrast to the sliding, hierarchical scale of humanity/normalcy in *The Fifth Child*, most of the central characters in *Sing Fox to Me* have some sort of disability or difference: Samson has Down syndrome, and Jonah's oxygen at birth was limited; he does not have an explicit diagnosis in the narrative, but repeated reference is made to his small, thin body, and in Kanake's exegesis of an earlier version of the novel for her PhD, she explains that Jonah has 'significant issues to do with social development' (Kanake, 2014, 351). In the same commentary, she also suggests that Clancy has dementia (Kanake, 2014, 351), which in the published version of the novel might be interpreted from his confusion over past and present, and he also walks with a limp. River, as mentioned above, experiences some degree of cognitive disturbance, and Mattie – daughter of Murray and Tilda – is deaf, and she uses sign language (as does Samson, although he is hearing and he also uses spoken language as well). Moreover, there is a veritable bestiary of non-human animals, and human-animal comparisons woven through the narrative; more than can be done justice in the scope of this chapter, but it should be noted here that non-human animals with disabilities also feature prominently: Queenie, Clancy's dog, is elderly and has physical limitations due to her age, and King, Murray's tame kookaburra, cannot fly.

Samson's narrative perspective is self-conscious and sensitive, as are his connections to non-human animals; on travelling to the mountain for the first time, he remembers an incident at their house in Queensland, where an amphibian is uncovered in the garden. Although Samson quietly identifies the creature as a 'burrowing frog' based on his memory of a poster he has seen at school (Kanake, 2016, 297), the rest of his family persist in referring to it as a 'toad', and David unceremoniously kills the frog by running it through the head with a shovel. Samson reflects: 'If they could have, his parents would have run his extra chromosome through as well' (Kanake, 2016, 297). Back in the present moment, when the family arrive at Clancy's house, David instructs Samson to '[u]se full sentences, and keep your tongue inside your mouth' (Kanake, 2016, 340): 'Samson thought of the burrowing frog shattering into bloody lumps beneath the shovel-head. He bit his tongue again, only this time on purpose' (Kanake, 2016, 343). At times when Samson contemplates his difference to his peers, the 'toad' metaphor returns, embodying 'the extra chromosome' (Kanake, 2016, 3049). The toad is figured as undesirable – comparable to Down syndrome in an ableist society – but crucially, this is founded on a misrecognition, for Samson's own knowledge of wildlife is ignored by the shared perception of the rest of his immediate family, which is motivated by fear, loathing, and disgust. In the context of Australia, toads deemed as disposable pests might be related to the case of the cane toad, an imported species in the twentieth century, another consequence of centuries of Western colonialism that has destabilized the indigenous ecosystem.[7] Samson's claiming of his additional chromosome as animal in this context serves to expose the inextricable connections between human and non-human animals in the history of colonial exploitations, but also how fearful assumptions about all who are devalued by normative society construct misunderstanding and prejudice.

---

7 The cane toad was introduced to Queensland, Australia, in 1935 as an import from South America to protect sugar cane crops. For further information, see White, Russo, and Shine (2018).

The fatal consequences of colonial misunderstanding and prejudice are writ large across the story of the Tasmanian Tiger; when British colonialists claimed the island as territory in the early nineteenth century, the thylacine was swiftly identified as a menace to livestock and thousands had been killed for bounty as the century draws to a close. As David Owen has identified, fictions of the Tiger's ferocity abounded throughout this period,[8] but just as pertinent are white, Western accounts of the thylacine's 'low degree of intelligence', 'belonging to a race of natural born idiots' (cited in Jarvis, 2018). The colonial ideology that indigenous non-human animals are primitive, stupid, and dangerous offers a toxic reflection of the attitude towards the Aboriginal people of Tasmania as well. Lyndall Ryan identifies how the genocide of Tasmanian Aborigines by European colonialists was justified by white settlers claiming that 'the Aborigines themselves were responsible for their near demise by virtue of their "innate inferiority" and inability to "compete successfully with Europeans"' (Ryan, 2012, 216). Kanake herself terms the Australian setting of her novel as 'disabled', the bush is aligned with intellectual disability as an absolute 'Other' (Kanake, 2014, 343), and the metaphor of the lost tiger at the heart of the text is conscious of the consequences of the oppressive conflation of racism, ableism, and speciesism in colonial history.

Jonah, following River's footsteps, becomes obsessed with the tiger, namely the tiger skin that Clancy keeps locked away in River's bedroom. Jonah tries to befriend Queenie the dog and King the kookaburra, yet perceives himself to be rejected by both: he smothers King, enraged by what he interprets as the bird's mocking laughing at him (Kanake, 2016, 1484) and accidently impales Queenie when she lunges at him in the bush (Kanake, 2016, 2300). Jonah's adoption of the tiger skin is poignant in the sense that he believes he experiences interanimal connection; he longs for recognition from the tiger skin, gazing into its eyes and questioning: 'You like me the best […] don't you?' (Kanake, 2016, 2113). Jonah finally claims tiger – putting on the skin that seems uncannily to take him over, blurring their identities (it might be said that the tiger finally claims him) – and he escapes from Clancy's house and into the bush. He becomes a shadowy, symbolic figure, part-tiger, part-boy, still lurking around the outskirts of the mountain home at the novel's conclusion. Although the boundaries between human and non-human animal are transgressed by both River and Jonah, these claims of tiger are motivated by trauma. In River's case, the illness and death of her mother, but also the absence of her beloved Murray who their parents have decided to send away: towards the end of the novel, we learn that George was actually River's father and hence her burgeoning relationship with Murray would have been incestuous (Kanake, 2016, 2735). A further connection between River and Jonah is their killing of other, non-human animals: Clancy remembers how River would leave these corpses on their lawn (Kanake,

8 See Owen (2003) for a cultural history of the Tasmanian Tiger.

2016, 2933); and Jonah's killing of non-human animals even predates his time on the mountain, as Samson believes his brother is responsible for the death of fruit bats back at their home in Queensland (Kanake, 2016, 2372). It is possible to interpret such interspecies associations as reverting to the long-established conflation of cognitive difference and animality, yet surely it is significant that it is the *tiger* – shrouded as it is in colonial myth, terror, prejudice, and exploitation – that is their shared focus. The tiger skin is an artefact of colonial oppression of non-human animals, and their recognition/identification is a misrecognition: the tigers were never what their fevered, human-animal imaginings have conjured, and thus human appropriations of the tiger tend towards the destructive and predatory.

On the subject of mythical creatures, there is a delicious irony in the novel's non-human reimagining of one of the chief originators of so many aspects of the metanarrative of Down syndrome. In a family discussion about the origin of pejorative terms such as 'retard' and 'mong', David explains: '"Mongoloid came before Langdon Downs", [...] and Samson imagined two giants fighting like Godzilla and King Kong' (Kanake, 2016, 1212). In Samson's mind, the racism and ableism of 'Mongolian idiocy' takes on the characterizations of a non-human monster, but Langdon Down himself is conceptualized as the fictional monster-gorilla. Samson's imaginative connections thwart the binary system of speciesism, for both Godzilla and King Kong are monsters of *human* invention (not dissimilar to the fantasied monstrosity of the Tasmanian Tiger). Jonah is quick to remind Samson of Down syndrome's historic conflation with 'the Mongol hordes [...] they were bloodthirsty savages' (Kanake, 2016, 1212) but Samson's mother denies him immediate access to the 'Encyclopaedia Britannica', where he might find out more about this connection (Kanake, 2016, 1223).

Yet on the mountain, Samson's meeting with Murray and his learning about the Aboriginal Dreaming via the Rainbow Snake offers a more productive animal-mythic identification for Samson. After an argument with Mattie, Samson wishes 'he could change his chromosomes, fill in the lines on his palms and reshape his eyes' (Kanake, 2016, 2231), expressing a desire to rid himself of the physical signs of his Down syndrome, and he begins to imagine himself as becoming part of the Rainbow Snake. This vision returns when Samson sets off on his own search of the mountain to find Jonah, and imagines the Rainbow Snake inside of him, swallowing 'the toad', meaning that he 'wasn't disabled or handicapped or special anymore' (Kanake, 2016, 3060). I do not think this should be interpreted as the narrative attempting to get rid of, overcome, or compensate for Samson's Down syndrome, as Samson also acknowledges here that he 'had never really minded his outsides':

> The toad heard him, and Samson felt it move through the Rainbow Snake, and the Snake moved too. Slowly, it let go of them both, leaving Samson the same, but with enough rainbow left to decide how he felt

inside. This was his extra chromosome now. It was every colour and thin as mist.

(Kanake, 2016, 3060)

I argue that what changes is the connotations around Samson's claiming animal; the additional chromosome of Down syndrome is no longer a persecuted, misunderstood pest, but a powerful spirit-animal that predates colonial exploitation of indigenous human and non-human animals, and troubles the boundaries of colonizer/colonized, disabled/non-disabled, and human/animal. Samson's appropriation of the Rainbow Snake could be considered a cultural appropriation, to some degree, and yet the novel's exposition of the tangled histories of racist science, speciesism, and ableism is always attuned to differences and inequalities, and the profound points of connection between how indigenous humans, non-human animals, and people with disabilities have been maligned. In the quotation above, the authority of the reference textbook (symbolically named after the home of the British Empire) is discarded, and the experiential, alternative knowledge of the Tasmanian Aborigines is privileged. The promise of *Sing Fox to Me* is the imaginative potential of how interconnectedness between people with Down syndrome and animals might be reappropriated.

Concluding discussion

This chapter considers a range of non-human animals in its exploration of the metanarrative of Down syndrome as proximity to animality; I try to move beyond a focus on 'higher' non-human animals, even as I recognize that the hierarchical ordering of humans and non-human animals tended towards comparisons with apes, monkeys, intellectual disability, and 'savage races'. My discussion of Lessing's and Kanake's engagements with the Down syndrome-animality metanarrative seeks to identify the ideological pitfalls – and potentials – of such comparisons. However, I confine my analysis to fictional representations of both Down syndrome and non-human animals; I do not wish to wade in on the merits of the 'Endangered Syndrome' campaign, and would rather have commentators with Down syndrome such as Francie Munoz and Dylan Harman continue that particular debate.

Is fiction a safer space to imagine the progressive possibility of such claims for both people with intellectual disabilities and non-human animals, rather than in the material conditions and oppressions of lived experience, of the normative social order? Again, I am probably not the person to answer this question, and Elizabeth Davies is not around to be part of this ongoing conversation. Nevertheless, her tales of Georgina and Super-Dog's interspecies connection have now reached an audience beyond our childhood bedroom; this narrative does not dismantle the assumed authority of that school textbook, but it offers an alternative story.

References

Barr, S. (2018) Campaign Comparing People with Down's Syndrome to Endangered Animals Sparks Controversy. [online]. *The Independent*. 9 November. Available from: https://www.independent.co.uk/life-style/downs-syndrome-endangered-animals-campaign-controversy-canada-a8626581.html [accessed 31 August 2020].

Bérubé, M. (2010) 'Equality, freedom, and/or justice for all: A response to Martha Nussbaum', in E. F. Kittay and L. Carlson (eds.) *Cognitive Disability and Its Challenge to Moral Philosophy*, Oxford: Wiley-Blackwell.

Brown, D. (2018) Woman Speaks Out against Campaign Comparing People with Down Syndrome to Animals. [online]. *CBC*. 7 November. Available from: https://www.cbc.ca/news/canada/toronto/campaign-down-syndrome-endangered-list-1.4896518 [accessed 5 February 2021].

Canadian Down Syndrome Society (2018) Endangered Syndrome. [online]. Available from: https://www.endangeredsyndrome.com/ [accessed 31 August 2020].

Carlson, L. (2010) *The Faces of Intellectual Disability: Philosophical Reflections*, Bloomington and Indianapolis: Indiana University Press.

Crookshank, F. G. (1931) *The Mongol in Our Midst: A Study of Man and His Three Faces*, 3rd edition, London: Kegan Paul, Trench, Trubner and Co Ltd.

Crome, L. and Stern, J. (1972) *Pathology of Mental Retardation*, 2nd edition, Edinburgh and London: Churchill Livingstone.

Darwin, C. (1871) *The Descent of Man*, New York: A. L. Burt.

Gelb, S. A. (2008) Darwin's use of intellectual disability in the descent of man, *Disability Studies Quarterly Spring* 28 (2) [online].

Haraway, D. J. (2008) *When Species Meet*, London and Minneapolis: University of Minnesota Press.

Ireland, W. W. (1877) *On Idiocy and Imbecility*, London: J and A Churchill.

Jarvis, B. (2018) The Obsessive Search for The Tasmanian Tiger. [online]. *New Yorker*. 2 July. Available from: https://www.newyorker.com/magazine/2018/07/02/the-obsessive-search-for-the-tasmanian-tiger [accessed 31 August 2020].

Kanake, S. (2019) 'The down syndrome novel: A microcosm for inclusion or parental trauma narrative', in B. Hadley and D. McDonald (eds.) *The Routledge Handbook of Disability Arts, Culture, and Media*, Oxon: Routledge.

Kanake, S. (2016) *Sing Fox to Me*, Victoria: Affirm Press.

Kanake, S. (2014) Sing Fox to Me: An Investigation into the "Use" of Down Syndrome in both the Down Syndrome and Gothic Novel. PhD Thesis. Queensland University of Technology, Brisbane, Queensland, Australia.

Kaposy, C. (2018) *Choosing Down Syndrome: Ethics and New Prenatal Testing Technologies*, Cambridge and London: MIT Press.

Keevak, M. (2011) *Becoming Yellow: A Short History of Racial Thinking*, Princeton and Oxford: Princeton University Press.

Kittay, E. F. (2010) 'The personal is philosophical is political: A philosopher and mother of a cognitively disabled person sends notes from the battlefield', in E. F. Kittay and L. Carlson (eds.) *Cognitive Disability and Its Challenge to Moral Philosophy*, Oxford: Wiley-Blackwell.

Kuhse, H. and Singer, P. (1985) *Should The Baby Live? The Problem of Handicapped Infants*, Oxford: Oxford University Press.

Langdon Down, J. (1866) 'Observations on an ethnic classification of idiots', in Clincial Lecture Reports, London Hospital, 3: 259–262.

Langdon Down, J. (1887) *On Some of the Mental Affections of Childhood and Youth*, London: J. and A. Churchill.

Lessing, D. (1988) *The Fifth Child*, London: Jonathan Cape.

McBride Johnson, H. (2003) Unspeakable Conversations. [online]. *The New York Times Magazine*. 16 February. Available from: https://www.nytimes.com/2003/02/16/magazine/unspeakable-conversations.html [accessed 31 August 2020].

McDonagh, P. (2008) *Idiocy: A Cultural History*, Liverpool: Liverpool University Press.

Merton, T. A. (1968) *Mankind in the Unmaking: The Anthropology of Mongolism*, Sydney: Bloxham and Chambers.

Minich, J. A. (2016) Enabling whom? Critical disability studies now. *Lateral*, 5 (1). Available from: http://csalateral.org/issue/5-1/forum-alt-humanities-critical-disability-studies-now-minich/ [accessed 6 September 2020].

Owen, D. (2003) *The Tasmanian Tiger: The Tragic Tale of How the World Lost its Most Mysterious Predator*, Baltimore: Johns Hopkins University Press.

Perry, D. M. (2018) People with Down Syndrome are not Endangered Animals. [online]. *Pacific Standard*. 16 November. Available from: https://psmag.com/education/people-with-down-syndrome-arent-endangered-animals [accessed 31 August 2020].

Ryan, L. (2012) *Tasmanian Aborigines: A History Since 1803*, Sydney: Allen and Unwin.

Shuttleworth, G. E., and Potts, W. A. (1910) *Mentally Deficient Children: Their Treatment and Training*, 3rd edition, London: H. K. Lewis.

Singer, P. (2015) *Animal Liberation*, 3rd edition, London: Bodley Head.

Singer, P. (1994) *Rethinking Life and Death: The Collapse of Our Traditional Values*, New York: St. Martin's Griffin.

Singer, P. (2010) 'Speciesism and moral status', in E. F. Kittay and L. Carlson (eds.) *Cognitive Disability and Its Challenge to Moral Philosophy*, Oxford: Wiley-Blackwell.

Smith, K. (2011) *The Politics of Down Syndrome*, Alresford, Hants: Zero Books.

Snyder, S. L. and Mitchell, D.T. (2006) *Cultural Locations of Disability*, Chicago and London: University of Chicago Press.

Stechyson, N. (2018) People with Down Syndrome are an "Endangered Species", Says Advocacy Group. [online]. *Huffpost*. 11 November. Available from: https://www.huffingtonpost.ca/2018/11/06/down-syndrome-endangered-species_a_23581477/?guccounter=1&guce_referrer=aHR0cHM6Ly93d3cuZ29vZ2xlLmNvbS88&guce_referrer_sig=AQAAAFjWczg5mJ3fNFLBEsFl8_XXaGPqCVQjW9jgxS5xDHvMUP9fX5oK_E0uLteuw2Rfnq48Abeba0ZnufsgO9nHVF9ivWVDGSkx3NdDj2LkSVY4aCYjKyqDt_l9IIwbQExItzpMm0w2dYo_Ph4y6QDKQ94CIpm8kvvWK1IcymvZdlV6 [accessed 31 August 2020].

Taylor, S. (2017) *Beasts of Burden: Animal and Disability Liberation*, London and New York: New Press.

Tredgold, A. F. (1920) *Mental Deficiency: Amentia*, 3rd edition, New York: William Wood and Company.

Wanshel, E. (2018) Controversial Campaign Calls People with Down Syndrome "Endangered Species". [online]. *Huffpost*. 10 November. Available from: https://www.huffingtonpost.co.uk/entry/down-syndrome-endangered-species-canada_n_5be5c35ee4b0769d24ccd03a?ri18n=true&guccounter=1&guce_referrer=aHR0cHM6Ly9jb25zZW50LnnlhaG9vLmNvbS88&guce_referrer_sig=AQAAADMi8Sn1L-IM2Uf3HyUjAudxajMV5OzsNEE9lhaTnNnlKoBE8ACi3VzrP7Um3AoXlfDRp1n5L7ntb37oO6Ft8DsfnbjXq1tfYTbuQ8d1SN4KTyGQzALY3uSAqqesNk9H7qCFCeP4YJ5geIDS5Yq57kJqsTVqkmbBK6C6OZqG92O9 [accessed 31 August 2020].

White, P., Russon, A., and Shine, R. (2018) We've cracked the Cane Toad genome, and that could help put the brakes on its invasion. [online]. *The Conversation.* 19 September. Available from: https://theconversation.com/weve-cracked-the-cane-toad-genome-and-that-could-help-put-the-brakes-on-its-invasion-103362 [accessed 31 August 2020].

Wright, D. (2011) *Downs: The History of a Disability,* Oxford: Oxford University Press.

9

THE METANARRATIVE OF DWARFISM

Heightism and Its Social Implications

Erin Pritchard

Preliminary Discussion

It is my contention that probably no other minority group's identity has been influenced more by cultural representations than dwarfism. Dwarfism is 'not just a physical condition; it is a social and cultural metaphor' (Massie and Mayer, 2014, 55). There are numerous stereotypes and tropes associated with people with dwarfism, which are constructed by heightism within, for example, the media. Heightism is defined as 'unfair treatment based on height, *especially*: prejudice or discrimination against short people' (Merriam-Webster, 2020). Heightism is evident in prejudiced behaviour, cultural representations, and attitudes towards people with dwarfism. According to the metanarrative identified and explored in this chapter, heightism results in people with dwarfism being thought humorous, child-like, and asexual.

As a woman with dwarfism, I am aware of the social implications of the metanarrative. Growing up, I was exposed to various images of dwarfism, including films such as *Snow White and the Seven Dwarfs* (1937) and *Charlie and the Chocolate Factory* (1971). Dwarfs were never shown as fully human or as people experiencing the disabling realities of dwarfism. Although I shared the same impairment as the dwarf characters, I could not relate to them, but I knew that my body was similar to theirs, and that was how people saw me. I felt uncomfortable because their impairment was exposed as different, something to be stared at, or laughed at, and I did not want this to be what represented me; yet it did and continues to do so. I am often called names relating to these characters, which demonstrates a clear social association that affects my psycho-emotional well-being. Using these experiences to exemplify the implications of the metanarrative of dwarfism is my response to the volume's critical concept of assumed authority. In other words, this chapter's critique aids in challenging the metanarrative of dwarfism in order to create space for a better social identity.

The first part of the chapter focuses on methodology. I explore the benefits of using an autoethnographic approach, of drawing on my own experiences as a woman with dwarfism to demonstrate how the metanarrative of dwarfism shapes social encounters. Autoethnography, according to Richards (2008), is important in research that aims to reconstitute identity. Dwarfism is just one part of my identity, but to many people it is my *only* identity, and their view of it is often misconstrued by the related metanarrative. I explore the importance of using my experiences to provide a valid account of such impact on society.

The chapter is then divided into three analytical discussions, each focusing on a different strand of the metanarrative, the first of which is the terminology associated with dwarfism. I explore the use of heightist terminology employed by normates (Garland-Thomson, 1997) when writing about people with dwarfism. I demonstrate how terms used in the media such as *big* and *tall* subconsciously reinforce dwarfism as inferior. Ironically, these terms are often used when someone is trying to write positively; however, due to heightist attitudes, they only serve to keep people with dwarfism in a subordinate place within society. Finally, the discussion demonstrates how the media actively uses terms associated with smallness when writing negative stories featuring people with dwarfism.

In the second analytical discussion, I focus on one of the most well-known stereotypes associated with dwarfism, which is humour. I use the character Mini-me, featured in two of the Austin Power's films, to demonstrate how dwarf characters are often used as comedic fodder. The discussion shows how the entertainment industry has a strong influence on the ways people with dwarfism are constructed and subsequently perceived within society. My identity is misinformed by these misrepresentations of dwarfism, often leading me to be treated accordingly: to be ridiculed and mocked. While the entertainment industry is responsible for these representations, I draw on *Maybe the Moon* and a scene in the 2003 film *Elf* to demonstrate how culture also exposes the entertaining stereotype of dwarfism and its social implications.

The last analytical discussion focuses on sexuality and how it is constructed within *Maybe the Moon* and *Mendal's Dwarf.* Using the critical concept of the unforbidden relationship (Bolt, 2019), this discussion explores how the representations both focus on intimacy between people with dwarfism and their average-sized partners, and the sociocultural attitudes that construct dwarfism as asexual. I argue that such asexuality resonates with the way people with dwarfism are deemed subhuman. I also draw on sociocultural attitudes within the media towards dwarfism and sexuality before sharing some of my own experiences to demonstrate how this strand of the metanarrative plays out.

Methodological Discussion

My interest in the metanarrative of dwarfism is influenced by my own experiences as a person with dwarfism. As a result, I have chosen to use autoethnography as a way to explore the social implications of the metanarrative. This method 'allows researchers to draw on their own experiences to understand a particular phenomenon or culture' (Mendez, 2013, 280). In this chapter, I challenge dominant heightist assumptions replicated within the strands of the metanarrative of dwarfism. However, by drawing on some of my experiences I also demonstrate how I am able to relate to some of the representations that challenge the metanarrative.

Autoethnography allows me to demonstrate how the metanarrative of dwarfism constructs the social experiences of a person with dwarfism without involving participants. This approach is beneficial because people with dwarfism can be considered an over-researched group. While I do not mean this in an academic sense, people with dwarfism are often approached by various media sources wanting to know their experiences of living with dwarfism, often for voyeuristic purposes. Richards (2008, 1720) suggests 'one way of resisting objectification by others is by writing about oneself'. Sharing my social experiences of the metanarrative of dwarfism aids in providing a first-hand account, which I interpret as a person with dwarfism and thus challenge how others construct me.

It has long since been argued that disability research is often conducted by non-disabled academics and thus fails to represent disabled people's lived experiences (Kitchin, 2000). While I do not completely agree with this contention, as non-disabled academics can be useful allies, from experience I am aware that too often disabled people's voices are silenced by the majority of non-disabled people, including professionals. The majority of academic work on dwarfism has been written by average-sized people.[1] These pieces of valuable academic work are written *about* as opposed to *by* people with dwarfism, which can subtly change their meaning. Research carried out by non-disabled researchers can be hampered by subtle forms of cultural ableism (Svendby et al., 2018). For example, Kruse (2002) recognizes that as a six-foot man he relies on his participants with dwarfism to share their experiences; thus, the reader is dependent on Kruse's interpretation of them. In some papers (e.g. Ablon, 1990; Kruse, 2002), dwarfism is argued to be more of a difference than a disability. I disagree as I have encountered numerous disabling experiences related to my dwarfism, whether we take the medical or social model approach to it. As Richards (2008, 1717) points out, 'an expert on the lived experiences of disability is the person experiencing it'. Outsiders can only ever be onlookers, so they never truly know what it is like to be a person with dwarfism, subjected to the psycho-emotional impact of the metanarrative.

---

1 There is the exception of the report about the medical and society experiences of people with dwarfism led by Tom Shakespeare, as a well-known academic with dwarfism, and co-written with two average-sized academics.

As a disabled academic, I feel empowered to be able to work in disability studies; I am given a platform to raise awareness, often by utilizing my own experiences. Autoethnography is a form of emancipatory research, which gives voice and improves a person's position within society (Richards, 2008). Using my voice I empower myself by challenging dominant assumptions, constructed by the metanarrative, which I experience on a daily basis.

As research within disability studies favours research carried out *by* and *with* disabled people, research that also reflects on the disabled researcher's own experiences should be equally valid. The use of 'autoethnography allows personal experiences to become valid data' (Smith, 2005, cited in Taber, 2010, 13). Autoethnography is beneficial in providing a voice for disabled people but also, more specifically here, to disabled academics. Williams and Marvin (2015) point out that non-disabled academics have the advantage of working in institutions that are designed for them. However, an advantage that autoethnography provides to disabled academics is the ability to use their own experiences as a form of research, which aids in levelling the playing field.

Analytical Discussion 1

Bigger Is Better

The terms we use are important in constructing how we identify somebody and their place within society: 'Language matters for our understanding of disability because it is through the words we use that our expectations and assumptions are shaped. These, in turn, impact upon the extent to which people are valued' (Mallett and Slater, 2014, 91). The words used in the media are part of the metanarrative of dwarfism. While disability hate speech is recognized as language which is degrading, harassing, or stigmatizing, which affects disabled people's dignity, reputation, and status within society (Sherry et al., 2020), the subtler everyday forms have been given limited recognition. Language has the power to define cultural groups (Haller et al., 2006) and it can be argued that the subtler forms, including those within the media, provide the foundations for ensuring people with dwarfism remain within an inferior position in society.

Before I examine the terms used in the media, I explore the various terms used to denote the condition that is commonly referred to as dwarfism. There are numerous terms used to refer to a person with dwarfism, including but not limited to *dwarf, person with dwarfism, little person, person of small stature*, and *person with restricted growth*. It is important to think deeply about which term is most appropriate to use as some are loaded with problematic connotations, such as the mythic, or they construct people with dwarfism as child-like. For example, *little person* is a term favoured in North America; however, it is also a term used to refer to children and thus can be considered infantilizing. I remember looking for a greeting card for my friend who had just had her first child, and came across a card saying, 'Congratulations on your brand-new *little person*'. While there was no offence intended, the card aided in reinforcing the connection between dwarfism and immaturity. People with dwarfism are already infantilized, due to their small stature, so to connect them further to children through the choice of the name given to their impairment only reinforces this form of representation.

It must be pointed out, however, that the term *dwarf* is disliked by some people with dwarfism due to its mythical connections and because of slurs such as 'poison dwarf' – a term used to describe an unpleasant person. Osensky (2018) points out that words used to describe taller people are much more flattering than words used to describe smaller people. Thus, the reason why there are numerous terms used to describe someone with dwarfism and the contention behind them may not be so much to do with cultural differences, but rather that it is impossible to agree on a positive term when those associated with shortness are always negative.

The various terms used to denote smallness are often associated with inferiority. The language we use is 'institutionally ableist' (Bolt, 2014, 16), or more precisely, in relation to dwarfism, *heightist*. Osensky (2018) points out that idioms associated with size mostly convey the message that 'bigger is better'. Idioms associated with smallness are often used to denote bad traits. These include but are not limited to *small minded* (i.e. narrow minded), *small fry* (i.e. unimportant), and *short changed* (i.e. to be conned). However, words associated with being big and tall denote goodness, such as *big hearted* (i.e. kind and generous) and *walking tall* (i.e. showing pride in oneself). In various human interest stories about people with dwarfism, particularly those which are laden with inspiration porn, in magazines and newspapers, an obvious binary is exposed that constructs tall as good and small as bad. Ironically, articles aiming to promote a positive perception of dwarfism do the exact opposite when they use phrases such as *walking tall* and *big hearted* to celebrate the achievements of someone with dwarfism. These only emphasize the normate writers' underlying heightism. For example, I put the terms *walking tall* and *dwarf* into Google and was instantly presented with an article 'Rico walking tall after Dwarf Sports Association Games success' (Palmer, 2019). The article is about a young boy with dwarfism succeeding in sports, something which of course should be celebrated, but in a way that does not undermine his dwarfism. The use of the phrase *walking tall* reinforces subliminal messages that smallness is bad and that, to be good and admired, Rico must overcome his dwarfism through being metaphorically recognized as tall. Of course, no matter how good Rico is at sports, he will never be tall; however, his admirable achievement must be celebrated with compliments that construct him as tall and thus superior. These articles expose everyday heightism in society, as the phrase *walking small*, although more accurate, would not be as complementary. Osensky (2018) points out that we always 'look up to someone', but never want to 'stoop to their level'. It is almost as if the average-sized writer is accepting us into their world. We have passed the challenge, proved ourselves worthy, and can now enter their average-sized kingdom and be admired as 'honorary' tall people.

When there is an article that is about a person with dwarfism doing something socially unacceptable, however, such as committing a crime, idioms associated with smallness are used repeatedly, which reinforces the belief that small is bad. For example, in an article about a man with dwarfism being arrested for breaking and entering, it was reported that he went on a 'mini crimewave'; that he was a 'mini blighter' and a 'diminutive criminal' (Tozer, 2008). The constant use of these synonyms reinforce the novelty factor of his height and are used in a mocking way. Mockery towards dwarfism is another strand of the metanarrative associated with humour and aids in placing people with dwarfism in an inferior social position.

Analytical Discussion 2

A Little Childish Humour

When thinking about a person with dwarfism, the first point of reference is often an entertaining character, perhaps someone seen in a film or storybook. There is a cultural fascination (Shakespeare et al., 2010), where people with dwarfism are often used as comedic fodder within films and television shows, as well as humorous oddities that can be hired out for celebratory events. People with dwarfism are rarely seen in society,[2] but they are prominent within the entertainment industry. This imbalance gives the entertainment industry more control over how people with dwarfism are represented and subsequently perceived within society. Representations of dwarfism are constructed by the average-sized person; however, it is dwarf entertainers, through their consent to perform, who aid in keeping the heightist metanarrative alive.

An unfortunately well-known film character with dwarfism is Mini-me, who was played by the late Verne Troyer. Automatically the name *Mini-me* focuses on the characters short stature. Reductive labels are often used to denote disabled characters and frame their impairments as their key characteristic (Garland-Thomson, 1997; Bolt, 2014). Mini-me features in the films *Austin Powers the Spy Who Shagged Me* (1999) and *Austin Powers in Goldmember* (2002). These are popular action spy comedies, spoofs of the iconic James Bond films. Mini-me is first introduced as a clone of Austin Powers's arch-nemesis, Dr Evil. He is described as an exact clone of Dr Evil, but one-eighth his size. Along with his name, the description of him automatically places emphasis upon his short stature.

Being Dr Evil's clone reflects historical perceptions of dwarfs, where they often played diminutive mimics of average-sized characters (Adelson, 2005). This mimicking suggests that dwarfs have limited personality traits. He is not his

---

2 Dwarfism is considered a rare impairment. There are approximately 250,000 people with Achondroplasia, the most common form of dwarfism, worldwide (Horton et al., 2007).

own person but instead provides the comic fodder that would not be expected from the average-sized Dr Evil. Mini-Me has been described as 'a thirty-two inch dwarf who bites and generally terrorises the staff at World domination headquarters … this is a movie in which a midget [*sic*] bites the star in the crotch and then gets picked up, swung around, and bashed into a pole … the different parts of a messy comedy have to be good' (Denby, 1999, cited in Adelson, 2005, para. 41). Throughout the two films, Mini-me (or more specifically his height) is used for comedic purposes. Being picked up and swung around relates to derogatory entertainment, such as dwarf tossing.

Dr Evil's relationship with Mini-me sometimes mimics those between royalty and court dwarfs, where the latter were often kept as pets or playthings. For example, Mini-me is kept on a leash like a dog and his height is associated with immaturity to provoke humour. Disability infantilization, as identified by Bolt (2014), is a stereotype often associated with dwarfism. The use of infantilization creates an incongruous encounter. Although Mini-me is short in stature, he is still an adult, yet Dr Evil constantly infantilizes him, which is evident when he talks to him in a baby voice and in one scene carries him in a papoose. In another scene, Mini-me is dressed up as a baby and is pushed around in a pram. When I went to the cinema to see *Austin Powers: The Spy Who Shagged Me*, I noticed that the preteen next to me was cooing at Mini-me, a character played by an actor who was obviously old enough to be her father. However, his short stature, lack of voice, and dependency on Dr Evil aided in constructing him as child-like. People with dwarfism are often infantilized, which renders them inferior within society as immaturity is often associated with powerlessness.

The association between height and humour has problematic implications for how people with dwarfism are perceived and treated. I am assumed not only to be an entertainer but also to be a figure of fun whom it is acceptable to mock (like a typical dwarf entertainer). This mockery is a heightist trap that keeps people with dwarfism in an inferior place within society. If I do not play along, I challenge the stereotypical perception of a dwarf, which results in me being labelled an 'angry dwarf'. However, I am just a person who, like anyone else, does not enjoy being mocked by others.

To counteract the humorous stereotype, it is important to explore how culture can also expose and challenge this strand of the metanarrative. In Maupin's novel *Maybe the Moon* (1992), the protagonist Cadence Roth shares her life via a series of diary entries, as a struggling actress with dwarfism. Amstead Maupin focuses on realistic portrayals of marginal characters, including dwarfs (Gaustad, 2010). Numerous parts of the story allow it to seem semi-autobiographical for anyone with dwarfism, such as the representation of being a spectacle, being bullied by strangers, being seen as asexual, and the numerous physical barriers encountered. Ironically, the one part where the majority will not find it semi-autobiographical is Cadence's employment within the entertainment industry.

The key part of Maupin's story is that Cadence works in the entertainment industry and makes constant references to her previous work, where she fulfilled the role of an Elf. *Maybe the Moon* shows how the entertainment industry capitalizes on height (i.e. impairment) for use in prosthetics. Again, the height of people with dwarfism is their only reason for being part of the show. What is interesting is that Maupin demonstrates that there is more to Cadence than just filling a prosthetic suit. Maupin entwines his novels within a larger societal framework (Gaustad, 2010). Based on the metanarrative it is easy to assume that all people with dwarfism depend on the entertainment industry as a form of employment. There are multiple contributing factors to this heightism. Because dwarfism is a rare impairment, but prominent within the entertainment industry, it creates a false impression that all people with dwarfism must work in that field (i.e. the only place we are seen). People with dwarfism are not common enough to be seen working in everyday occupations, such as teaching, but the media provides a large platform that exposes those who do work in the entertainment industry. A personal example of related assumed authority was when I was about seven years old and my mother was asked by a doctor if I had ever thought about joining the circus.

There are, of course, occupations that are off limits to people with dwarfism, which applies to most people with physical impairments, yet it is not assumed that, for instance, wheelchair users must rent themselves out in order to make a living. For example, when a casting company decided to use average-sized actors for the roles of the dwarfs in a pantomime production of *Snow White and the Seven Dwarfs*, Peter Burrows, who co-owns Willow management dwarf acting agency, complained that it puts people with dwarfism out of work (Khan, 2016). This implies that people with dwarfism rely on the entertainment industry; put another way, though, it is Peter Burrows who relies on people with dwarfism to work in that industry in order to run his company and make a living.

In *Maybe the Moon*, Cadence strives to be an actress but, as a dwarf, is only offered roles such as props or a children's entertainer. After being dropped by her agent, she begins working for an entertainment company that specializes in children's parties. It is no surprise that the children want the dwarf, as Cadence points out: 'I'm a novelty, so it's easy enough to imagine the scenario: "Can I, Mommy, please, please? Zachary had the midget lady for his birthday"' (Maupin, 1992, 84). The book demonstrates that dwarf entertainers are wanted only for the novelty factor of their height, as opposed to any talents they may possess. The choice of the term *midget* also reinforces the novelty factor, given its origins within the freak show. This part of the book struck a chord with reality for me, as I can recall an interaction with a mother who approached me when I was out shopping, asking me to come to her daughter's birthday party dressed as Hello Kitty. She enthusiastically told me how I would make a better Hello Kitty than a regular entertainer as her daughter did not like the 'big one'. My stature would thus be beneficial for providing a small Hello Kitty, probably a truer-to-form replica of the Japanese cartoon character. I do not work in the entertainment industry, but the mother assumed that I did because I am a dwarf. She even went on to tell me how her daughter found people like me (i.e. dwarfs) hilarious. This was because the only exposure her daughter had had to people with dwarfism was within the media. This example of assumed authority demonstrates why it is problematic to expose particular tropes of the metanarrative of dwarfism to children, as it shapes their reality and how they respond to people with dwarfism: 'they learn about disabled people through books, films and legends' (Shakespeare, 1994, 2). A person with dwarfism is easily recognizable, and if a child has no point of reference outside the metanarrative, then that perception is likely to influence new understandings of society.

An example of cinematic representation that challenges the humorous stereotype of dwarfism, however, is the 2003 Christmas film, *Elf*. Instead of playing one of Santa's elves, the film casts an actor with dwarfism in a different role. Peter Dinklage plays the bestselling children's author Miles Flinch, who also happens to have dwarfism. His character is revered and somewhat feared due to his high-powered position. In one scene, he is in a boardroom meeting that is interrupted by Buddy the Elf, played by the average-sized actor Will Farrell. It is Buddy's naivety and child-like persona that allows him innocently to confuse Miles for a real-life Elf, which Miles mistakes for mockery. What is interesting is that the average-sized person is constructed as child-like as opposed to the person with dwarfism. As a woman with dwarfism, I found this to be a relatable scene as I am used to people comparing me with mythical creatures, such as elves, for comic effect. For example, around Christmas time people sometimes shout across the street that they have seen a 'real-life Elf' in order to generate laughs from their friends. This is another form of assumed authority, which demonstrates how the construction of dwarfism as a subhuman figure of fun, which is often infantilized, influences notions of asexuality.

Analytical Discussion 3

(A)sexual Little Thing

People with dwarfism are often deemed asexual, oversexed, or seen as a fetish. In relation to the construction of asexuality, any relationship between a person with dwarfism and an average-sized person is considered a 'forbidden relationship' as it crosses the normative divide (Bolt, 2019). In relation to heightism, the notion of the forbidden relationship and dwarfism can be thought of as the intention to prevent the small body from reproducing. This discussion unpacks the forbidden relationship within *Mendal's Dwarf* and *Maybe the Moon*, demonstrating that it is not a biological cause, but rather sociocultural factors, influenced by heightist assumptions. I demonstrate how in both novels attitudes from average-sized people create the unforbidden relationship, which I further exemplify through drawing on my own experiences, as well as attitudes expressed within the media.

Mendal's Dwarf, by Simon Mawer, is a story based on Benedict Lambert, or Ben, a geneticist with dwarfism. Benedict is the great-great-great nephew of Gregor Mendal, a Monk who did genetic experiments on plants, which led to the Nazi's concept of eugenics. Tomoiaga (2011) suggests that both characters are situated on the margins of society due to their social and physical conditions. The novel adopts a personal tragedy point of view of disability, as Benedict dedicates his work to looking for a cure for his condition. However, his longing for a relationship with Ms Jean Pricey is thematic throughout the book.

While Jean falls in love with Ben, she cannot cope with marrying him or having his child, which emphasizes the forbidden relationship. Tomoiaga (2011: 255) points out that Ben experiences a 'long period of rejection on the part of women, who cannot see themselves involved with him, even though he is intelligent, and funny, and full of sexual energy'. Instead, Jean forms a relationship with an average-sized man. This exposes Kaplan's (2017, 6) suggestion that disabled men are commonly judged as sexual non-contenders as they do not fulfil traditional male gendered roles, which mandates physical strength. *Mendel's Dwarf* exposes how Ben is perceived as undateable due to his dwarfism:

> 'I'm in love with you', I told her. I was looking at her knees. I know a great deal about knees, the peculiar form of then, the awkwardness, the plain ungainliness of them. But these knees were slender and elegant, the delicate contour of each patella like a nacreous burial mound of all my hopes.
> 'I knew you'd do this', she said quietly.
> 'What do you mean?'
> She was almost in tears. 'Can't you see it's impossible?'
> 'Of course it's impossible', I retorted. 'It's the impossible that attracts me. When you're like I am, who gives a toss about the possible? You are the most beautiful girl I've ever known – correction: the most beautiful woman I've ever *seen*, which includes every edition of *Penthouse* over the last ten years – and I want you to be in love with me too'.
> 'But I *can't* be'.
> 'I'll say it for you: you can't love me because I'm hideous and deformed, a freak of nature, and people would stare. Very well, love me in private. I won't push it. I don't get many moments like this and I'm playing off the cuff, but I'll offer you this: nothing at all. No obligations, no commitments, nothing. I just want to hear you admit it. You love me'.
> 'This is bloody ridiculous'.
> 'Don't use that kind of language. It doesn't go with the English-rose look. I'll make one concession. You can say this: "I *would* love you if you weren't a shrunken monster"'.
>
> *(Mawer, 1997, 55)*

Emphasis is placed upon Ben's line of vision, which reminds readers of his short stature, the cause of the forbidden relationship. Jean is the English rose, while

Ben is the 'shrunken monster'. A binary is created, similar to beauty and the beast. Ben is rejected due to heightism, which is constructed by sociocultural notions of dwarfism that reinforce the notion of the forbidden relationship. Jean is in love with Ben but rejects him because of his dwarfism. Ben is fully aware of this fact and the behaviour in society that their relationship would produce, such as staring. It is not unusual for people with dwarfism to be stared at anyway, but when holding hands with a person much taller, the incongruous sight encourages even more of this behaviour. Accordingly, Jean ends up in a relationship with an abusive partner, which is deemed more acceptable within society than dating a person with dwarfism.

Maybe the Moon exposes the sociocultural attitudes surrounding people with dwarfism who form intimate relationships with average-sized people. Cadence forms a relationship with an average-sized man, which challenges the notion that people with dwarfism only date each other. What is most interesting is how Maupin exposes the average-sized person's prejudice towards dwarfism and sexuality. This takes place towards the end of the book when Cadence's diary is offered to a screenwriter:

> How wed are we to Cady's romantic life? The sex scenes made me extremely uncomfortable, and I can assure you I won't be the only woman who'll feel that way... the central romantic relationship would be between Renee and Neil ... I would find it far more intriguing if Cady were acting as a sort of witty mediator between the full-sized lovers. We don't want to know who she fucks. We really don't.
>
> *(Maupin, 1992, 330)*

The screenwriter's reply demonstrates that she cannot accept the notion that people with dwarfism can date average-sized people, which she finds grotesque. This representation resonates with social attitudes towards dwarfism and dating. I once overheard a co-worker at a call centre asking someone if it was weird to fancy a dwarf (not me, but the actor Peter Dinklage). *Maybe the Moon* exposes not only that people with dwarfism can actually date average-sized people, but also the resulting heightist attitudes of other people. Bonnie (2004, 125) states that 'society at best finds the thought of a disabled person being sexual repulsive and at worst presumes we are asexual'. That is why it is deemed more appropriate to focus on the relationship between two average-sized people (i.e. Renee and Neil) and leave Cadence as the 'witty mediator', which subtly exposes the normate's conception of people with dwarfism as humorous but asexual. Maupin challenges the presumption that someone with dwarfism cannot have sex, or is emotionally incapable, while exposing how average-sized people hold these views and how they play out within society.

One of the most striking parts of the book is when Cadence and her room-mate Renee come into contact with a group of teenage boys. People with dwarfism receive a lot of unwanted attention, especially from groups of teenagers (Pritchard, 2014). The scene revolves around the teenagers who are driving alongside Renee and eventually notice Cadence in the passenger seat:

> 'Shit, man, she's not a kid with her'.
> 'Nah, it ain't a kid. What the fuck is that?'
> 'You won't fucking believe this, man. She's even got a friend for you!'
> 'Ha ha…you see that?'
>
> *(Maupin, 1992, 41)*

Renee is constructed as sexual, while Cadence is infantilized and used as a joke. To further the latter's asexualization, Cadence is not given a gendered pronoun, instead referred to as 'that'. If any member of the group were to date her, he would become a laughing stock. I relate to this representation when I remember dating a man who I had met through a mutual friend. We were planning our first date when he texted me to tell me that, although he thought I was beautiful and intelligent (his words), he found it hard to date me as his friends thought it 'funny' that he was intimate with a dwarf. I do not know what he meant by 'funny' as I dumped him before I could ask. Did he mean we must have looked funny together due to our opposing heights or due to the cultural baggage that my body carries? Both of these reasons are influenced by sociocultural understandings of dwarfism, which ended our relationship. This outcome demonstrates the humorous strand of the metanarrative evident in the media, but also the infantilization of dwarfism.

People with dwarfism are often infantilized due to their small stature. Historically, people with dwarfism were kept as pets. These two conceptions, if connected to sexuality, result in notions of paedophilia or bestiality, two forms of repulsive sexual behaviour. The American comedian and presenter Chelsea Handler, when asked on a talk show if she would ever sleep with a person with dwarfism, responded 'No, as it would be child abuse'. This absurd comment is unsurprising since Chelsea went on further to say, 'I love little people. I want to tackle them. I see them and I want to hold myself down. I bite Chuy [Bravo] sometimes'. Chuy Bravo is a late dwarf entertainer who worked as Chelsea's sidekick. Therefore, the implication is somehow that, while sleeping with a dwarf is child abuse, biting a middle-aged man is affectionate.

Concluding Discussion

Autoethnography is a beneficial research method for understanding how the metanarrative of dwarfism impacts upon the identity and standing of people with dwarfism in society. While most people have grown up surrounded by representations of dwarfism, few have experienced the social implications. Autoethnography is a useful research method for disabled academics, who can draw on experiences for research purposes. This method aids in identifying the assumed authority of many average-sized people, one of the social manifestations of the metanarrative of dwarfism.

The metanarrative of dwarfism is bolstered by heightism, from the terminology we use to the infantilizing way people with dwarfism are deemed asexual. Heightism needs to be taken as seriously as other 'isms', such as racism, sexism, and disablism. In other words, we need to question how we represent people with dwarfism in everything from the entertainment industry to media and culture more broadly.

Engaging with problematic language, which is common within many articles about dwarfism, helps to demonstrate the wide-ranging metanarrative that is underpinned by heightism. Here I include articles that aim to raise awareness but are underpinned by heightist assumptions, in order to demonstrate how deeply ingrained the metanarrative of dwarfism is within the psyche. Over time, I have come across too many of these articles, especially as many are shared by certain organizations for people with dwarfism, aiming to raise awareness about the impairment. However, they reinforce problematic representations that construct smallness as undesirable. On the other hand, there continue to be numerous articles that use subtle ableist language to mock people with dwarfism and reinforce the notion that small is bad (using small terms to denote badness). For articles to be positive, then, they need to ensure that there are no underlying heightist assumptions. Even the negative articles should refrain from mockery, as the mockery affects all people with dwarfism, as opposed to just the dwarf in the article.

The rarity of dwarfism and its contrasting abundance in cultural representations is problematic in allowing a false representation to be constructed and rarely challenged. The popularity of dwarfism in the entertainment industry, but rarity elsewhere, provides a strong foundation for the humorous strand of the metanarrative to influence social encounters between people with dwarfism and other members of society. Focusing on the character Mini-me is important as he is a well-known character, but unlike other such dwarfs in films he is given a prominent role, which makes his representation even more significant.

Consideration must be given to representations that both reinforce and challenge the metanarrative of dwarfism in order to provide a more nuanced approach to understanding different social implications. I am used to coming across representations of dwarfism that actively create a fictional and very problematic representation of dwarfism. However, some of the more nuanced representations are intriguing. Representations within *Maybe the Moon, Elf* and *Mendel's Dwarf* are more true to life and relatable. Nevertheless, in some cases the writers still fail to resist inclusion of certain parts of the metanarrative that prove problematic.

Both *Maybe the Moon* and *Mendal's Dwarf* are obvious choices when focusing on sexuality and dwarfism, as one of the main themes throughout both books is the intimate relationship with an average-sized person. Unlike many other representations, the two stories construct people with dwarfism as sexual. However, in both stories, a binary is created in which the dwarf is constructed as grotesque and their average-sized love interest (or main friend) is constructed as beautiful. Importantly, both stories show how it is the sociocultural construction of dwarfism that impacts their relationship, as opposed to their actual dwarfism.

References

Ablon, J. (1990) Ambiguity and difference: Families with dwarf children. *Social Science and Medicine*, 30 (8): 879–887.

Adelson, B. M. (2005) The changing lives of archetypal 'Curiosities' – and echoes of the past, *Disability Studies Quarterly*, 25 (3).

Bolt, D. (2014) *The Metanarrative of Blindness: A Re-Reading of Twentieth Century Anglophone Writing*. Ann Arbor: University of Michigan Press.

Bolt, D. (2019) *Cultural Disability Studies in Education: Interdisciplinary Navigations of the Normative Divide*. Abingdon: Routledge.

Bonnie, S. (2004) Disabled people, disability and sexuality. In Swain, J., French, S., Barnes, C. and Thomas, C. (eds.), *Disabling Barriers – Enabling Environments* (2nd ed). London: SAGE, 125–132.

Gaustad, S. (2010) Maupin, Amistead. *American Fiction: A2*. Vol. 2.

Garland-Thomson, R. (1997) *Extraordinary Bodies: Figuring Physical Disability in American Culture and Literature*. New York: Columbia University Press.

Haller, B., Dorries, B. and Rahn, J. (2006) Media labelling versus the US disability community identity: A study of shifting cultural language. *Disability and Society*, 21 (1): 61–75.

Horton, W. A., Hall, J. A. and Hecht, J. T. (2007) Achondroplasia. *The Lancet*, 370 (9582): 162–172.

Kaplan, R. (2017) Non-normative sex and bodies in *Game of Thrones*: How extreme bodies question the nature of sex and sexual images. *Kultur und Geschich*, 18: 1–18.

Khan, A. (2016) Why are pantos casting tall people as dwarves? *The Guardian* [online]. Available from: https://www.theguardian.com/stage/shortcuts/2016/nov/21/dwarf -actors-taller-actors-steal-panto-roles (accessed 16 April 2020).

Kitchin, R. (2000) The researched opinions on research: Disabled people and disability research, *Disability and Society*, 15 (1): 25–47.

Kruse, R. (2002) Social spaces of little people: The experiences of the Jamisons. *Social and Cultural Geography*, 3 (2): 175–191.

Mallett, R. and Slater, J. (2014) Language. In Cameron, C. (ed.), *Disability Studies: A Student's Guide*. London: SAGE, 91–94.

Massie, P. J. and Mayer, L. S. (2014) Bringing elsewhere home: *A Song of Ice and Fire*'s ethics of disability. In Fugelso, K. (ed.), *Studies in Medievalism*. Cambridge: D.S. Brewer, 45–59.

Maupin, A. (1992) *Maybe the Moon*. London: Black Swan.

Mawer, S. (1997) *Mendal's Dwarf*. London: Abacus.

Merriam-Webster (2020) 'Heightism' Merriam-Webster [online]. Available from: https ://www.merriam-webster.com/dictionary/heightism (accessed 25 March 2020).

Mendez, M. (2013) Autoethnography as a research method: Advantages, limitations and criticisms. *Colombian Applied Linguistics Journal*, 15 (2): 279–287.

Osensky, T. (2018) *Shortchanged: Height Discrimination and Strategies for Social Change*. Lebanon: NH: ForeEdge.

Palmer, K. (2019) Rico walking tall after Dwarf Sports Association Games success. *Essex County Standard* [online] Available from: https://www.gazette-news.co.uk/news/17623322.rico-walking-tall-after-dwarf-sports-association-games-success/ (accessed 03 February 2020).

Pritchard, E. (2014) The social and spatial experiences of dwarfs in public spaces. Unpublished PhD thesis, Newcastle University.

Richards, R. (2008) Writing the othered self: Autoethnography and the problem of objectification in writing about illness and disability. *Qualitative Health Research*, 18 (12): 1717–1728.

Shakespeare, T. (1994) Cultural representation of disabled people: Dustbins for disavowal. *Disability and Society*, 9 (3): 283–299.

Shakespeare, T., Thompson, S. and Wright, M. (2010) No laughing matter: Medical and social experiences of restricted growth. *Scandinavian Journal of Disability Research*, 12 (1): 19–31.

Sherry, M., Olsen, T., Vedeler, J. S. and Eriksen, J. (2020) Introduction. In Sherry, M., Olsen, T., Vedeler, J. S. and Eriksen, J. (eds.), *Disability Hate Speech: Social, Cultural and Political Contexts*. London: Routledge, 1–17.

Svendby, R., Romsland, G. I. and Moen, K. (2018) Non-disabled ableism: An autoethnography of cultural encounters between a non-disabled researcher and disabled people in the field. *Scandinavian Journal of Disability Research*, 20 (1): 219–227.

Taber, N. (2010) Institutional ethnography, autoethnography, and narrative: An argument for incorporating multiple methodologies. *Qualitative Research*, 10 (1): 5–25.

Tomoiaga, L. (2011) The ethics of science and the other as a picaroon: Simon Mawer's *Mendal's Dwarf*. *Buletin Stiintific, Fascicula Filologie*, XX (A): 253–265.

Tozer, J. (2008) Mini crimewave: The dwarf bugler who squeezed through tiny holes to help gang steal scrap metal. *Daily Mail* [online]. Available from: https://www.dailymail.co.uk/news/article-1037204/Mini-crimewave-The-dwarf-burglar-squeezed-tiny-holes-help-gang-steal-scrap-metal.html (accessed 30 April 2020).

Williams, J. and Marvin, S. (2015) Impairment effects as a career boundary: A case study of disabled academics. *Studies in Higher Education*, 40 (1): 123–141.

PART III

Chronic Conditions and the Emergence of Disability

10

THE METANARRATIVE OF CHRONIC PAIN

Culpable, duplicitous, and miserable

Danielle Kohfeldt and Gregory Mather

Preliminary discussion

The experience of pain is ubiquitous, a central trait of what it means to be human (Scarry, 1985). Pain that persists or recurs for more than three months, however, is regarded as an *abnormal* protracted response to disease, infection, or failure to heal properly (Merskey and Bogduk, 1994). In other words, chronic pain is pathologized. Yet, chronic pain is not uncommon. About 20% of the world's population are chronically pained (Goldberg and Summer, 2011), and the experience is so widespread that the International Classification of Diseases of the World Health Organization deemed it necessary to create 38 diagnostic codes spanning seven unique categories of chronic pain conditions (Treede et al., 2015). Despite the efforts of medical science, an empirical understanding of the aetiology of chronic pain remains elusive. There is not a single unitary experience of chronic pain, which may be constant or intermittent, fluctuating and unpredictable, sometimes disabling and sometimes not, the outcome of an identifiable or unidentifiable cause. The subjective, embodied experience of chronic pain is uniquely personal; there is no typical chronically pained subject. Yet, chronically pained people are subject to the norms, values, discourses, and social and legal policies that underpin the construction of disability. Thus, we argue that people who live with chronic pain do share some common, socially patterned experiences, shaped by the metanarrative of chronic pain (Bolt, 2020).

Julian Rappaport (1995) observes that metanarratives are 'those over-learned stories communicated through mass media or social institutions that touch the lives of most people, such as television, newspapers, public schools, churches, or social network gossip' (803). Metanarratives are dominant cultural understandings granted legitimacy as truth. Metanarratives are remarkably pernicious because they operate beyond and outside the confines of interpersonal dynamics.

Indeed, metanarratives are ideological – systematically informed, controlled, and perpetuated by dominant groups – and therefore function to uphold structures of power. As Black feminist scholar Patricia Hill Collins (2000) asserts, a metanarrative is not just one of many possible ways of interpreting the world, but the only way. The assumed authority chronically pained individuals encounter within interpersonal relationships with normates (Garland-Thomson, 1997) is upheld by those ideologies.

Metanarratives of disability are readily apparent in popular cultural representations but differ in the degree to which they are critiqued or simply asserted. Kugelmann, Watson, and Frisby (2019) distinguish between first-hand, insider representations, and those created by chronic pain outsiders. They found that media created by people with first-hand experience of chronic pain tended to advance a more structural analysis of the causes of chronic pain and to suggest collective approaches to care. Likewise, first-person chronic pain narratives on social media (e.g. memes, photos, blogs) can challenge and transform conventional illness narratives, with implications for communicating pain outside biomedical contexts (González-Polledo, 2016; González-Polledo and Tarr, 2014). Magnet and Watson (2017) examine graphic memoirs by disabled women who experience pain and depression, and show how the graphic-comic medium is uniquely positioned to both expose and trouble normative expectations. Taken together, these studies suggest that first-person media representations of chronic pain tend to frame it as a problem with sociopolitical structural roots and ramifications rather than simply a matter of individual suffering.

The comics medium has existed since at least the 1830s (Groensteen, 2009; Harvey, 2009), and, like other forms of popular media (e.g. television, film, magazines), comics serve as cultural texts that produce and reproduce stories about particular groups (Harvey, 2009; Kukkonen, 2013; McCloud, 1994; Smith, 2015; Smith and Alaniz, 2019). Historically, comics deployed physical disabilities as visual shorthand to convey malice, depravity (Alaniz and Smith, 2019), or extrahuman abilities – the 'supercrip' (e.g. *Daredevil*). Thus, consistent with other forms of popular media, comics have systematically depicted disabled characters in dehumanizing ways (e.g. as monstrous, in need of saving, or heroic) that serve to perpetuate denigrating cultural stereotypes about disability. Despite comics' poor track record of critical disability representation, this popular form of media has the capacity to usurp normative assumptions of disability (Wegner, 2020). With their juxtaposition of gestural images and text, comics are uniquely positioned to intervene in the metanarrative of chronic pain (Brophy and Hladki, 2014; Køhlert, 2019), and are especially promising when posed by individuals with first-hand experience of chronic pain. If pain is outside language, as Elaine Scarry (1985) famously argued, then graphic mediums may provide an alternative means of conveying pain that does not depend on precise linguistic articulation. Magnet and Watson (2017) argue that, the possibility of interrupting contemporary ableist depictions of disability through comics – especially in the genre of visual autobiography in which people with disabilities write about themselves and their lives in pictorial form – remains a helpful corrective to mainstream and commercial representations.

(Magnet and Watson, 2017, 251)

This chapter explores three strands of the metanarrative of chronic pain as depicted in contemporary autobiographical webcomics created by chronically pained women (*Chronic Pain Is a Party*; *Doodle Thru*; *My Chronic Pain Diary*). These strands include the chronically pained individual as culpable, duplicitous, and miserable.

Methodological discussion

We approach this chapter from the perspective of two chronically pained individuals with an interest in the disruptive and transformative potential of comics to 'provide their tellers with an opportunity to counter objectification … and assert subjectivity or agency in a marginalizing and ableist society' (Køhlert, 2019, 126-127). Thus, we have sought out comics created by people who experience chronic pain (*Chronic Pain Is a Party, Doodle Thru*, and *My Chronic Pain Diary*). Our aim is to identify key themes in the comics' depiction of mundane social encounters between people with chronic pain and normates.

Social encounters depicted in comics can expose taken-for-granted assumptions about chronic pain that are otherwise implicit. Illustrations of social encounters are especially potent contexts for identifying metanarratives because they reveal the incongruity between expectations of normalcy and impairment. Thus, chronic pain comics are positioned to reveal the implicit cultural assumptions – metanarratives – that organize and animate social relations. Therefore, we narrow our focus to only those panels that depict or make reference to social encounters. In total, we have reviewed 181 *Doodle Thru*, 135 *Chronic Pain Is a Party*, and 90 *My Chronic Pain Diary* single-panel webcomics created between 2016 and 2020. All are single-panel autobiographical comics created by women who experience chronic pain as the result of multiple illnesses and impairments. One woman is Latina and two are White. All three webcomics depict the protagonist character in romantic partnerships with cisgendered men. Two creators reside in the United States and one lives in Ireland.

We have applied inductive, thematic analysis (TA; Braun and Clarke, 2006) to examine the metanarrative of chronic pain in the webcomics. TA is a systematic analytical approach that seeks to identify patterns in data. Consistent with TA, we have engaged in an iterative process that involved immersing ourselves in the data (i.e. viewing and reviewing each comic), noting similarities and incongruities between our own experiences and those depicted in the comics, and identifying recurring assumptions and ideas. We have prioritized those that overlapped with our own experiences with chronic pain. Finally, we have constructed three broad thematic categories, each representing a unique thread of the overarching metanarrative of chronic pain.

Because our lived realities inform our analyses, we describe our experiences with chronic pain in order to demonstrate the point that, although we have quite distinct histories of pain, the metanarrative unifies our encounters in the social world. I (i.e. Danielle) started experiencing neck and back pain early in life. There are photos of me at age four or five wearing a foam cervical collar to treat a pulled muscle (I was jumping on my bed – an activity I continued for years, almost always resulting in the need for the neck brace). Within the first two years of entering the tenure track, I began having episodes of intense neck and back pain, during which I could not work for days or weeks at a time. For the past few years, the pain has been chronic, which for me means pain every day. Despite a filing cabinet drawer full of MRI and CT scans, physical therapy assessments, rheumatologist consultations, and neurological evaluations, the source of my pain remains elusive. Doctors call this kind of pain 'idiopathic', which is the medical science equivalent of throwing their hands up in the air and shrugging. Workplace accommodations allow me to sustain research, teaching, and service activities at my university.

The metanarrative of chronic pain is based in part on the assumption that pain is temporary, so chronic pain is always suspect, particularly if the cause is non-apparent. Due to the lack of identifiable pathology for my pain, medical practitioners expect me to recover. Therefore, my medical assessments for workplace accommodations include a date range, after which I should no longer need accommodations. If the pain endures beyond that date (as it always has), Title IX policies in the United States dictate that I must submit a new form, signed by a medical professional, confirming I am still in need of such accommodations. It is not enough for me simply to report that I still experience chronic pain; validation must come from an authority, which requires that I schedule an appointment, travel to the hospital, pay for the visit (my health insurance requires a 'co-pay' of $25–$40 to see a doctor), and repeat the process of explaining where, how bad, and how often it hurts, in order to obtain a signature. The metanarrative lurks behind the rationale for these processes. Because chronic pain is suspect, the formal requirement (i.e. burden) to prove and reprove impairment seems completely reasonable.

One experience, in particular, illustrates the threads of the metanarrative of chronic pain that become obvious in social encounters with normates. For the past several years I have presented my research on popular culture fandom at the Comics Arts Conference, held concurrently with San Diego Comic Con. I and my colleagues divide our time between attending talks on academic scholarship and attending talks by science fiction and fantasy authors and creators. One year, during a particularly bad pain day, I was unable to sit during an author panel, but standing was tolerable. I moved to the back of the large, mostly empty room and stood near the wall. Almost immediately a room attendant approached and asked me to take a seat. I explained that I needed to stand because of a back problem. The attendant reported that fire codes require all participants to sit so as not to block exit paths. At this point I explained that I have a 'back condition' that causes chronic pain and am unable to sit for long periods of time. I held up the back-support pillow that has become my constant companion in an attempt to prove my point. The attendant frowned and expressed how sorry she was that I have pain, and explained that disabled seating was located at the front of the room. When I replied that I was happy they provided disabled seating but that I needed disabled standing, I was told, politely but firmly, to sit down or leave.

My encounter at the convention highlights key points related to the metanarrative of chronic pain. First, I was hesitant to disclose that I was in pain because I am wary of being perceived as a complainer. I saw chronic pain as my problem to deal with, and standing was my strategy for coping. Once I disclosed my chronic pain, the room attendants reacted by wincing and expressing pity, suggesting they felt uncomfortable. Yet, I was not perceived as disabled and therefore denied reasonable accommodations. In fact, the accessibility options offered were not appropriate for my needs – the room attendants were unable to reconcile disability with someone who needed to stand rather than sit. Of course, it should be noted that ableism is a structural form of discrimination. The Title IX policies that require extra paperwork, and the fire codes that prohibit standing, disproportionately burden disabled people when enforced by employees simply following procedures.

Shortly after this experience, I encountered chronic pain scholarship by Emma Sheppard, Patricia deWolfe, and Alyson Patsavas. The fact that it took me so many years to understand the causes and consequences of chronic pain as structural, and not only personal, speaks to the thread of the metanarrative related to culpability – chronic pain was my responsibility to address, a belief I had internalized. I felt guilty requesting workplace or other accommodations, because I did not yet think of myself as 'actually disabled'. Just as deWolfe (2002) began to identify as disabled only after she could not open a door at her university due to limitations from pain and realized it was not the pain but the door that was disabling her, it was not until I experienced disabling policies and social structures like those described above that I began to identify with and use the term *disabled*.

My (i.e. Greg's) journey with disability and chronic pain began in 2007. In my teens, I was drawn towards the metal scene, both due to the fact that the genre served as an outlet for my suburbanite rage, as well as my misinterpretation that violence and blood equated to 'more masculinity'. At age 17 I attended a metalcore concert where a man hit me from behind as I attempted to exit the mosh pit at an *As I Lay Dying* concert, breaking my neck and crushing 80% of the humeral head of my shoulder. I am fortunate to have had access to over a decade of medical interventions: five surgeries, stem cell and hormone treatments to regrow tendon and bone, pain management clinics, and a gamut of alternative treatments that have taken me across the country. Ultimately, my experiences with disability and chronic pain would end up dictating my pursuit of a graduate degree in Human Factors/Ergonomics due to my intimate understanding of how life-changing ergonomic design can be for folks who sustained serious injury.

I believe there is a widespread misunderstanding of the body's ability to fully recover after traumatic injury. For most individuals, pain is a fleeting sensation – a warning or message to inform or modify behaviour. Media depictions of the heroic protagonist recovering from spinal injury through grit and determination contribute to the metanarrative that chronic pain is a failure of the individual to take responsibility for their own healing.

In addition, due to the association between chronic pain and assumptions of duplicity, I now bring a thick folder of medical documentation with me almost everywhere I go in order to 'prove' my legitimacy. As a young man who is (sometimes) able to walk, drive, and attend school with appropriate accommodations, I often encounter individuals who assume I am fleecing the system. I have experienced outright harassment when people witness me stepping out of my car from a disabled parking spot, despite my disabled parking placard. Engaging in activities that conflict with assumptions about how disabled people ought to demonstrate our pain for others fuels the metanarrative of chronic pain as duplicitous.

Analytical discussion 1

Culpability

Chronic Pain Is a Party, created by Poly González, offers anecdotal snapshots of life with chronic pain. Throughout the webcomic, González navigates a slew of ableist interactions that suggest personal culpability. For example, one panel entitled 'when people just can't understand' features González in conversation with an incredulous peer who asks, 'but how come are you still in pain?' A bubble above González's head reveals an inner thought, 'here we go again', an indication that such questioning is hardly novel. González, who experiences chronic pain related to endometriosis, replies, 'em, well yes, you see there is no cure for chronic diseases'. An open-palmed hand gestures towards the woman, signalling that González is in teaching mode, reciting a well-rehearsed, politely delivered defence with a half-smile that belies her frustration. Her peer's inquiry demands an explanation for protracted pain, implying at once that long-term pain is abnormal, and that it is taking too long to recover. In turn, González must defend the chronicity of her pain by leveraging the parlance of biomedicine (i.e. disease, cure). The ideology of ability (Siebers, 2017) insists on manageable bodies amenable to treatment, back to some baseline of normalcy before pain. Under the ideology of ability, failure to control our own body entitles normates to an alibi. As deWolfe (2002) notes, 'undertones of blame frequently lurk in this approach: it is taken for granted both that it is our duty to overcome illness (Herzlich and Pierret, 1984, 283–288), and that it is always in our power to do so (Duff, 1994, 41)' (deWolfe, 2002, 262). Thus, a chronically pained body is presumed to be a failure of self-control (Sheppard, 2020).

The metanarrative of chronic pain as culpability constructs chronically pained individuals as in need of intervention (which is not the same as in need of *care*, an interdependency framework disability and feminist scholars have promoted), thus engendering advice from those who inhabit (temporarily) able bodies. Therapeutic suggestions have the effect of both policing chronically pained bodies and infantilizing them, without addressing the sociocultural, economic, or political structures that cause or perpetuate chronic pain (Kugelmann, Watson, and Frisby, 2019). All three of the comics speak to the frequency of (mostly) well-intentioned, unsolicited input from family, friends, co-workers, doctors, and strangers about the aetiology of and/or the right treatment for pain. The ongoing, indefinite nature of chronic pain violates the 'overcoming disability' imperative, eliciting recommendations, chastisements, or accusations. Jill Brook, the creator of *Doodle Thru*, and diagnosed with Myalgic Encephalomyelitis/Chronic Fatigue Syndrome (ME/CFS), depicts a doctor outfitted in a white lab coat, clipboard in hand, stating, 'ME/CFS patients just need to exercise more'. The doctor is positioned in the upper left corner of a line graph illustrating the relationship between confidence on the Y-axis and knowledge on the X-axis, indicating his blend of high confidence and low knowledge. The panel is captioned, 'the Dunning-Kruger Effect in action!' The Dunning-Kruger Effect describes the phenomenon of 'meta-ignorance', in which 'poor performers in many social and intellectual domains seem largely unaware of just how deficient their expertise is' (Dunning, 2011, 247). Brook's suggestion that the doctor's confidence outpaces his knowledge of her illness speaks to the assumed authority conferred to supposed experts despite ignorance of their own incomplete knowledge. Implicit in the doctor's recommendation is the sociocultural construction of the chronically pained person as lazy. Lack of exercise is the cause and suggests an easy cure. Attempts to help 'fix' chronic pain are, again, animated by the metanarrative that *you* are the cause of *your* own suffering.

Moreover, the metanarrative linking chronic pain to personal responsibility suggests that the real problem is not chronic pain but the failure of the individual to remediate the pain properly. In his conceptualization of the ideology of ability, Siebers (2017) notes the common assumption that 'disability can be overcome through will power or acts of the imagination' (316). Failure to do so predictably results in victim blaming, a point made explicit by Brook in another comic. This time, Brook draws herself breaking the fourth wall, looking at and speaking directly to her reader. Comics about disability have deployed this technique as a way of disrupting the hegemonic gaze, staring back at the audience as a way to redirect attention away from the disabled body and onto the normate (Garland-Thomson, 1997; Køhlert, 2019). Brook's body is in a supine position, with her legs propped up on a large document emblazoned with the title: 'Chronic Illness Victim Blaming Worksheet'. She compels the reader to make explicit their unspoken assumptions about her condition, stating, 'I'll make this easy for you … Go ahead … I've heard it all'. The worksheet includes multiple choice and fill in the blank options:

> She/he has this life-altering illness because she/he ate too (much/little/poorly), exercised too (hard/often/seldom), worked too (much/little/hard), and/or made these bad life choices: [three blank numbered lines are provided], and that's why this would never happen to me.

Alongside the worksheet, a quote describes the psychology of victim blaming: 'When people want to believe that the world is just, and bad things won't happen to them, empathy can suffer (The Atlantic, Oct. 5, 2016)'. If disability is an outcome of defective character and poor decision making, it follows that in a fair society chronic pain is not only preventable but also deserved. The disabled body – in this case, the body in chronic pain – creates an irreconcilable tension between the social fiction that good things happen to good people and the inevitability of disability.

Taken together, the comics described above illustrate that people who live with chronic pain are subject to surveillance by normates and to their assumed authority. Such an asymmetric relationship is tenable only under the condition that chronic pain is the result of an individual failing to manage and control one's body. When pain persists, responsibility lies solely with the person in pain. Likewise, we are absolved from collective responsibility to enact care. Here we might recall that metanarratives are ideological (Collins, 2000; Martín-Baró, 1994); their social function is served when they effectively maintain the defensibility of the existing social order. Chronic pain stands in opposition to the neoliberal impetus to perfect the self, to focus one's attention on the project of self-improvement. Locating pain within an individual's control reflects the deep ruptures in care fostered by a neoliberal context that demands not that we support one another but that we leave each other alone (Dutt and Kohfeldt, 2018; Held, 2006).

Analytical discussion 2

Duplicity

Assumptions that the body is controllable,

> also pervade interactions between sick people and their families, friends and neighbours, as doubt is cast on the *bona fides* of those who fail to recover. The long-term sick may be suspected of seeking attention, or of avoiding normal responsibilities or relationships.
>
> *(deWolfe, 2002, 262)*

Credibility as a source of knowledge about one's own experiences is not equitably distributed. Indeed, race, gender, age, and social class intersect with disability to position some groups as more 'trustworthy' than others in clinical encounters for pain management (Buchman, Ho, and Goldberg, 2017; Patsavas, 2014). Women, BIPOC, and other historically subordinated groups are more likely to have the existence and severity of their pain questioned, and to be perceived by healthcare providers as malingering (Boddice, 2015; Wailoo, 2014). The act of downgrading the authenticity of chronic pain has been described as a form of epistemic violence, 'a type of violence that attempts to eliminate knowledge possessed by marginalized subjects', and functions to 'damage a given group's ability to speak and be heard' (Dotson, 2011). For chronically pained individuals, 'prejudicial stereotyping causes the listener to attribute a reduced level of credibility to a speaker's testimony than they otherwise would have given if the prejudice was not present' (Buchman, Ho, and Goldberg, 2017, 35). Given the chance to disclose their experiences, the perceived reduction in credibility effectively silences the person with chronic pain when their testimony is not taken seriously. Several panels from the webcomics series illustrate how epistemic injustice is accomplished via the metanarrative of duplicity.

In one panel from *Chronic Pain Is a Party*, the severity of González's account of chronic pain is diminished in a medical encounter. A male doctor greets her with, 'So, it says here you live with chronic pain?' González responds, 'that's right Dr'. In turn, the doctor states, 'well, it's really not that big deal you can still work don't you?' González's reaction to the doctor's flippant remark is communicated by a scribbled jagged spiral line inside a thought bubble, indicating a nonverbal emotional response we read as anger and frustration. The illustration is accompanied by the caption, 'when you're asked to stop whining'. Medical doctors occupy a position of social influence and therefore have access to the power to shape collective cultural understandings. Thus, downgrading the severity and impact of a patient's pain in a way that suggests she is whining is uniquely significant when enacted by a doctor. Furthermore, the feminization of 'whining', a behaviour associated with petulant children, undergirds the doctor's question. Steeped in a subtext of doubt, his rhetorical question exposes suspicions that González is exaggerating. In turn, González is unable to elaborate her testimony, as her doctor's question elides verbal response. In effect, she is silenced.

Similarly, a *Doodle Thru* panel depicts a woman preparing for a doctor's appointment by adorning herself in a dress tie, moustache, and John Deere cap. The caption states, 'Tina was curious where her doctor's appointment would lead if "neurotic woman" were off the table'. The impact of Brook's webcomic relies on the routine delegitimization of women's knowledge about their own bodies, a well-documented and common experience among disabled women (Fine and Asch, 1988). In the context of medical care, the roles of doctor and patient are freighted with historical inequities and power imbalances. Patsavas (2014) notes the gendered repudiation of pain women endure in medical encounters:

> I bring with me an individual history of doctors dismissing my experience of pain and a collective history of women in pain being locked up and/or

> thrown out of offices for "hysterical behavior", just as the doctor brings with him a history of seeing thousands of other patients expressing pain and a collective history of a medical system that trains doctors to view pain and people in pain as suspect.
>
> *(Patsavas, 2014, 215)*

Chronic pain is always suspect because it rarely emanates from a visible injury, and because of its oscillating, unstable nature. Thus, doubts about the veracity of chronic pain claims are anchored in the 'ableist model of cure' that assumes you can only be either 'successful and fixed or broken and fucked' (Lakshmi Piepzna-Samarasinha, 2018, 231). The notion that chronically pained people may work (as the doctor in González's comic indicated) violates that binary. As Buchman, Ho, and Goldberg (2017) point out, 'when chronic pain impedes the production of clinical knowledge by defying the easy objectification that is at the core of the epistemology of Western biomedicine, it becomes subject to doubt and scepticism' (34). Chronic pain is notorious for evading identifiable anatomical pathology. Indeed, 'many, if not most kinds of chronic pain cannot be correlated with any underlying pathology. The epistemic structure of Western allopathic medicine – its claims to truth and veracity – depends on frameworks of clinical correlation and pathological anatomy' (Buchman, Ho, and Goldberg, 2017, 34).

Analytical discussion 3

Misery

Very often the comics depict chronically pained people as suffering and miserable, illustrating another thread of the metanarrative of chronic pain. The comics, however, propose that such misery is experienced not (only) as a result of pain, but in relation to social-structural obstacles, including social stigma, infantilization, and coping with exclusion from friends and family who would prefer to avoid spending time with so-called complainers. Pain is far from pleasant, but we often suffer added harms imposed by external forces. For example, in one issue of her webcomic *My Chronic Pain Diary*, Ciara Chapman draws herself as a diminutive figure, taking up barely one quarter of the page, with her head bowed (Chapman, 2019). She is drawn in black and white, while everything around her is in bright colour. A bird twice her size is perched above her, menacingly watching as she works at a table top. Line after line of the phrase 'Hurry up!' is scrawled across the background over 100 times. Thoughts surrounding Chapman include: 'Why is this taking so long?' and 'I'm doing everything I can'. The image illustrates the power of imposed norms around pace and productivity to contribute to the internalization of a sense of falling behind.

The sense of being surveilled by normates is made more explicit in a second panel featuring Chapman spotlighted in a circle of light, surrounded by colourful, larger than life creatures. She is shown from behind, her colourless silhouette evocative of Lewis Carroll's Alice. Four large human-like but not quite human figures loom over her. Their long arms point at her. Printed on their arms are the phrases, 'where are you going?', 'what are you doing?', 'what does your doctor say?', and 'but who will stay with you?' The accompanying caption conveys the infantilization Chapman experiences as she encounters this line of questioning: 'Over time, my loss of independence is making me feel smaller, and smaller, and smaller, and smaller'. As disability and feminist scholars have argued, the neoliberal imperative to achieve autonomous, independent selfhood is at odds with a relational, liberatory ethics of care that values interdependence (Dutt and Kohfeldt, 2018; Patsavas, 2014). Thus, the prospect of needing care is associated with a loss of esteem and perceived value. Moreover, the care that is offered for chronic pain is often experienced as scolding for behaviour perceived as inconsistent or inappropriate for someone in pain.

Finally, the metanarrative of chronic pain as misery contributes to the assumption that people who live with chronic pain are complainers and therefore to be avoided. Siebers (2017) explains how the ideology of ability creates the social conditions under which a,

> loss of ability translates into loss of sociability. People with disabilities are bitter, angry, self-pitying, or selfish. Because they cannot see beyond their own pain, they lose the ability to consider the feelings of other people. Disability makes narcissists of us all.
>
> *(Siebers, 2017, 316)*

In *Chronic Pain Is a Party*, a panel entitled 'when "friends" diminish your feelings' portrays González and a friend seated across from one another talking over coffee. The friend asks, 'so, really how r u?' González replies, 'not so well'. Her friend retorts, 'well you do have a boyfriend, a good one actually'. 'Yeah, so?' asks González. The friend asserts, 'then you have no right to complain'. A bubble below González contains her unspoken thoughts: 'but I'm not complaining, I'm just sharing my feelings because you asked'(González, 2019) The perception that chronically pained people are complainers is particularly damaging to social relations, as normates avoid interactions with those they consider miserable. Yet, people who experience chronic pain are placed in a double bind where they either disclose their pain and risk perpetuating a stereotype or self-silence and downplay or hide their pain. Neither option is appealing. Indeed, the misery González depicts in her comic emanates not only from pain, but also from the reactions of other people, revealing how 'social arrangements and atmosphere' contribute to the experience of pain (deWolfe, 2002, 261). The ableist reactions to the characters in these comics illustrate what Magnet and Watson (2017) describe as an 'everyday form of trauma to which people with disabilities are subjected' (258).

Concluding discussion

The threads of the metanarrative of chronic pain depicted in the words and images of the *Chronic Pain Is a Party, Doodle Thru*, and *My Chronic Pain Diary* illuminate the complexity of chronic pain as those of us with pain navigate social institutions and individual relations. Autobiographical comics about chronic pain are an invitation to de-ideologize taken-for-granted assumptions about life with chronic pain by offering a more complex personhood for those who experience intractable pain. As a form of life writing, the webcomics explored in this chapter ought to be considered alongside other autobiographical comics that depict disabled bodyminds. Notable examples include Al Davison's *The Spiral Cage*, Alison Bechdel's *Fun Home*, and Allie Brosh's *Hyperbole and a Half*, graphic novels offering longform explorations, and mostly conventional narrative style and character development (if unconventional stories). Self-published, open-source, single-panel webcomics may not carry the same prestige but, nonetheless, convey important knowledge about the experience of chronic pain.

In capturing the first-person lived realities of chronically pained individuals, attending to autobiographical comics aligns with calls from feminist and critical disability scholars to privilege work by disabled people in our scholarship. Garland-Thomson (2005) calls for undertaking a 'project of narrative recuperation' (1560), in which the stories of disabled women are given audience. She also asserts that a feminist disability studies advances theory from the perspectives of disabled women subjects, taking the form of life writing that 'protests the disability system' (1569), rather than simply the telling of a 'disability memoir or illness narrative'. The comics described in this chapter do just that. Furthermore, Sami Linton (1998) calls for the creation of cultural narratives grounded in disability experiences. Indeed, citing Linton, Dirth and Adams (2019) characterize disabled experience as 'both a marginalized cultural identity and an epistemic perspective with disruptive analytical potential' (260).

The concept of epistemic violence serves as a theoretical frame to help organize the disparate threads of the metanarrative illustrated in the comics. Taken together, the comics we analyze portray a pervasive and persistent silencing of women in chronic pain. Interfacing with medical professionals, family, and friends often produces a denial of one's suffering or encouragement to work on 'getting better'. From our personal experience, encounters with normates can be silencing, especially in situations where you are asked to prove your disability status. We have both experienced the frustration of our first-hand descriptions of our impairments being inadequate to access resources or accommodations. Instead, a formal authorization from someone presumed qualified to speak on our behalf (i.e. a medical professional) is necessitated. Carel and Kidd (2014) argue that 'ill persons are vulnerable to testimonial injustice through the presumptive attribution of characteristics like cognitive unreliability and emotional instability that downgrade the credibility of their testimonies'. There is more to testimonial injustice than simply not being listened to. We are positioned such that we *must* disclose information about our 'conditions' in order to access resources (e.g. disabled seating, standing desk) or justify actions that seem incongruous with our outward appearance (e.g. appearing young, or appearing non-disabled). In a sense, we are constantly made to speak, but our 'testimonies' are elicited through coercion and control only to be met with disbelief, suspicion, or avoidance. In addition, our disclosures often adopt and parrot the parlance of the medical profession. We are not sharing our own personal, messy, complex lived experiences, but rather giving normates what they want to know in a language they can understand – the language of Western biomedical epistemologies. Ironically, we are forced to perpetuate the legitimacy of the biomedical model by employing it (strategically) to justify our rights and experiences, which seems to be another class of epistemic violence. In this case, autobiographical comics about chronic pain offer an alternative to biomedical representations of patients in need of treatment or neoliberal subjects responsible for their own healing through financial investment in pharmaceutical interventions.

Finally, on a hopeful note, denigrating metanarratives are actively resisted by oppressed groups. We have found plentiful counter-narratives within the chronic pain comics. We think it is worth noting that while our intention was to foreground the metanarrative of chronic pain, many of the comics employ humour to call out the absurdity of the metanarrative. Even the titles of the comics themselves, most obviously *Chronic Pain Is a Party*, are subversively humorous, recasting the experience of intractable pain from tragedy and misery to comedy and even joy. The comics creators break down binaries by asserting the possibility that we can be simultaneously in pain and laughing, doodling, even partying. A counter-narrative manifest within the comics is that pain does not make one abject, humourless, or without joy. The metanarrative of chronic pain, aligned with the ideology of ability, tells us that pain is joyless, so to assert humour even in the experience of pain produces a tension that unveils cracks in the façade of the metanarrative.

References

Alaniz, J. and Smith, S. T. (2019) Introduction: Uncanny bodies, in S. T. Smith and J. Alaniz (Eds.), *Uncanny Bodies: Superhero Comics and Disability*. University Park: Pennsylvania State University Press.

Boddice, R. (2015) *Pain: A Very Short Introduction*. Oxford: Oxford University Press.

Bolt, D. (2020) The metanarrative of disability: Social encounters, cultural representation and critical avoidance, in N. Watson and S. Vehman (Eds.), *Routledge Handbook of Disability Studies* (2nd Edition). New York: Routledge.

Buchman, D. Z., Ho, A., & Goldberg, D. S. (2017) Investigating trust, expertise, and epistemic injustice in chronic pain. *Bioethical Inquiry*, 14: 31–42.

Braun, V., and Clarke, C. (2006) Using thematic analysis in psychology. *Qualitative Research in Psychology*, 3: 77–101.

Brophy, S., and Hladki, J. (2014) Visual autobiography in the frame: Critical embodiment and cultural pedagogy, in S. Brophy and J. Hladki (Eds.), *Embodied Politics in Visual Autobiography*. Toronto: University of Toronto Press.

Carel, H. and Kidd, I. J. (2014) Epistemic injustice in healthcare: A philosophical analysis. *Medicine, Health Care and Philosophy* 17: 529–540.

Chapman, C. (2019) *My chronic pain diary*. Available from: https://www.mychronicpaindiary.com/.

Collins, P. H. (2000) *Black Feminist Thought: Knowledge, Consciousness, and the Politics of Empowerment*. New York: Routledge.

deWolfe, P. (2002) Private tragedy in social context? Reflections on disability, illness and suffering, *Disability and Society* 17 (3): 255–267.

Dirth, T. P. and Adams, G. A. (2019) Decolonial theory and disability studies: On the modernity/coloniality of ability. *Journal of Social and Political Psychology* 7 (1): 260–289.

Dotson, K. (2011) Tracking epistemic violence, tracking practices of silencing. *Hypatia* 26 (2): 236–257.

Dunning, D. (2011) The Dunning–Kruger effect: On being ignorant of one's own ignorance. *Advances in Experimental Social Psychology* 44: 247–296.

Duff, K. (1994) *The Alchemy of Illness*. London: Virago Press.

Dutt, A. and Kohfeldt, D. (2018) Towards a liberatory ethics of care framework for organizing social change. *Journal of Social and Political Psychology* 6 (2): 575–590.

Fine, M. and Asch, A. (Eds.) (1988) *Women with Disabilities: Essays in Psychology, Culture, and Politics*. Philadelphia: Temple University Press.

Garland-Thomson, R. (1997) *Extraordinary Bodies: Figuring Physical Disability in American Culture and Literature*. New York: Columbia University Press.

Garland-Thomson, R. (2005) Feminist disability studies. *Signs* 30 (2): 1557–1587.

Goldberg, D. S. and Summer, J. M. (2011) Pain as a global public health priority. *BMC Public Health* 11 (770): 1–5.

González, P. (2019) *Chronic pain is a party*. Available from: http://www.facebook.com/chronicpainisaparty.

González-Polledo, E. (2016) Chronic media worlds: Social media and the problem of pain communication on Tumblr, *Social Media + Society* 6 (1): 1–11.

González-Polledo, E. and Tarr, J. (2014). The thing about pain: The remaking of illness narratives in chronic pain expressions on social media. *New Media and Society* 18 (8): 1455–1472.

Groensteen, T. (2009) Why are comics still in search of cultural legitimization? in J. Heer and K. Worcester (Eds.), *A Comics Studies Reader*. Jackson: University Press of Mississippi.

Harvey, R. C. (2009) How comics came to be, in J. Heer and K. Worcester (Eds.), *A Comics Studies Reader*. Jackson: University Press of Mississippi.

Held, V. (2006) *The Ethics of Care: Personal, Political, Global*. Oxford: Oxford University Press.

Herzlich, C. and Pierret, J. (1984) *Malades d'hier, maladies d'aujourd'hui: De la mort collective au devoir de la guérison*, (E. Forster, Trans.) Baltimore: Johns Hopkins University Press.

Køhlert, F. B. (2019) *Serial Selves: Identity and Representation in Autobiographical Comics*. New Brunswick: Rutgers University Press.

Kugelmann, R., Watson, K., and Frisby, G. (2019) Social representations of chronic pain in newspapers, online media, and film. *PAIN* 160: 298–306.

Kukkonen, K. (2013) *Contemporary Comics Storytelling*. Lincoln: University of Nebraska Press.

Lakshmi Piepzna-Samarasinha, L. (2018) *Care Work: Dreaming Disability Justice*. Vancouver: Arsenal Pulp Press.

Linton, S. (1998) *Claiming Disability: Knowledge and Identity*. New York: New York University Press.

Magnet, S. and Watson, A. (2017) How to get through the day with pain and sadness: Temporality and disability in graphic novels, in E. Ellcessor and B. Kirkpatrick (Eds.), *Disability Media Studies*. New York: New York University Press.

Martín-Baró, I. (1994) *Writings for a Liberation Psychology* (A. Aron and S. Corne, Trans.) Cambridge: Harvard University Press.

McCloud, S. (1994) *Understanding Comics: The Invisible Art.* New York: Harper Perennial.

Merskey, H. and Bogduk, N. (1994) *Classification of Chronic Pain* (2nd edition), Amsterdam: International Association for the Study of Pain (IASP) Press.

Patsavas, A. (2014) Recovering a cripistemology of pain: Leaky bodies, connective tissue, and feeling discourse. *Journal of Literary and Cultural Disability Studies* 8 (2): 203–218.

Rappaport, J. (1995) Empowerment meets narrative: Listening to stories and creating settings. *American Journal of Community Psychology* 23 (5): 795–807.

Scarry, E. (1985). *The Body in Pain.* Oxford: Oxford University Press.

Sheppard, E. (2020) Chronic pain as emotion. *Journal of Literary and Cultural Disability Studies* 14 (1): 5–20.

Siebers, T. (2017) Disability and the theory of complex embodiment: For identity politics in a new register, in L. J. Davis (Ed.), *The Disability Studies Reader* (5th edition). New York: Routledge.

Smith, S. T. (2015) Who gets to speak? The making of comics scholarship, in M. K. Czerwiec, I. Williams, S. M. Squier, M. J. Green, K. R. Myers, and S. T. Smith (Eds.), *Graphic Medicine Manifesto*, University Park: Pennsylvania State University Press.

Smith, S. T. and Alaniz, J. (Eds.) (2019) *Uncanny Bodies: Superhero Comics and Disability.* Pennsylvania: The Pennsylvania State University Press.

Treede, R. D., Rief, W., Barke, A., Aziz, Q., Bennett, M. I., Benoliel, R., Cohen, M., Evers, S., Finnerup, N. B., First, M. B., Giamberardino, M. A., Kaasa, S., Kosek, E., Lavand'homme, P., Nicholas, M., Perrot, S., Scholz, J., Schug, S., Smith, B. H., Svensson, P., … Wang, S. J. (2015) A classification of chronic pain for ICD-11. *Pain* 156 (6): 1003–1007.

Wailoo, K. (2014) *Pain: A Political History.* Baltimore: Johns Hopkins University Press.

Wegner, G. (2020) Reflections on the boom of graphic pathography: The effects and affects of narrating disability and illness in comics. *Journal of Literary and Cultural Disability Studies* 14 (1). 57–74.

11

THE METANARRATIVE OF DIABETES

Should you be eating that?

Heather R. Walker and Bianca C. Frazer

Preliminary discussion

From public service announcements on the subway to a punchline in a sitcom, references to diabetes saturate the media landscape in the United States. However, despite this prevalence, the general public has far from a comprehensive or accurate understanding of the condition. Diabetes itself is a non-apparent autoimmune and/or metabolic condition expressing itself in multiple forms. Each form describes the body's ability (or inability) to produce or utilize the essential hormone insulin in order to regulate blood glucose levels. According to the CDC, 30.3 million people in the United States – about one out of every ten – have some form of diabetes. Technological advancements[1] of the twentieth and twenty-first centuries have transformed diabetes from a fatal condition to a chronic one, but have also ushered in new forms of surveillance and control. Though advances have made diabetes more manageable for diabetics, the stereotypes and misinformation about it remain pervasive. Not only do these stereotypes propagate the metanarrative we unpack in this chapter, they also infiltrate the healthcare settings upon which diabetics[2] rely to remain alive.

We live in a social environment that understands diabetes as a consequence of gluttony and inactivity – an individual problem rooted in personal choice. The common inquiry 'should you be eating that?' prevails as a reminder that the person with diabetes makes choices, often poor ones, that means she deserves her

---

1 These advancements include the discovery of insulin, at-home blood glucose monitors, insulin pumps, and continuous glucose monitors.
2 We have decided to use identity-first terminology throughout this chapter as opposed to person-first terminology. We use the term *diabetics* to cover all forms of diabetes, of which there are many. With that said, we acknowledge that diabetic communities are not monolithic.

condition – for it was her bad choices that got her there. Health-related research on diabetes focuses on individual management and prevention that justify a culture of surveillance. Furthermore, research projects that focus on social contexts that reproduce stigma are few and far between. Bias against diabetes persists in spaces where diabetes is abstract and the assumptions, or the metanarrative, about it are presumed to be common sense and natural.

This chapter delves into three pervasive strands of the metanarrative that maintain the social conditions of diabetes, namely: (1) people with diabetes do not take care of themselves; (2) to achieve health, diabetics just need to follow three simple rules; and (3) diabetics are an economic drain on the health system. The chapter analyzes multifaceted and interdisciplinary evidence, such as the Netflix TV show *Sweet Magnolias*, the play *The Cake*, news media comments, television series, social media viral memes, and poignant research studies in order to illuminate the current social landscape of diabetes and what is being done to counter it.

Methodological discussion

Thematic and textual analyses are two practical approaches to identify the metanarrative of diabetes. Both methods focus on describing and interpreting media such as film, TV, news, social media, and ads (McKee, 2003). With thematic analysis, researchers investigate for 'recognizable reoccurring topics, ideas, or patterns (themes) occurring within the data that provide insight into communication' (Hawkins, 2018). This style of observation is useful for spotting strands of the metanarrative that shape and reproduce popular notions of diabetes. As authors, we apply textual analysis to content from entertainment, news media, and social media. Textual analysis is the means by which researchers interpret the 'language, symbols, and/or pictures present in texts' (Hawkins, 2018). Textual analysis is useful in this research because it allows writers to 'make an educated guess at some of the most likely interpretations that might be made of that text' (McKee, 2003). Entertainment, media, and the knowledge translation of research shape ideology about diabetes by presenting the beliefs about it as uncontested and obvious. Through textual analysis, we name, interpret, and critique the messaging about diabetes conveyed by language, images, and symbols. We contest what these texts present as natural, obvious, and true about people with diabetes.

One limitation with this form of interpretation is that 'no approach tells us the "truth" about a culture' (McKee, 2003). In other words, the meanings and symbols embedded within these texts are multifaceted and multilayered. Our interpretations may not cover every aspect of what they communicate. However, as interpreters, our perspectives are grounded in our separate social science and humanities training, as well as both of our lived experiences with diabetes.

Similar to metanarratives of disability at large or other specific conditions, the metanarrative of diabetes fails to account for the complexities of lived experience and diabetic embodiment. As women who have a collective 47 years of lived experience with diabetes, we ourselves have cycled through various internalizations of the metanarrative we unpack in this chapter. We have felt the blame, shame, and disappointment that live and breathe life into this metanarrative. The experiential knowledge we each bring to this analysis enriches and deepens our understanding of the power the metanarrative has, even over our own lives and histories. Some of the evidence we critically examine in this chapter was stumbled upon, happenstance of living with this disease for so long. As we go about our lives with diabetes, we are confronted tirelessly with mounting examples of the destructive play of these metanarrative strands. At each encounter, we are left to negotiate internally: Do we give the free labour of correcting or countering the metanarrative, or do we reserve our limited energy and let the metanarrative go unchallenged? Because of this eternal negotiation, in addition to identifying and unpacking the three strands of the metanarrative of diabetes we identify here, we offer community-generated counter-narratives that have made headway in addressing the harm of diabetes stereotypes. Our hope is that by extending counter-narratives we can more effectively poke holes in the metanarrative that remains tightly gripped around the public imagination of diabetes.

Analytical discussion 1

Diabetics do not take care of themselves

The first strand of the metanarrative states that people with diabetes earned their diagnosis and presumed ill-health through poor lifestyle choices. It puts forward a conception of the diabetic as a person both unable and unwilling to 'take care of themselves'. Underlying this metanarrative strand, which is perhaps the most pervasive of the three we unpack, is *choice* and its surveillance by non-diabetic persons. In the case of diabetes, the surveillance of choice is most apparent around food and fat embodiment. In an era where the self-care industry is booming,[3] the ascribed identity of the diabetic as lazy, unmotivated, and uncaring appears even more blameworthy. Further, the portrayal of diabetes, ever entangled in fat embodiment, calls upon thin, non-disabled people to observe, judge, and intervene in the dietary and physical micro-decisions diabetics make. By virtue of their thinness and able-bodiedness, outsiders are imbued with moral authority to express worry and fear for the health of their loved ones.

---

3 The self-care industry has been proliferating in American culture as a social practice since at least 2016. However, the concepts of self-reliance upon which self-care rely date much further back. Anthropologist Jordan Kisner's article on the politics of the self-care movement and industry warn that the 'risk of promoting individual self-care as a solution to existential anxiety or oppression is that victims will become isolated in a futile struggle to solve their own problems rather than to collectively change the systems causing them harm' (Kisner, 2018). Kisner's warning is further substantiated in the case of diabetes where the diabetic is seen as the antithesis of self-care.

This power dynamic illuminates Simon Williams's formulation of health as a moral performance (Williams, 1998). Williams argues that within Western middle-class culture and late capitalism, health is the ability to 'oscillate precariously between bodily discipline and corporeal transgression'. We might imagine, for example, a thin young person walks into a bakery and orders two pastries. Their indulgence is not only understood and unquestioned but also celebrated. They are enjoying life, we imagine. We see them partaking in an act of humanness they have earned through good health. Now we consider the same scenario, only the pastry purchaser has diabetes. This person is not celebrated, but rather, we imagine them as immoral and unwilling to control their corporeal desires for the sake of health. Even though the behaviour performed by each person is the same, one is given the latitude of full humanhood, while the other is denied a crucial aspect of it. If we imagine the diabetic person in this scenario is also fat, the surveillance and subsequent judgement is amplified.

What is more, fatness is used metaphorically to explain diabetes. They are inextricably entangled. Scholars from fat studies attest that fatness is evidence of biodiversity, not necessarily poor health (Mollow, 2017). The metanarrative pathologizes fatness as a choice and, by extension, contends that fatness and diabetes are the consequences of poor choice. This circular logic reinforces the metanarrative strand that diabetics 'don't take care of themselves' so strongly that the connection goes unquestioned even in media representations of diabetes that take the disease more seriously.

One contemporary pop culture example of this metanarrative can be found in the US-based Netflix original series *Sweet Magnolias* (Anderson, 2020). The first season, which aired in the United States in May of 2020, features three adult, cisgender women living in a small, rural southern town. The whole town attends religious services and is portrayed as pious and moral – though situationally conflicted. By the end of the first episode, the creators establish a recurring scene in which the three women spend time together over dinner and margaritas. All three women engage in the same dietary choices. Throughout the first few episodes, the show also establishes Dana Sue's character. She is characterized as a tough, no-nonsense, strong woman type – the single mother of a teenage daughter. Dana Sue exhibits some mild signs of stress early in the series but is shown to have time to own a restaurant, serve as main chef there, make plans to co-own a forthcoming business, and maintain relationships with her daughter, friends, and co-workers. The show does not surveil her food choices, but rather points to social factors that contribute to mounting situational stress. In Episode 5, Dana Sue's stressors seem to collide, and she faints. She is taken to the hospital where she is told by a doctor that she has had a 'hyperglycaemic event'.

The doctor takes this moment to remind Dana Sue that her mother died of diabetes and that if she does not 'cooperate' – a metonym for compliance – then she will be facing a similar fate. In the language of the metanarrative, the doctor's statement resounds of 'just start taking care of yourself and you won't die like your mother did'. This dramatic portrayal of diabetes is situated not in the unique actions of Dana Sue, but in her fat embodiment. In other words, the audience is given no other evidence of her personal dietary and health choices aside from a collective behaviour in which her thin friends also engage. Thus, the audience is left to surveil the fat character's choices on the basis of her fatness alone, and judge those behaviours more harshly on the threat of diabetes. The audience becomes an authority over Dana Sue, expected to watch her behaviours and judge the success or failure of them – more so than they do her thin counterparts. In sum, this example demonstrates how fat embodiments of diabetes associated with choice face scrutiny that thin, non-disabled embodiments do not.

Dana Sue's case also provides context to analyze the directionality by which such surveillance is transmitted between non-disabled people. When Dana Sue's doctor begins her diabetes journey with a threat (i.e. you'll die like your mother if you continue to not take care of yourself), he does so in front of Dana Sue's daughter. In so doing, he effectively bestows authority of surveillance upon her daughter through fear. This plotline, which begins and ends within this singular episode, concludes with a begrudging statement on the part of Dana Sue to comply with standard health behaviours – again, none of which she is shown to not exhibit prior to her fainting incident. As is demonstrated by Dana Sue's storyline, the authority to surveil seems to be directionally transmitted from healthcare providers to lay people in the real world.

The shareability of images and articles across social media has lent itself to the creation of a media environment that emboldens non-disabled persons' sense of authority to surveil the choices made by both people with diabetes and fat embodiment. We might take, for example, an image produced and shared by a physician on Facebook in 2019.

The image is of a person's legs wearing blue jeans from the shin down. One foot is adorned with a black sneaker and the other foot has been photoshopped to look like an ice-cream cone. The leg image is laid over a grey background. The text in the image reads, '*It's sweet, but it isn't worth it. [subtext] Every 30 seconds, a leg is amputated due to diabetes*'. The professional look of the meme/photo lends authority to the image, along with the use of statistics.

This image was shared thousands of times, with sharers both making light of amputations and pointing to the error of choice in those diagnosed with diabetes. As we see exemplified by this image, the metanarrative strand that folks with diabetes 'don't take care of themselves' extends into the realm of earned physical disability – in this case, amputation. The image asserts that eating ice-cream cones – again a celebrated activity when performed by thin non-disabled people – is a choice that can lead to amputation when performed by diabetics. The text accompanying the image argues that the ice cream is not worth the risk of amputation, and implies that choosing ice cream over that known risk signals an unwillingness to take care of oneself.

The metanarrative is strengthened each time this image is shared as the authority to surveil is transmitted to each non-disabled person who encounters it. Simply seeing the image transmits the responsibility and authority to surveil to all persons who meet at least one of the following criteria: they are non-disabled, they do not have diabetes, and they have never had an amputation or the threat of one. The transmission of authority seems to be justified directionally because the content was generated and initially shared by a physician.[4] This image traffics in both the first and second metanarrative strands we have selected for this chapter. The first regards blame for choices made in the past, and the second regards choices that could and should be made in the future.

Analytical discussion 2

Just follow the three simple rules

The second strand of the metanarrative of diabetes also regards choice; however, it does so within imagined futures. This metanarrative posits that diabetes prevalence and symptomatology will be reduced when diabetics follow a shortlist of three health-related rules: (1) eat well, (2) exercise often, and (3) lose weight.[5] The diabetic then is characterized as the antithesis of these simple rules. Said another way, the diabetic is equated to a lack of ability to perform the rule-based behaviours. This metanarrative also functions to assert an authority unto non-diabetics to surveil the dietary and physical movements of individuals with diabetes, reduce the diabetic experience, and disregard the complex agency and embodiment of diabetic populations.

Today, no one would be hard-pressed to find a sitcom, film, television series, musical theatre performance, or public social media campaign that references or makes a joke of diabetes. In popular Western-based series like *Parks and Recreation, Friends, New Girl*, and so on, references to diabetes are casually and repeatedly used for comic relief. For example, in the Season 10 finale of the *Great British Bake Off*, celebrity judge Paul Hollywood casually referred to a contestant's chelsea buns as 'diabetes on a plate' (Kanter, 2019).[6] These casual and seemingly innocuous references to diabetes exemplify an extension of the second strand of the metanarrative by showing diabetes/diabetics as the antithesis of the three rules. This means that the personification of diabetes relies on a public imagination that equates diabetes to eating poorly (i.e. consuming large amounts of sugar), being physically inactive, and having fat embodiment. Rather than selecting and analyzing one media portrayal of diabetes that exhibits this

---

4 Social media contagion and virality does not require that the original sharer's information remain with the shared image. In this case, however, the doctor's identity was shared along with the image, which emphasized the authority of the message.

5 A common portrayal of the three rules can be found at the bottom of this CDC infographic: https ://www.cdc.gov/diabetes/pdfs/library/socialmedia/diabetes-infographic.pdf. With that said, a Google image search of 'diabetes infographic' will generate hundreds of thousands of results, the majority of which articulate a version of these three rules.

6 The joke was removed from the episode on Netflix and UK streaming services after UK- and US-based audience backlash arose across social media.

metanarrative, we instead turn to a poignant research study which entered these rules into the public imagination as the only acceptable imagined future for diabetics.

The Finnish Diabetes Prevention Study (DPS), which has been cited well over 20,000 times since its publication in 2002, was the first longitudinal mass-cohort study to show that type 2 diabetes could be *prevented*, and that the most effective strategy for doing so was through lifestyle changes (Diabetes Prevention Program Research Group, 2002; Lindström *et al.*, 2003). However, the intervention used to achieve these results was multifaceted, intensive, and involved more touch points than most healthcare systems' can sustain. Participants, who all had one-to-one tailored interventions, were paid to see nutritionists frequently, join activity groups, and take part in regular education sessions over a three-year period. Researchers reported that 'In addition, there were voluntary group sessions, expert lectures, low-fat cooking lessons, visits to local supermarkets, and between-visit phone calls and letters' (Lindström *et al.*, 2003). Taken together, the lifestyle of the participants became wrapped around the intervention, surrounded on all sides by medical authorities and surveillance.

While the intervention is complex and highly individualized, many researchers and clinicians who have read and cited this study interpret the results as a simplified reiteration of the three ubiquitous rules. Further, as is made evident by innumerable media campaigns and infographics about diabetes floating around the internet, lifestyle is perceived as the solution to the problem of the diabetic body – by virtue of the three rules. It is through the process of oversimplification that the agency of the diabetic becomes reduced to and indeed predicated upon these rules. For if the diabetic cannot follow them, not only are they 'not taking care of themselves', they are also giving up a future of potential health.

In capitalist systems like the United States, health insurance plans would not likely pay for people without a diagnosis (prediabetes), or with one for that matter, to partake in highly intensive programmes akin to the tailored intervention offered by the DPS, even if the infrastructure was there to support and surveil them. And so, what is left is the expectation of individual behaviour change without the institutional or programmatic support necessary to achieve those behaviours with regularity, the result of which has ever more shifted the work of surveillance into the realm of the individual. The ultimate form of surveillance, in the case of diabetes, then, occurs in its transference into self-surveillance. Because the medical establishment presents these three rules as so simple, the diabetic has nowhere to look but inward to find a cause of failure. For if diabetes really is as simple as following these rules, the one struggling inevitably asks, 'why can't *I* do this?' This process of internalized Othering is one mechanism that maintains the strength of the metanarrative, especially in populations of persons with diabetes who do not have access to any counter-narratives.

Researchers explore this internalization of the metanarrative and resulting self-othering in a California-based health-centre study (Chaufan, Constantino and Davis, 2013). They specifically sought to understand participants' beliefs about inequitable social contexts as *normal, natural,* or *inevitable.* Researchers found that staff tended to explain a diabetes diagnosis as *a failure of the individual.* Staff persons believed that diabetes is a signal of a defective person who is either ignorant of self-care strategies or unwilling to make changes necessary to manage diabetes effectively (Chaufan et al., 2013). Participants tended to internalize similar attributions. They believed that if they were better educated and made better choices, their health would be better. Even when prompted during interviews with questions related to structural inequalities, participants reverted back to individual attributions and solutions. They looked at themselves, their habits, their diets, and their cultural practices as the problem that needed to be fixed. This implies that participants believed that the 'proper locus of intervention' ought to occur exclusively at the individual rather than the social level (Chaufan, Constantino, and Davis, 2013, 161). It also implies that the result of their self-surveillance is new or renewed self-blame.

This strand of the metanarrative was admittedly the most challenging for us to analyze. Both of us have struggled with internalization of failure throughout our lives with diabetes. For us, it took entrance and entrenchment into disability studies scholarship to be liberated from the deeply embedded ableist ideologies underlying this metanarrative. While counter-narratives certainly exist, such as Health at Every Size, which posits that there is not any one metric of health that is achievable for everybody (ASDAH, 2009), their discoverability is limited. Informed by our collective lived experiences and knowledge, we can assume even the most convincing counter-narratives are subverted by the metanarrative.

Analytical discussion 3

Show me the money

The third strand of the metanarrative is the belief that diabetes is an economic drain on the health system and wider economy. Popular culture offers up this theme in multiple locations – across film, TV, and live performance. One example is a scene from Bekah Brunstetter's play *The Cake* (Brunstetter, 2018). Brunstetter is perhaps best known for writing and producing the TV show *This Is Us.* Her 2015 dramaedy *The Cake* is based on the true events of a baker in Colorado who refused to make a wedding cake for a same-sex couple. In the play, the baker is conflicted about making a wedding cake for her friend's daughter who is getting married to a woman. *The Cake* had an Off-Broadway run in New York and has been produced at regional theatres all over the United States.

In an early scene, the fiancé arrives at the bakery and begins a casual, over-the-counter conversation about the ethics of selling sugary treats. The fiancé, Macy, asks the baker, Della, if she has considered her 'social responsibility to provide products with less sugar' (Brunstatter, 2018, 10). Before Della can protest, Macy voices her concerns: 'The latest is that sugar is more addictive than cocaine. And yet it's in all of our foods, and so basically there's a new generation of young Americans who are practically *born* with diabetes' (Brunstatter, 2018, 10). This argument centralizes the belief that sugar causes diabetes, and thus frames diabetes as the result of addiction to and consumption of sugar. The comment erases genetic components of diabetes and solely implicates *out-of-control* behaviour as the cause of diabetes – a conception that belies the first two strands of the metanarrative.

Macy continues her argument that there are long-term consequences of eating sugary foods. In her final point, Macy catastrophizes a dystopic future populated by people with diabetes: 'In forty years we're going to have a bunch of people who can't provide for themselves, they'll be so fat they can't leave their houses' (Brunstatter, 2018, 10). Here, Macy uses ideas of diabetes and fat bodies interchangeably, and then contends that such bodies cannot leave their houses to work and generate income. She ends her argument by saying, 'so basically we'll be supporting them with our taxes, those of us who aren't dead from cancer' (Brunstetter, 2018, 10). Macy paints a picture of the public having to take on added burden to support those who make dangerous choices, like eating too much sugar, whose bodies then cannot be productive members of a capitalist economy and society. While the play is a 'drama-edy' and the conversation can be interpreted as comic relief, its threads underlie the stigmatizing metanarrative of diabetes. The two women engage in an ethical debate about sugar consumption before the more poignant conflict is introduced: Will Della make a wedding cake for Macy and support this same-sex marriage? However comedic the scene is played by the actors, the ideologies underpinning them extend far beyond attempted humour; they are exhibited by and held with sincerity by people with legislative power in the United States.

Members of the US Republican Party showcased the fear that people with diabetes are an economic drain on the healthcare system in their 2017 effort to repeal the Patient Protection and Affordable Care Act (ACA). This story unfolded across the news media when Mick Mulvaney, the then White House Budget Director, discussed plans to roll back parts of the ACA. He defended his plan by saying, 'We have plenty of money to provide that safety net so that if you get cancer you don't end up broke … That doesn't mean we should take care of the person who sits at home, eats poorly and gets diabetes' (Leonard, 2017). Here, the metanarrative builds on the construction of the diabetic as gluttonous and lazy – tacking on an imagined consequence that if diabetics continue to fail at performing the three rules, they are effectively refusing to be productive members of the capitalist economy. This logic Others people with diabetes and actively disregards other social, cultural, economic, health, and bodily factors involved. As the result of 'their' refusal to take care of themselves, Mulvaney argues that 'we' should not allocate money for 'their' healthcare.

However striking this example may seem, linking productive value to the economy and worthiness of care is not a new argument to deny people with disabilities rights, care, and dignity. An ideology of productivity in capitalist systems imparts citizenship and the protections and benefits available to them only unto those perceived as productive. For decades disability rights activists have fought for accommodations in order to access and contribute to the workplace, while simultaneously fighting to de-stigmatize non-productivity. However, even after the gains of the Americans with Disabilities Act (ADA), the government posted a Myths and Facts section of its website to defend against the fear that 'the government [was] being bamboozled into providing accommodations for those who are undeserving' (Herndon, 2002).

Politicians tend to frame who is deserving and who is not through the innocence-blame binary. Mulvaney alluded to the person with cancer as innocent of any immoral behaviour, while pointing a finger at the person with diabetes as guilty of immoral behaviour and thus ill-deserving of healthcare coverage. This representation of diabetes is akin to the racist myth of the 'Welfare Queen', where the imaginary spectre of someone taking advantage of the government and living luxuriously is used to cut social support programmes and further stigmatize disabled populations.

One counter-narrative that undercuts the logic of this metanarrative is the stance that diabetics bear the biggest burden under the insulin crisis. The term *insulin crisis* came about as a result of 'high insulin prices' and 'cost-related insulin underuse' (Luo and Gellad 2020). Between 2002 and 2013, pharmaceutical companies increased the price of insulin over 300% (Luo and Gellad, 2020), which has created a widespread affordability problem resulting in the rationing of insulin. Practices like insulin rationing, which have been fatal, have devastated the United States so much that grassroots efforts, such as the #Insulin4all social media movement, have come to fruition. While the metanarrative suggests that the public will be responsible for an unjust financial burden, the reality is that people with diabetes are dying and engaging in an underground market because they cannot afford the high cost of diabetes drugs and supplies (Litchman *et al.*, 2020). This metanarrative strand is linked with the previous ones in that it perpetuates the notion that it would be unjust for the taxpayer to contribute to the healthcare coverage of people who 'cannot control' themselves and refuse to follow the three simple rules. This counter-narrative demonstrates that the social landscape of diabetes is incredibly complex with many choices beyond the control of the individual. However, as observed with other counter-narratives, the broader metanarratives prevail.

Concluding discussion

As we have shown throughout this chapter, the three strands of the metanarrative of diabetes function together to reduce the autonomy of a person with diabetes, minimize their authority over their own choices, and affirm outsider authoritative surveillance regarding lifestyle that is predicated on misunderstandings of diabetes. The resulting stereotypes, woven into several examples of media, including TV, commercial theatre, news media comments, social media posts, and health and medical research, vigorously cut through emergent counter-narratives with relative ease. Similarly, the belief that these tropes are self-evident and accurate holds each in place without being otherwise challenged. As the first two metanarrative strands hold each other up based on ideology around individual choice, the third strand is the logical result of a social contract that appears to reward individual hard work and discipline. Thus, the third metanarrative strand works as a justification for less social responsibility of people who are perceived to *make bad choices wilfully.*

What makes these three metanarrative strands particularly insidious is the underlying assumption built into them: that people's health status is always and directly a result of their choices, their will, and their agency. Futures imagined for the diabetic body, then, are both grim and perceived as *deserved*, a marked difference from existing cripistemologies (Kafer, 2013). Existing cripistemologies, such as the cripistemology of pain (Sheppard, 2019), explore the ways in which experiential knowledge interact with normative discourses and metanarratives – understanding the disabled person as uniquely qualified to provide a particular form of expertise to inform that cripistemology (Johnson and McRuer, 2014). The three metanarrative strands we identify here collectively suggest that the obstacle of a good life with diabetes is not even diabetes, but rather is the self. Because normative discourses and the metanarrative of diabetes are shrouded in blame of the individual and because they conceive of a painful imagined future for the diabetic as deserved, existing cripistemologies have yet to expand enough to capture the particularities of diabetes as a disability. While this chapter serves to enter diabetes as disability into conversation with disability studies rhetoric and contemplations, much more is needed.

What has made our readings of the metanarrative of diabetes remarkably well-suited for further exploration within disability studies is the complex entanglement of social and embodied experiences with the disease. For, the same self-surveillance we describe as being a precursor to self-Othering and internalized stigma can be and often is experienced as a form of liberation from the authoritative surveillance of the medical establishment and its rigid three-rule system. That is to say, the physical, emotional, and mental burden may be reduced when the diabetic person performs the self-management rituals and practices they have been imprinted with throughout the duration of their diabetic life.

Self-management as performance becomes not only a form of physical liberation but also an act of defiance. When the diabetic engages in an act of self-management in accordance with the three rules, they defy the first strand of the metanarrative: that singular lived experience demonstrates that diabetics do take care of themselves. When the diabetic engages in an act that intentionally betrays the three rules, they defy the second strand of the metanarrative and threaten the validity of the stigmatizing question, 'should you be eating that?' For the answer of 'should' is irrelevant because the act is already being done. The diabetic, as an agent of their own health, is openly declaring themselves the sole arbiter of choice. This logic, ever so problematically, doubles as a tool of liberation and a reification of the ubiquitous three metanarrative strands. Diabetes and its embodied experiences are riddled with logical dilemmas and conundrums such as this.

A solution, we posit, would require the public imagination of diabetes to shift in three ways: first, towards a more complex understanding of choice – namely that *choice* is constrained by race, ethnicity, zip code, class, gender, size, ideological beliefs, and more; second, towards an awareness of the broader social landscape of diabetes, including but not limited to the insulin crisis, access to insulin, and the metanarrative that inspires self-Othering and internalized blame; and third, towards a willingness to question assumptions built into the metanarrative and its tools of reproduction. To get there, scholarship of diabetes-as-disability ought to initiate dialogue with a counter-question to the ever pervasive 'should you be eating that?' We propose that, to begin unpacking the cripistemology of diabetes, scholars should engage the public in critical thinking and ask, 'why not?'

References

Anderson, S. J. (2020) 'Sweet Magnolias', United States: Netflix.

Asdah (2009) *Health At Every Size SM Fact Sheet, Association for Size Diversity and Health*. doi: 10.1038/oby.2009.191.

Brunstetter, B. (2018) *The Cake*, New York: Samuel French

Chaufan, C., Constantino, S. and Davis, M. (2013) "You must not confuse poverty with laziness": A case study on the power of discourse to reproduce diabetes inequalities. *International Journal of Health Services* 43 (1): 143–166.

Diabetes Prevention Program Research Group (2002) Reduction in the incidence of type 2 diabetes with lifestyle intervention or metformin. *New England Journal of Medicine* 346 (6): 393–403.

Hawkins, J. M. (2018) Thematic analysis, in M. Allen (Ed.), *The SAGE Encyclopedia of Communication Research Methods*. Thousand Oaks: SAGE.

Herndon, A. (2002) Disparate but disabled: Fat embodiment and disability studies. *NWSA Journal* 14 (3): 120–137.

Johnson, M. and McRuer, R. (2014) Cripistemologies. *Journal of Literary and Cultural Disability Studies* 8 (2): 127–148.

Kafer, A. (2013) *Feminist, Queer, Crip*, Bloomington, IN: Indiana University Press.

Kanter, J. (2019) 'The Great British Bake Off': Paul Hollywood Joke Cut From Episode, Deadline. Available at: https://deadline.com/2019/10/great-british-bake-off-paul-hollywoods-diabetes-joke-cut-1202768195/.

Kisner, J. (2018) The politics of conspicuous displays of self-care. *New Yorker*. Available at: https://www.newyorker.com/culture/culture-desk/the-politics-of-selfcare.

Leonard, K. (2017) Mulvaney agrees with 'Jimmy Kimmel test. *Washington Examiner*. Available at: https://www.washingtonexaminer.com/mulvaney-agrees-with-jimmy-kimmel-test/article/2622843.

Lindström, J. et al. (2003) The Finnish Diabetes Prevention Study (DPS): Lifestyle intervention and 3-year results on diet and physical activity. *Diabetes Care* 26 (12): 3230–3236.

Litchman, M. L. et al. (2020) The underground exchange of diabetes medications and supplies: Donating, trading, and borrowing, Oh My!. *Journal of Diabetes Science and Technology* 14 (6): 983–986.

Luo, J. and Gellad, W. F. (2020) Origins of the crisis in insulin affordability and practical advice for clinicians on using human insulin. *Current Diabetes Reports* 20: 1–8. doi: 10.1007/s11892-020-1286-3.

McKee, A. (2003) 'What Is Textual Analysis?', in SAGE Publications Ltd (ed.), *Textual Analysis*, London: SAGE Publications Ltd.

Mollow, A. (2017) Unvictimizable: Toward a fat black disability studies. *African American Review* 50 (2): 105–121.

Sheppard, E. (2019) Chronic pain as fluid, BDSM as control. *Disability Studies Quarterly* 39 (2).

Williams, S. J. (1998) Health as moral performance: Ritual, transgression and taboo. *Health: An Interdisciplinary Journal for the Social Study of Health, Illness and Medicine* 2 (4): 435–457.

12

THE METANARRATIVE OF CANCER

Disrupting the battle myth

Nicola Martin

Preliminary discussion

Metanarratives of cancer seem to be laced with battle language, which suggests that if the affected person puts up a good enough fight they will be able to defeat the disease. My personal narrative disrupts this unscientific and oppressive notion. Cancer killed John, my athletic vegan 25-year-old son, on 12 December 2012 after he had endured a year of gruelling treatment. Metanarratives around grief and bereavement seem to be built on the idea that grief is time limited and time will heal. Failure to follow a particular trajectory towards accommodation of the loss can result in the acquisition of a diagnosis of 'Complicated Grief' (White, 2013). As a bereaved mother I dispute this idea. There is nothing complicated about my grief apart, perhaps, from my resulting indifference to my own cancer diagnosis in 2016. Complicated Grief is categorized clinically as lasting to a debilitating degree for two or more years (White, 2013). Undoubtedly, my grief will last for the rest of my life. I simply have a broken heart. It is not difficult to imagine. Cancer is a monster which lurks in the collective imagination and every parent's worst fear is the death of their child. I rather resent the role of Sleeping Beauty's 13th fairy that my frightening life experiences have forced upon me. She is the one who appeared uninvited and cursed Sleeping Beauty at her christening. Fairy tales can be very grim. Winston Churchill would certainly not be my role model but his expression 'keep buggering on' resonates more with me than the 13th fairy's approach of spreading gloom over everything. He was a bereaved father.

Metanarratives of cancer are laced with terror as well as battle language. On a personal level my own brush with cancer did not terrify me. Cancer is a broad church. Mine was stage one A and curable. I am in remission. John's was stage four, fatal and absolutely terrifying. I wish we could have swapped places.

Although I am expected to balance my experience with his in this personal narrative, doing so feels impossible because we did not get an equal dose. Noticing two spots of post-menopausal bleeding, going to the GP on the insistence of my partner, diagnosis, surgery (three times over one year), and recovery does not compare with being handed a death sentence − Mine was Cancer Lite. I was certainly messed up physically by the operations and have been left with residual physical impairments. John had multiple rounds of debilitating chemotherapy which was ultimately pointless. Metanarratives around having a positive attitude and therefore somehow being able to defeat cancer offend me deeply. I got cancer, received effective treatment, and carried on. My son never really had this option.

When I returned to work eight weeks after my second operation, I was a mess. My hands were numb, I walked with a stick and could not stand up straight. Unable to push open the heavy doors, I kept getting stuck behind them and had to rely on passers-by to rescue me. Some sort of phased return to work was arranged by occupational health, but I just plodded on until I had to have further surgery. Following another eight-week absence, I returned to my job, overdid it and ended up back in hospital with dangerously high blood pressure. Pain and fatigue were considerable for about two years after my final surgery.

Psychologically I was preoccupied with the idea that I should not be alive when my son was dead. Without a doubt the worst thing was telling people about my diagnosis. John had died less than four years earlier and I had been reassuring my children that there was no reason to assume that cancer would pay another random visit to our house. Having swallowed my feelings since my son was diagnosed in order to function, I had developed an overwhelming desire not to be a nuisance. While he was ill, I was terrified of not being able to cope and I had got used to wearing a mask of capability which looked as if it was about to slip. I also nurtured the idea that John's death was my fault. My worries were not about myself but about causing yet more pain to others.

There is little else to say about my cancer. Perhaps people look at me and think 'cancer survivor'. I do not know. What I do know is that I really do find the battling metanarrative of cancer unacceptable. It is not a case of my fighting and winning and my son giving up and losing. He said, 'People will think I didn't try hard enough'. He did. It was never a fair fight. A ticking time bomb is another of those military metaphors of which I disapprove, but I must admit to feeling that one day cancer will explode and kill me. Realistically the odds are in my favour and old age should get me first. Although in legal terms a cancer diagnosis equates to disability, despite my resulting physical limitations it is grief which impacts on my identity and day to day life to a disabling extent. Metanarratives of disability only really encompass grief when the tipping point is reached and 'Complicated Grief' or similar labels can be applied. The medicalized labelling of psychological pain is problematic on many levels. Unfortunately, labels often act as gateways to services and legal protections through equalities legislation. Accessing mental health support without going through some sort of diagnostic process is tricky, especially when services are under pressure. In my fortunate situation, compassion and empathy from friends and family did not dry up after a prescribed period of mourning. Metanarratives of grief are punctuated with suitable timelines over which the bereaved person should not stray. My friends and family disagree and so do I.

Methodological discussion

Methodology feels like a grand word in this context. I am telling my story from my perspective with reference, as appropriate, to theory and scholarship. Autoethnography fits this approach. My positionality is clear. There is no such thing as objective truth and this narrative is mine alone. The analytical frame I adopt involves theorizing grief, loss, and cancer in relation to disability, then considering my experiences through intersectional personal and professional lenses, before wrapping things up with some sort of conclusion which I hope is not too trite. *Life goes on* might be an appropriate cliché if this story was just about me, but the problem is that John's life did not go on. From this point in the telling, my cancer is a minor character and grief is the main story, because that is just how it is.

Analytical discussion 1

Applying grief, loss, and bereavement theory

Metanarratives around grief, including Complicated Grief, are not all about bereavement but are always associated with loss. The experience of loss could relate to something like children growing up and leaving home, or missing out on a bonus at work. Life events such as these can be felt acutely even if they seem insignificant from the outside. Insecure early attachments and childhood trauma can result in ambiguous feelings of loss in adulthood (Bowlby, 1969, 1982; Freud and Strachey, 1964). Jung refers to 'individuation' as the achievement of 'a true integrated self' (Kotzé, 2014, 16) and contends that the process can be disrupted by childhood trauma. Being built on a firm footing of love and safety from early in life, and having strong social support, makes it easier apparently to deal with life's challenges. My childhood was not traumatic and I was built on solid foundations of attachment. I got to the age of 53 before a monster called. Despite my best efforts, I cannot say the same for my children, who were in their early 20s when their lives were knocked sideways by John's cancer diagnosis. He was sick for a year, during which time I was in such a deep pit of denial that I was almost impossible to reach. In this respect, I feel I failed as a mother and this feeling is hard to shake. Metanarratives around good enough parenting are built on notions of creating security through firm, loving attachments and keeping the precious child safe.

Throughout John's treatment I expected someone to materialize, who was tasked with looking after his mental health and I hoped there would be some consideration of the mental health of the rest of the family too. This did not happen, despite the rhetoric of organizations like Macmillan who proudly display the slogan 'no one should fight cancer alone' (Macmillan, 2020). It should have. Since we lost John, the rest of us have had various encounters with bereavement counselling, some more successful than others. At least some sort of mental health support was on the agenda. We needed it sooner.

Denial was originally identified in 1970 by Kübler-Ross as a stage of grieving. She conducted research with terminally ill patients and their families and identified a more or less stable pattern of five stages of grief: denial, anger, bargaining, depression, and acceptance (Kübler-Ross, 1970). Guilt, isolation, and hope were also part of the mix and Kübler-Ross concluded that progress through the stages was not necessarily linear or time-limited. Her work was not just about bereavement; she was also interested in the perspectives of dying people. I am still preoccupied with John's suffering during the year he was sick. Days before the end he said, 'I thought it would be all right mum'. You and me both, son.

Various stage theorists followed suit after Kübler-Ross and described variations on her original theme. Parkes and Prigerson (2010) used terms like *numbness, pining, disorganization,* and *reorganization.* In an attempt to gain some sort of control we were actually more organized than ever before in our household while John was sick. We did not let things fall apart organization-wise afterwards either. There were even days when the dishwasher and the washing basket were both empty. The surface of our pond was calm, but just underneath we were frantically paddling to keep afloat.

Reorganization in the Parkes and Prigerson (2010) model involves accommodating 'Continuing Bonds' with the person who has died. That is the easy part for us and is made easier because we still have Max. Although they are identical twins, my sons are really different, but Max's beautiful face is a reminder of his brother. I am not able to look at photographs of John, but I don't need to as he is always in my imagination. Not all grief theorists are as positive as Parkes and Prigerson about Continuing Bonds. Some view the idea as symptomatic of 'Complicated Grief', particularly if the feeling that the loved one is somehow not really dead seeps into the mix (Field et al., 2005; Klass et al., 2014; Scott, 1997; Stroebe et al., 2010). I know my son is dead but that does not mean that I have reached Kübler-Ross's (1970) magical state of 'Acceptance'. It is totally unacceptable to me that a 25-year-old should lose his life and I am troubled about having survived cancer when he did not. Worden (2018) discusses addressing the tasks of grief in stages, which include working through the pain, adjusting to the new situation, and emotionally relocating the deceased in the past. Recently I was at a conference and I commented that working at Sheffield Hallam University was the best time of my life. An innocent delegate offered the opinion that it was such a shame to hear me talk like that because it was as if I had shut the door on the idea of better things ahead. He did not know my situation and I did not say anything. In reality that is exactly what I have done. When I had three living children my life was better. I am leading a diminished life. Metanarratives around bereavement imply that the journey of grief comes to an end at some point, which is often referred to as acceptance. Kübler-Ross (1970), however, talked about 'Chronic Sorrow' and acknowledgement of this idea is important. That is where I live. Amazingly, it is possible to function with a broken heart.

Nobody has diagnosed me with 'Complicated Grief', but the internet reliably informs me that I tick all the boxes. I disagree with the internet because my grief seems simple to me. White (2013) would certainly describe it as complicated. Features include a tendency 'to push the pain away' (17), avoid going out and making contact with people, stopping exercising, and developing poor eating and sleeping habits'. All these things persisted for me for about three years and I am still a chronic insomniac. My one visit to John's grave was on Christmas Eve 2012 on the day of his funeral. It was pouring with rain. I have no plans to return because I do not trust myself to be in that space and not lie down beside him in the dirt. The idea of him being there in all weathers troubles me. By now my lovely son must be a skeleton. I am horrified by this thought. White calls it 'Avoidance'. I call it a coping mechanism. Grief is worse in the middle of the night. In my dreams John is usually alive but often has cancer. Sometimes he is dead but still here and nobody is quite sure. I want to dream about him, and I constantly imagine conversations we might have together. This all seems perfectly reasonable to me, but I imagine the *Diagnostic and statistical manual of mental disorders* (*DSM-5*) (American Psychiatric Association [APA], 2013) would disagree. Even if Continuing Bonds are indicative of Complicated Grief, John is not someone I can relocate in the past and I have no wish to do so. My love for my son occurs in the present tense. To me this seems remarkably uncomplicated. Of course, my bond with him continues. I am his mum. Metanarratives of parenting are underpinned by the idea of permanent unconditional love. Dissonant notes are sounded when the child has died. This situation subverts the whole order of things and makes others feel uncomfortable and afraid. I do not want to evoke this reaction.

Post-traumatic stress disorder (PTSD) and Complicated Grief, according to White (2013), often walk hand in hand. He describes the symptoms of PTSD as lasting more than six months and involving 'intrusive repeated images and mental pictures related to the death and/or its consequences' (White, 2013, 16). While this is still part of my experience, I no longer run a full-colour moving picture of John's death in my internal peripheral vision, but I do always have his image in my mind.

On 13 September 2018, Oxford University's Dr Anke Ehlers delivered a lecture at the Royal Society in London entitled 'Haunted by Memories'. Ehlers used terms like 'intrusive memories', 'triggers', and 'flashbacks' to explain PTSD. All these ideas are familiar to me, but what I found most interesting was the idea of 'Derealization', which she discussed in relation to a self-portrait by Frida Kahlo. The artist painted it after the near-fatal bus crash which left her disabled. Kahlo described the sensation of looking in on her body from the outside. My memories of the hospice and of John's funeral are like this.

In his memoir *Reasons to Stay Alive*, Matt Haig described derealization as feeling 'detached from oneself' (Haig, 2015, 187). 'I derealised. The string that holds on to that feeling of selfhood, the feeling of being me, was cut, and it floated away like a helium balloon' (Haig, 2015, 187). I know that state.

I used to say that I no longer felt like a real person. The word *dehumanizing* crept into my vocabulary to express my anger that nobody medically qualified realized that I was in a florid sense of denial throughout John's treatment. I felt that if someone medical had spoken to me about my son's terminal prognosis, I would perhaps have been more use to him and the rest of my family. Perhaps they did in euphemistic terms, using words like: 'We are going to have to have some difficult conversations'. None of that penetrated my shell. Grief theory is complicated and convoluted because these angry emotions also come with a side order of inevitable guilt.

Ehlers also talked about the feeling of wanting to die. No one is supposed to admit to that one, but I wanted to die when John died. In fact, I wanted us all to die because I could not imagine our family without him there. Owning up to this would probably have landed me in hot water in relation to mental health services, but I had the sense to keep it to myself. As far as I know, PTSD is not recorded in my medical records, but seven years after the death of my son I still feel as if I am walking beside myself. My engagement with the world is split between keeping on buggering on and managing the constant acute awareness of John's permanent absence. Generally, I function in this state. Sometimes I just run out of steam. The idea that this terrible thing must be happening to another family rather than mine preoccupied me while John was ill, and I still cannot reconcile my sense of self with the identity of bereaved mother.

Haig (2015) provides a list of symptoms of clinical depression to which I can relate, and reminds us that anxiety and guilt are often depression's bedfellows. Depressive indicators include fatigue, low self-esteem, slowing of movement and speech, appetite disturbance, irritability, introversion, and anhedonia (i.e. 'the inability to experience pleasure in anything'). While I have never been told that I have this diagnosis, I do recall a trip to my GP to discuss my insomnia, at the insistence of my partner. She asked me why I wasn't sleeping, and within 2 minutes of telling her, I found myself back in the waiting room with a prescription for antidepressants, which made me feel somewhat invisible and also not really worthy of her attention.

Haig's description of his guilt about being depressed reveals a degree of complexity which I did not experience and a metanarrative laden with value judgements:

> If you feel the same amount of depression as someone would naturally feel in a prisoner of war camp, and are instead in a nice semidetached house in the free world, then you think 'Crap, this is everything I ever wanted, why aren't I happy?
>
> *(Haig, 2015, 164)*

Compounding depression and anxiety by overlaying a big dollop of guilt only makes matters worse, but it would be a mistake to think that these reactions can be consciously controlled. My guilt is extremely tangible, because I firmly believe that if I had got John to the doctor about his migraines, they would have carried out blood tests and found and fixed his cancer. This is of course nonsense, but Complicated Grief and PTSD do not traditionally walk hand in hand with rational thinking.

Anxiety symptoms include restlessness, a sense of dread, feeling constantly on edge, difficulty concentrating, irritability, impatience, and distractibility (Haig, 2015, 58). Physical signs include dizziness, drowsiness, pins and needles, palpitations, dry mouth, sweating, shortness of breath, stomach ache, nausea, diarrhoea, headache, excessive thirst, frequent urinating, period problems, and insomnia (Haig, 2015, 156). Stress makes matters worse, and low self-esteem is common in people experiencing grief and PTSD. Although I can relate to all of this, I have somehow managed to choke my anxiety into submission, or more accurately suppression. It may come back and strangle me later. In order to function, I have to keep troublesome ideas tightly controlled and have developed an uncanny capacity to do so. *DSM-5* (APA, 2013) will undoubtedly have a label for this. John is an identical twin. He shares all his DNA with Max. I have chosen not to think about the possibility of the monster calling on our family again. Freud might classify this response as 'reaction formation' (Freud and Strachey, 1964; Granek, 2010). It feels like one of my more useful defence mechanisms.

Scholarship informed by the lived experiences of bereaved mothers is in short supply and dads hardly get a look in at all. In 1997 Dr Judith Bernstein conducted a study with around 50 others similarly bereaved. She called the resulting book *When the bough breaks: forever after the death of a son or daughter*. The word *forever* is pivotal and prolific in metanarratives of child loss by bereaved parents. None of Bernstein's participants had any expectation of getting over their loss. They were doing their best to muddle through.

In 2017, Sara Ryan published an autoethnographic account of her experience of the sudden and preventable death of her son, Connor (Ryan, 2017). The manner of Connor's death meant that the family then had to endure a protracted inquest. John's death was unavoidable, and Connor's was not. We experienced kindness from family and friends following our loss and were generally ignored by the medical establishment. Sara and her family endured a lengthy ordeal at the hands of the legal profession. We both talk about PTSD, which Ehlers associates with sudden death. I experienced John's death as sudden because I had not accepted its inevitability. Connor's sudden death was different. It is not helpful to apply what Sara Ryan calls 'that grief theory bollocks' (which was largely conducted with populations other than bereaved parents) to every loss of every child. Although there are numerous studies which gaze in a medicalized way at the symptoms people in my situation display, there is very little insider perspective scholarship which takes a more nuanced view.

Disability adopts a peculiar place in the metanarrative about the loss of a child. In 2017, the story of terminally sick baby Charlie Guard was all over the news. Charlie's parents were unable to accept medical opinion that their baby was profoundly disabled and dying. Charlie was their beautiful boy, and of course, they were doing everything in their capacity to persuade the doctors to save him. Empathy for the young couple appeared to me to be in short supply. Having taught children with multiple and profound impairments and life-limiting conditions, I understand that love is unconditional and permanent. Researchers need to talk directly to bereaved families before applying labels like 'Complicated Grief'. They need to include parents of disabled children in these conversations and set aside any ableist assumptions.

Labelling the particular flavour of psychological reaction is only going to be useful to bereaved families if doing so results in some sort of useful intervention. Access to help without having to negotiate a medicalized gateway would be simpler. People able to pay can bypass referral and diagnostic obstacles, which hardly seems fair. Others who cannot afford to 'go private' may be able to access up to six sessions of Cognitive Behavioural Therapy (CBT) on the National Health Service in the UK. CBT is designed to challenge the client to think more positively about life events (Pearce, 2019). It would have been useless to me. There is nothing positive about the death of a young man of 25. Grief theorists agree that there is no quick fix, but long-term psychological therapy is only really available to people who can pay. I have not come across any research about psychological interventions with parents hospitalized after the death of their child.

Research into how bereaved families find help is lacking. The chances of being able to source mental health assistance while in thrall to PTSD, Complicated Grief, depression, anxiety, derealization, profound loss, and other flavours of unimaginable psychological pain are vanishingly slim. Resources could be signposted much more clearly. Peer support is available from charities such as The Compassionate Friends (TCF). Service providers, such as the GP, do not have access to any sort of directory which would name organizations such as TCF.

Research ethics are a bit of a minefield. I have contributed to research from my perspective as a bereaved mother. The location of the interview was, disconcertingly, in a psychiatric hospital. It was just a bookable university room but hardly a neutral space. The preamble and follow-up were rigorous, but I left feeling upset and patronized by the suggestion that I should go and have a nice cup of tea and a piece of cake afterwards. Questions like 'Do you know where your son is now?' floored me. Of course I know, but I could have done without the image of John in a cemetery. I just hope the findings translate into something of practical use.

Analytical discussion 2

Being at work

The previous section makes it quite clear that the loss of my son had a major impact on my mental health and the longer-lasting effects still persist, albeit in diminished proportions. In relation to being at work, it is clear to me both that work is not therapy and that having a job I love is an absolute lifesaver. Nevertheless, navigating the image I project in the workplace has become rather a complex balancing act between being honest and not freaking people out.

Roulstone and Williams (2014) observed that being open about disability at work carries a certain degree of ontological risk. Words like *cancer* and *bereaved mother* tend to conjure up uncomfortable images in people's imaginations (Dias et al., 2017; Tiedtke et al., 2017). Although honesty feels more important than attempting to curate myself in a favourable light in the hope of some future gain, I am aware that speaking openly about my grief might well lead people to draw their own conclusions about the state of my mental health. My protracted grieving and ticking time bomb cancer situation could well influence the way my colleagues see me and would probably make prospective employers think twice. If I were to apply for another job, I would not mention these inconvenient truths, despite being a fierce champion of the contention of the UK *Equality Act 2010* that disability is irrelevant to recruitment and reasonable adjustments are an entitlement for disabled employees. I recently heard from a prospective doctoral student who was troubled because cancer had been mentioned in their reference. This is not ok.

Undoubtedly, losing my son has influenced my subsequent career decisions alongside every other facet of my life. John died on 12 December 2012, and I went back to work on 03 January 2013. At the time I was Head of Disability and Wellbeing Services at the London School of Economics (LSE). Although I was able to act the part, I questioned my own integrity because the students' concerns seemed trivial to me in comparison to what happened to my son. Despite being nurtured and supported at LSE, I moved on. Academia UK popped up in the corner of my screen with an advert and I found myself sleepwalking into a new job in September 2013, without thinking it through. Amazingly, it was possible to go through the motions of an interview, and when asked if I was a firm candidate, my honest reply was, 'I don't know, my son died five months ago'. Somehow, in September 2013, I found myself as Principal Lecturer in Inclusive Education at London South Bank University (LSBU).

Currently, I am a professor of Imposter Syndrome at LSBU. I feel like a bit of a fraud. Professor of Imposter Syndrome is not my real title, but work is awkward because I know that I am the 13th fairy. Most of my teaching is in the Division of Education. Inevitably, child development is on the syllabus and I do talk about bringing up my children because it comes naturally to me to do so. In my head I am still a mum of three perfect adult children, Max, John, and Anna, 23 months apart, including identical twins.

Professionalism stops me from using work as therapy and I am very careful not to burden my students with my grief. If I am asked a direct question like 'How old are your twins?', I say: 'They were born in 1986'. It is problematic, I feel inauthentic and I wonder whether my colleagues, who all know, are quietly cringeing. My sense of self is impacted by my bereavement. I feel doubly stigmatized as that woman who lost her son to cancer, then got cancer herself.

Mothers are supposed to keep their children safe. I failed. The fact that I recovered is almost embarrassing.

In many ways I overcompensate at work. I feel like a pit pony. Every day I turn up and get on with it. Having dyspraxia presents its own challenges too, and I am often embarrassed and apologetic about all the things I am not very good at. Getting to grips with technology is not my forte and my short-term memory is very short term indeed, which does not make it any easier. Getting promoted to Professor shocked me. Before John died I was moving in that direction but afterwards I felt like a different person. Stuff on my CV which predated 2011 had become irrelevant to me.

Psychologically I knew I just had to keep going at work and at home. I knew I must not stop but I didn't really anticipate getting anywhere. Side by side in my head I experienced feelings of caring and not caring. During a conversation with my boss about whether something I had published was worthy of inclusion in the Research Excellence Framework submission, I remember thinking 'try to look as if you care'. Ambition had left the building and it was hard to see why any of it mattered. Only very recently I felt a twinge of annoyance with myself for not applying for a job which I had felt a hint of enthusiasm for and was probably right up my street. This is progress, maybe, of a sort.

As a researcher, I am wedded to the notion of 'nothing about us without us' (Charlton, 1998). Emancipatory principles (Watson, 2019) underpin everything I do as part of the Critical Autism and Disability Studies Research Group at LSBU. Our group is inclusive, and insider perspective is central to all our projects. We avoid the trap of milking insiders for their knowledge without even offering fair renumeration, and usefulness is always a primary concern. My experience, in relation to the study I described in the previous section, felt like being subjected to the medicalized gaze, rather than being an equal partner in an interaction with shared objectives towards making the world a better place for bereaved families. I am very committed to making sure that I do not make anyone feel like this.

Organizations such as TCF are sometimes approached by researchers and have to balance on a tightrope between the idea of not subjecting vulnerable people to possible harm, and contributing to something with the potential ultimately to be beneficial. When John first died, I was very vulnerable and would have talked to anyone about my experience of loss. Ethical protocols are there to protect vulnerable people. At work I am the ethics Rottweiler.

Currently, I am training part time to become a counsellor. It is quite possible that I will never practise, but I thought it might be interesting. I am acutely aware that my circumstances are relevant. Counsellors need to work ethically and to demonstrate congruence and unconditional positive regard. Comparing other people's experiences with my own and awarding myself the gold medal in the grief Olympics would not be helpful, but I might not be able to stop myself. Ethically, the therapist must make an informed judgement about their own competence and should signpost on if necessary. I imagine myself enacting counsellor behaviours such as active listening while thinking 'Too trivial' or 'Come on, Grandma was a hundred and three'. This is not unconditional positive regard. My experience of the death of my son is always going to be an influence. I would need to be absolutely honest with myself about how this may impact on my ability as a counsellor.

My interest in my colleagues and students is genuine. I feel like it is not my turn to climb the ladder of success but that I should be right there behind anyone who is hard working and ambitious. Encouraging other people actually gives me a sense of purpose. I would almost venture to suggest that I even feel like I might be a tiny bit good at it. Thank goodness for work. It gives me something to do which has a real purpose. At the end of every day I ask myself what I have done which has helped another person. If the answer is 'Nothing really', I will do something like fire off a random encouraging email. Maybe other people think this is part of my strangeness. Although I get good feedback about my contribution, derealization still stalks me. My sense of self left in late 2011 and has not returned fully. For this reason I could not possibly say what other people think of me because I just cannot work it out.

Analytical discussion 3

Keeping on buggering on

The most important thing in my life is my family, and the fact that I have two surviving children gives me a reason to keep buggering on. Work and personal life are not totally separate entities in my book. Work is good for me because it gives me a sense of purpose and is a major distraction. When writing, or even marking, I am mindfully absorbed in something other than my loss. I get the same feeling when I'm with friends and extended family and I am able to be supportive and engaged with their lives. My creeping lack of unconditional positive regard occasionally raises its ugly head and my inside voice says things like 'For goodness sake – it's only Australia – she'll be back' or 'So what? He can do his A levels again if necessary'. At least it is only my inside voice now, which is some sort of progress.

When John died I did not want to go anywhere or do anything ever again, but I had to because of my other son and my daughter. In relation to keeping on buggering on, I was going to work, seeing people, moving house, and apparently functioning as a sadder version of my usual self. In reality, my only concern was to keep going for my two other children and I was completely numb with grief. Carol Shields has the right words for this state of being:

> It happens that I am going through a period of great unhappiness and loss right now. All my life I've heard people speak of finding themselves in acute pain, bankrupt in spirit and body, but I've never understood what that meant. To lose. To have lost. I believed these visitations of darkness

lasted only a few minutes or hours and that these saddened people, in between bouts, were occupied, as we all were, with the useful monotony of happiness. But happiness is not what I thought. Happiness is a lucky pane of glass you carry in your head. It takes all your cunning just to hang onto it, and once it is smashed you have to move into a different sort of life.

(Shields, 2002, 1)

The fact is, after John, I regarded my happiness as completely unattainable, irrelevant, and undeserved. As well as my identity in the eyes of others shifting towards the tragic, in my own view I felt like a failure because I could not keep my son alive with my love. Seven years on and I am able to experience joy in muted colours. I no longer consider that what happened made a mockery of everything we ever did before as a family and everything we will ever do in the future. Socrates is associated with the expression 'an examined life is not worth living'. I have examined my life and I am living it with dignity, compassion, and love. Maybe my grief is still disabling and I am a worthy candidate for some of those labels from *DSM-5* (APA, 2013), specifically Complicated Grief. Maybe I am lucky enough to be surrounded with love and support and this takes the edge off.

It is possible to frame bereavement reactions in social model terms to an extent, in that good social support makes the whole vile experience more bearable and lack of social support makes it worse. Additional intersecting factors such as poor housing, unemployment, sickness, isolation, and money worries also contribute to making life feel like a bucket of shit. My life does not feel like a bucket of shit. One majorly shitty thing happened and some shit has stuck to my blanket, but it is still a nice blanket woven with love. My having cancer was not optimal, but I got off lightly there. I know other parents who have lost a child and have not been as lucky as I have in relation to social support, and have all sorts of other worries which I do not have about money, health, housing, and so on. Bereaved parents frequently talk about other people letting them down. Unwillingness to mention the name of the dead child, not marking anniversaries, crossing the road to avoid awkward encounters with surviving family members are all common experiences. None of these things apply in my case. It makes a huge difference. The fact that John's medical team did everything they could for him also helps. Unlike Connor Sparrowhawk, John's was not a death by indifference. My partner Mike says, 'At least we don't have to hate anybody'.

Often I imagine how John's life might have been. He would have graduated from Oxford four years ago. Maybe he would be working in a bookshop and married to a lovely man who shared his sense of humour. His sister, Anna is in America and I think he would have been a frequent visitor. Max and John would still look the same but different. John was always the less flamboyant dresser, although he might have changed in that respect. My three children were best friends. They inspire me. I am counting my blessings and know with absolute certainty that if I was given the choice of having John for 25 years or not, I would always choose to have that time with him.

Concluding discussion

I got over my cancer and filed it away. Some may regard this as unhealthy or a symptom of poor mental health. The Complicated Grief metanarrative undoubtedly floats around me but I reject its pathologizing connotations.

My work as a lecturer is a lifeline, but I am troubled by feelings of inauthenticity as I cannot exactly hit a bunch of students with the C bomb and expect them to come away unscathed, so I hide behind my professional cloak of invisibility in this regard. I do my best to be a decent person and a good enough employee. Encouraging other people motivates me more than other aspects of my work. Luckily, I do find my job distracting and interesting.

If I ever practice as a counsellor, I will wrestle my own self-obsession to the ground and work with the understanding that grief and loss come in all shapes and sizes. I will flex my empathy and positive regard muscles and keep them highly toned and be mindful of neither projecting my heartbreak on to others nor minimizing their losses by comparison with my own.

The majority of this personal narrative interrogates grief theory from the perspective of bereavement, and I acknowledge my own positionality as a bereaved mum. I only really know about my own grief. It is necessary to understand grief in detailed and subtle ways, rather than piling everyone into the Complicated Grief sack together and rolling us towards a mountain of pills.

Being surrounded by love is the best thing. Some people just know how to help because they are naturally kind and empathic. My family has not experienced people looking the other way. We are very lucky because we are secure and surrounded by kindness and always have been. Not everyone comes from a stable childhood and operates in a secure home with enough money and an army of people ready to help.

The intersection between prolonged profound grief and disability is complex. Applying a *DSM-5* (APA, 2013) label such as Complicated Grief to my situation does not strike me as a particularly productive thing to do. Having had cancer, I am notionally offered some protection by the *Equality Act 2010* as a disabled person. Politically I think this is a good thing. Emotionally, for reasons I explain in this chapter, I do not really associate cancer with myself because I closed the lid on that box some time ago.

References

American Psychiatric Association (2013) *Diagnostic and Statistical Manual of Mental Disorders: DSM-5*. Arlington, VA: American Psychiatric Association.

Bernstein, J. (1997) *When the Bough Breaks: Forever After the Death of a Son or Daughter*. Kansas City: Andrews McMeel Publishing.

Bowlby, J. (1969) *Attachment and Loss: Volume I: Attachment*. London: Hogarth Press and the Institute of Psychoanalysis.

Bowlby, J. (1982) Attachment and loss: Retrospect and prospect. *American Journal of Orthopsychiatry* 52 (4): 664.

Charlton, J. (1998) *Nothing About Us Without Us: Disability Oppression and Empowerment.* Berkeley: University of California Press.

Dias, N., Docherty, S. and Brandon D. (2017) Parental bereavement: Looking beyond grief. *Death Studies* 41 (5): 318–327.

Equality Act (2010) London: Stationery Office.

Field, N.P., Gao, B. and Paderna, L. (2005) Continuing bonds in bereavement: An attachment theory-based perspective. *Death Studies* 29 (4): 277–299.

Freud, S. and Strachey, J.E. (1964) *The Standard Edition of the Complete Psychological Works of Sigmund Freud.* London: Hogarth Press.

Granek, L. (2010) Grief as pathology: The evolution of grief theory in psychology from Freud to the present. *History of Psychology* 13 (1): 46.

Haig, M. (2015) *Reasons to Stay Alive.* Edinburgh: Canongate Books.

Klass, D., Silverman, P.R. and Nickman, S. (2014) *Continuing Bonds: New Understandings of Grief.* Abingdon: Routledge.

Kotzé, Z. (2014) Jung, individuation, and moral relativity in Qohelet 7: 16–17. *Journal of Religion and Health* 53 (2): 511–519.

Kübler-Ross, E. (1970) *On Death and Dying.* Oxford: Routledge.

Macmillan (2020) Macmillan Cancer Support. Available at: https://www.macmillan.org.uk.

Parkes, C.M. and Prigerson, H.G. (2010) *Bereavement: Studies of Grief in Adult Life* (4th edition). Hove: Routledge.

Pearce, C. (2019) *The Public and Private Management of Grief.* Cham: Palgrave Macmillan.

Roulstone, A. and Williams, J. (2014) Being disabled, being a manager: 'Glass partitions' and conditional identities in the contemporary workplace. *Disability and Society* 29 (1): 16–29.

Ryan, S. (2017) *Justice for Laughing Boy: Connor Sparrowhawk - A Death by Indifference.* London: Jessica Kingsley Publishers.

Scott, S.M. (1997) The grieving soul in the transformation process. *New Directions for Adult and Continuing Education* 1997 (74): 41–50.

Shields, C. (2002) *Unless.* London: Fourth Estate.

Stroebe, M., Schut, H. and Boerner, K. (2010) Continuing bonds in adaptation to bereavement: Toward theoretical integration. *Clinical Psychology Review* 30 (2): 259–268.

Tiedtke, C.M., de Casterlé, B.D., Frings-Dresen, M.H.W., De Boer, A.G.E.M., Greidanus, M.A., Tamminga, S.J. and De Rijk, A.E. (2017) Employers' experience of employees with cancer: trajectories of complex communication. *Journal of Cancer Survivorship* 11 (5): 562–577.

Watson, N. (2019) Agency, structure and emancipatory research: Researching disablement and impairment. In Watson, N. and Vehmas, S. (Eds.), *Routledge Handbook of Disability Studies* (2nd edition). Abingdon: Routledge.

White, C. (2013) *Living with Complicated Grief.* London: Sheldon Press.

Worden, J.W. (2018) *Grief Counselling and Grief Therapy: A Handbook for the Mental Health Practitioner* (5th edition). New York: Springer Publishing Company.

13

THE METANARRATIVE OF HIV AND AIDS

Losing track of an epidemic

Brenda Tyrrell

Preliminary discussion

In a moment of breaking the fourth wall, AIDS activist Sarah Schulman (2012, 45; emphasis mine) challenges her readers,

> *Do you know what I mean when I refer to 'AIDS of the past'?...* Where folks my age watched in horror as our friends, their lovers, cultural heroes, influences, buddies, the people who witnessed our lives as we witnessed theirs, as these people sickened and died consistently for fifteen years. *Have you heard about it?*

Not only is the result of this challenge illuminating and self-incriminating, but it also focuses on Schulman's personal narrative of HIV and AIDS. This approach keeps the reader grounded in the fact that HIV and AIDS is not simply a story, an overarching metanarrative with blank-faced individuals and ravaged bodies that get retold and reimagined the further we get away from Patient Zero. As she pleads with her readers not to forget the indeterminable loss of life, property, income, security, dignity, and compassion during the early years of the crisis, she confesses, 'I am driven by its enormous, incalculable influence on our entire cultural mindset and the parallel silence about this fact'. This chapter, too, is driven by AIDS of the past while, at the same time, leaning into how that past shapes and directs AIDS (and HIV) of the present and future.

On 5 June 1981, the Centers of Disease Control (CDC) released a statement in its *Morbidity and Mortality Weekly Report* (*MMWR*) on what would rapidly evolve into the HIV and AIDS epidemic. In a detached clinical tone, the statement announced that between October 1980 and May 1981, five young men, 'all active homosexuals' (Kaiser Family Foundation (KFF) @2018), obtained treatment for *Pneumocystis carinii* pneumonia at various hospitals in Los Angeles. The report continues to define the men by their social and sexual histories, listing not only their sexual orientation but also their purported drug uses. Not quite one month later, on 3 July 1981, *the New York Times* (NYT) published its first news article on the unfolding events. The NYT report is not the first coverage of the epidemic – both the *Associated Press* and *the Los Angeles Times* reported their findings on the same day and the *San Francisco Chronicle* reported its findings the next day (KFF@2018). Although the CDC and these doctors did not know it, these reports are only the beginnings of the newly emerging HIV and AIDS epidemic.

As it turns out, the world could not prepare for or predict the far-reaches of this epidemic or the systematic discrimination that happened to various populations, most notably gay men. From the first news articles about the epidemic, the patients are identified by their *sexual orientation*; indeed, as controversial activist Andrew Sullivan (1996) posits:

> In the past, plagues were often marked by their lack of discrimination, by the way in which they laid low vast swaths of the population with little regard for station or wealth or sex or religion. But AIDS was different from the beginning.

> As early as 1982, the CDC (KFF@2018) clarifies that the high-risk categories they set forth ('male sexuality, intravenous drug abuse, Haitian origin, and hemophilia A') should not be used to 'justify discrimination or unwarranted fear of casual transmission'. Despite this declaration, identifying these risk factors leads to a catastrophic othering which results in an assumed and natural link between homosexuality and HIV and AIDS. For example, Paula Treichler (1999, 53) reports that journalist David Black pithily reduces the risk factors into the '4-H Club' – that is, 'homos, heroin addicts, Haitians, and hookers', making the risk *factors* into *individuals* who purportedly practice risky behaviors. This early overarching metanarrative of HIV and AIDS comes at a high cost: by relegating this quickly emerging crisis to the gay population, and thus, not a concern for the unaffected population, a significant lack of support from health care providers and government agencies results, forcing community-based providers to establish their own health initiatives and outreaches. It is also important to recognize that the KFF timeline, while useful for mining data, is mostly focused on the United States, creating an inaccurate summary of the epidemic that features only one overarching metanarrative of HIV and AIDS, that of the United States being the most affected nation. Whiteside (2016, xiv) notes that 'The burden is not borne equally. It is the deprived and the powerless who are most likely to be infected and affected. AIDS is primarily a disease of the poor, be they nations or people'. Moreover, I argue, this practice leads to continued misunderstandings that the epidemic is nearing its end.

Notably, these swift and biased reactions mirror our current response to COVID-19. With the unexpected and swift emergence of the coronavirus, it is even more likely that the overarching metanarrative of COVID-19 will displace the landscape-changing effects of HIV and AIDS, as media, health care, various other entities, and even close friends continue to refer to COVID-19 as the worst pandemic in over a century (paraphrased). One reason for this may be in simple word choice – while COVID-19 is continually referred to as a pandemic, HIV and AIDS are still categorized as an epidemic. While this discrepancy seems minor, as discussed below, it has deep reverberations in the way the normate, heterocompulsory public considers the impact of COVID-19 and irresponsibly replaces it as the worst pandemic, some say, ever. Unfortunately, the negative impact that COVID-19 has had on the HIV and AIDS epidemic may be just as devastating, resulting in delayed medication delivery, inability to seek and receive medical care (due to stay-at-home orders, etc.), and so forth. Moreover, HIV and AIDS have a complicated relationship with illness and disability: The simple fact that individuals can carry the virus in their bodies long before it actually manifests as illness makes this virus especially dangerous and difficult to define as a disability.

This chapter considers the metanarrative of HIV and AIDS by examining three of its aspects. First, I discuss how the impact of certain words and acronyms inform the way the general public views HIV and AIDS, and how these same words and acronyms perpetuate the continued fear and stigmatization of those experiencing the virus. Within this discussion, I also analyze the use of the word *AIDS* in two science fiction texts, one early in the epidemic and one later, and discuss the linguistical power behind this word and how the science fiction trope of extrapolation allows the genre to imagine a future where 'the AIDS' is eradicated. Next, I compare two well-known authors, Schulman and Susan Sontag, and consider the effectiveness of Sontag's overarching metanarrative of HIV and AIDS when compared with the more individual narrative of Schulman in how the initial impact of the crisis is remembered. Finally, this chapter examines the ever-changing restrictions of US blood donation placed on gay and trans men and the impact of COVID-19 on those currently experiencing HIV and AIDS.

Methodological discussion

I must admit that when the volume editor asked me about my 'positionality' to this metanarrative, I scrambled to identify exactly what that is. What qualifies me, as one who does not experience HIV or AIDS, at least directly, to identify and critique this metanarrative? This question, I would argue, is one of the most contentious questions in the field of disability studies. Cripistemology scholars Johnson and McRuer (2014, 130) argue for 'the importance of challenging subjects who confidently "know" about "disability", as though it could be a thoroughly comprehended object of knowledge'. More importantly, for my work, cripistemology 'does not assume epistemic privilege for the disabled person' (130). In other words, one does not have to be identified as disabled to be experienced about it or to 'claim crip' when writing about it. Kafer (2013, 12) wonders what the impact would be on understanding the political nature of disability if we 'imagin[ed] a "we" that includes folks who identify as or with disabled people but don't themselves "have" a disability'. There is, of course, worry about misguided appropriation of this approach (McRuer, 2006); however, Kafer (13) insists that 'Claiming crip … can be a way of acknowledging that we all have bodies and minds with shifting abilities'. Along these same lines, I follow Kafer's (2013, 11) approach that 'do[es] not rely on a fixed definition of "disability" and "disabled person"' and her political/relational model (6) that intentionally blurs the distinctions between the medical and social models of disability. By challenging the seemingly unbreakable bond between impairment and disability, this chapter considers how this approach helps us think about those undiagnosed with HIV as able-bodied, even though they still technically have the virus and, more importantly, may inadvertently contribute to the spread of the virus.

Applying critical discourse analysis (CDA) to my work is also helpful because, as Margaret Price (2009) reminds us, CDA analyzes the inseparable connection between words and their societal impact. Price also clarifies the relationship between CDA and disability studies, positing that it 'concerns itself with human difference, and emphasizes the ways that people with disabilities are ostracized, medicalized, heroized, and otherwise pushed out of the societally-defined space' of what non-disabled folks might consider 'normal'. Given that much of my work is based in literature (words) and disability studies, and that this chapter addresses one such group of those historically ostracized, I utilize CDA to examine the language and rhetoric of HIV and AIDS as 'primary mechanism[s] of [power relationships]' (Price, 2009). Finally, I approach this chapter under the tutelage of Price and Shildrick's (2002, 64) resistance to the notion that 'there is some privileged standpoint from which disabled people alone can speak – as though theirs is the only "authentic" understanding of the specific embodiments in question'. In my particular case, I bring a view from behind what some might consider enemy lines – as part of the medical profession.

I was 16 years old, still in high school, and working at a care facility as a nursing assistant (NA) during the earliest years of the crisis. Initially, there was little knowledge on the spread of the virus or how to decrease the spread; but I (we) soon became aware that the days of gloveless resident cares were over. Wearing gloves then became a point of tension between administration and my fellow NAs as the availability of gloves decreased and the price soared; as that was nearly 40 years ago, I do not recall the exact price, but I do remember the phrase 'Five dollars a pair' floating around every time we asked for gloves. At first, we were only allowed one pair of gloves *per shift*, which meant washing our gloves (still on our hands) between residents which, as we know now, actually degraded the protective qualities. More significantly, the residents resented these new safeguards, feeling targeted, and repeatedly felt the need to assure us that they did not have 'the AIDS'.

As I entered the nursing profession several years later, one application question still stays with me: 'Check here if you will find taking care of a patient with AIDS ethically or morally challenging'. I left it blank, thinking 'of course I wouldn't, what nurse (or other medical professional) would?' However, when I took care of my first patient with full-blown AIDS, I was terrified. Questions flooded my mind as I prepared to enter their room for the first time: What if there were open areas on my skin that were so minusculely small that I couldn't see them? Or, what if there is blood in the urine and it spills or leaks through my gloves? I wanted so badly to double-gown, double-glove, double everything (single gown, glove, and mask were the standard protocols in the mid-1990s) but I resisted. And somehow, despite this overwhelming fear, I remembered that the patient I was about to encounter was still a person who deserved the best care I could provide and my respect and support. In my 18-plus years of nursing, I had two needle sticks – one was a needle slip and the other was because the sharps container was not emptied by the previous shift. Both times, I underwent about nine months of testing (each) before I was considered virus-free. The last time was especially difficult because I was also trying to start a family and there was a possibility that I might be pregnant. Although the pregnancy test came back negative, starting a family was put on hold until I tested virus-free. In sum, although the above represents one view from the medical lens, it also supports my concerns about the continued stigmatization of the virus because I, as a non-disabled person, experienced (and enacted) them myself.

A second factor that drives my interest in this metanarrative results from my research with science fiction and disability studies and the recent shift in science fiction critique to view HIV and AIDS as a more optimistic experience that creates a differently abled/minded (and superior) species. As rightly pointed out by several activists and scholars, this action runs the risk of forgetting the initial devastating effects of this pandemic on certain populations (which continues today for some), as well as the global reach of the pandemic. Schulman (2012, 14) calls this effect 'gentrification of the mind', which she explains thusly:

> Since the mirror of gentrification is representation in popular culture, increasingly only the gentrified get their stories told in mass ways. They look in the mirror and think it's a window, believing that corporate support for and inflation of their story is in fact a neutral and accurate picture of the world.
>
> *(28)*

Nearly a decade into the crisis, science fiction scholar Jeffrey A. Weinstock (1997, 83–84) recognizes this gentrification of the mind, noting the profound connection between the computer virus and AIDS that 'result[s] in the subsumption and problematic conflation of the mechanical and biological under the larger term *Virus*'. He continues that this 'virus rhetoric' is not problematic because it 'collapses the distinction between body and machine ... but, rather because [it] attempts to efface the lived-reality of human beings' (84).

In the years following the immediate impact of the virus, however, other science fiction scholars (Thomas, 2000; Lynch, 2001) put forth the notion that science fiction's depictions of the HIV and AIDS epidemic are an opportunity for the human population to develop and mutate into a being with heightened or superior skills than what currently exists. While this more expansive approach to HIV and AIDS appears to be a more positive and inclusive way to interpret the events that so dramatically changed the global landscape, it also requires us to ask, *should* we do that? This question is especially important when considering the lived futurity of those living with HIV and AIDS. And, significantly, individuals that remain undiagnosed; as Whiteside (2016, 22) reminds us, HIV is a lentivirus, a slow-acting virus, which means that the virus can remain dormant for a very long time. Whiteside (2016, 15) starkly notes:

> People infected with HIV remain so for the rest of their lives. The only way they leave the pool of HIV infection is by dying. This means the prevalence [i.e. absolute number of people infected] can continue rising even after the incidence [i.e. number of new infections over a given period of time] has peaked.

One can see the danger, then, of assuming that a cure, or simply preventing the transmission of the virus, will immediately end the epidemic and erase HIV and AIDS from our future.

Analytical discussion 1

The power (and erasure) of words

There is little doubt of the fear invoked by the initialism and acronym *HIV* and *AIDS*, which are at times carelessly tossed about in current conversations and often used interchangeably. However, it is important to remember two points about these shortened harbingers: First, they are two very different stages of the virus and preventing/treating/curing one does not necessarily result in the same results for the other. Moreover, the conglomeration of letters that make up each abbreviation succinctly identifies the function and result of each stage of the virus. The letters designated as AIDS or, in its long form, Acquired Immunodeficiency Syndrome, are what Whiteside (2016, 2) calls 'accurate[e]', it is acquired, which results in an immune system deficiency, and it is not a single disease, it consists of several – i.e. a syndrome. Named early in the crisis (1982), it is the result of the Human Immunodeficiency Virus (HIV), which proved harder to pin down and name, taking nearly five years to identify (1987). Second, the development of these acronyms represents more than simply a diagnosis; it represents part of the overall stigmatization of the virus itself. Indeed, in the early days of the crisis, the two are married with a slash (HIV/AIDS) because the acquiring of HIV led to death in 100% of the cases. It is not until later, after the development of a medicinal regime for HIV, that the two are separated into HIV *and* AIDS. While this action is, for the most part, a sign of success, it is also an easy way to forget that simply treating and preventing HIV does not automatically ensure a cure for AIDS.

When COVID-19 made its first appearance, I noticed that the *pandemic* descriptor was applied almost immediately. While I am not saying it is not a pandemic, I am left wondering why and how health organizations, the media, the government, and nearly everyone else determined that COVID-19 is a pandemic, but HIV and AIDS are not. An overwhelming number of artefacts refer to the HIV and AIDS crisis as an *epidemic* when, in fact, *pandemic* might be the more appropriate word choice. The CDC (@2012) defines an epidemic as 'an increase, often sudden, in the number of cases of a disease above what is normally expected in that population in that area'. To me, this definition creates two conflicting points about HIV: first, the disease *must already be present* in an area to have this sudden increase and, second, the outbreak is isolated in a *certain* population in a *certain* area. This is not the case with HIV. A pandemic, however, as defined by the CDC, is 'an epidemic that has spread over several countries or continents, usually affecting a number of people'. This definition clearly applies to both COVID-19 and HIV, as both viruses travel across borders indiscriminately. Although this distinction may seem trivial, it is important to remember the social and cultural weight that each word carries: individuals and groups are much more likely to pay closer attention to a pandemic, rather than epidemic, if one is aware of the disparate definitions. As a result, when two landscape-changing viruses exist at the same time, one (COVID-19) will not subsume the other (HIV).

While it was quite easy to write a fictional narrative involving HIV and AIDS in the early days of the epidemic, it was incredibly difficult to find an agent to accept it or an editor willing to publish it. Indeed, in the earliest days of the epidemic, using the word *AIDS* in print was clearly taboo. In her short story, 'The Way We Live Now' (1986), Susan Sontag does not mention the word *AIDS* once; however, there is little doubt that this is the condition that the character Max has acquired. In the publication history of his *Journals of the Plague Years*, Norman Spinrad reports that, although originally written in 1988, he was unable to publish the story as a short novel until 1995 because his agent surmised that 'no publisher will touch it with a fork. Because they know the distributors will shun it like the, uh, plague, too'. Spinrad (1995, 142) expands on her concern that the topic was 'too frightening' and 'that the public was in too deep a state of denial, out of which they had no desire to be roused'. Spinrad was not to be dissuaded, however, and the outline was finally published in 1995 – *sans* the word *AIDS*. All of this is not to say that science fiction writers remained complacent in the stigma of writing about AIDS and HIV. One clear example of this is found in William Gibson's *Virtual Light* (1993). In this novel, Gibson, widely recognized as the father of cyberpunk, which developed alongside the AIDS and HIV crisis, goes so far as to extrapolate a vaccine for 'the AIDS' (1993, 22) through the use of HIV-infected blood. Gibson's approach is singular: minor (and corporally absent) character J.D. Shapely first hovers in the background from the beginning of the book but, as the story unfolds and rushes to its denouement, Shapely's history and importance to the plot rapidly evolve into a full-blown character deserving the title of main protagonist.

The first appearance of Shapely is seen through the eyes of the main protagonist, Berry Rydell, who is lecturing his partner on the importance of getting the fictional vaccine to prevent getting 'the AIDS' (Gibson 1993, 22). As Rydell scoffingly notes, 'Prayer-hanky won't keep any AIDS off … Get yourself vaccinated, like anybody else' (22). While he is proselytizing, Rydell stares through his rear-view mirror at a 'street-shrine' dedicated to Shapely:

> Somebody had sprayed SHAPELY WAS A COCK-SUCKING FAGGOT in bright pink paint, the letters three feet high, and then a bright pink heart. Below that, stuck to the wall, were postcards of Shapely and photographs of people who must've died. God only knew how many millions had. On the pavement at the base of the wall were dead flowers, stubs of candles, other stuff.

In this quote, Gibson divulges several issues surrounding AIDS: first, and foremost, the growing mortality rate of the epidemic. The *MMWR* (KFF@2018) reports that in the United States AIDS was the number one cause of death in men ages 25–44 in 1992 (the year leading up to the publication of *Virtual Light*). Alongside of the trenchant death toll, Gibson also hints at the forgotten faces and lives behind the postcards and photos of the people who perished in the early days of the crisis. With the words 'SHAPELY WAS A COCK-SUCKING FAGGOT in bright pink paint, the letters three feet high', Gibson brutally identifies Shapely's lived reality by his sexuality and, in a larger context, the many other gay men being targeted and stereotyped as being deserving of or causing the epidemic. Ultimately, Shapely is murdered by 'fundamentalist Christians' (1993, 230); however, his impact on the world of the novel, as compared to Gibson's lived reality, cannot be understated because, as he reminds us: 'the live vaccine bred from Shapely's variant had saved uncounted millions' (350), a vaccine that we are still striving for today. Notably, his murderers' actions speak loudly to the fact that AIDS and HIV are initially identified as a '"gay plague" that, Weinstock (1997, 84–85) posits, is 'interpreted as divine judgement visited upon the heads of sinners'.

Along with identifying the clear connections Gibson makes to what he (contemporarily) sees happening around him, it is also important here to acknowledge Gibson's use of extrapolation as he creates a world that is able to find a vaccine for AIDS. We should keep in mind that *there is still no vaccine for HIV*. To some, after nearly 40 years of research advancements and no vaccine thus far, this approach may appear self-defeating. However, to others, it offers another lived reality to hope for; with writers like Gibson who keep 'the AIDS'

in the forefront, perhaps a future without epidemics is not such an extrapolation after all.

Analytical discussion 2

Sontag v. Schulman in competing metanarratives of HIV and AIDS

When thinking about the metanarrative of HIV and AIDS in terms of an
overarching metanarrative versus a more personal narrative, analyzing two high-
profile writers, Susan Sontag and Sarah Schulman, in conversation about HIV
and AIDS is quite revealing. Undoubtedly, most readers are somewhat familiar
with Sontag's *AIDS and Its Metaphors* (1989) that is housed alongside her other
well-known essay, *Illness as Metaphor*, in which she famously theorizes the role
of metaphor in illness. Writing nearly a decade later, Sontag briefly highlights
various aspects of *Illness*, Sontag (1989, 102) explains that understanding the
purpose of book carry high stakes because 'the metaphoric trappings that deform
the experience of having cancer have *very real consequences*: they inhibit people
from seeking treatment early enough, or from making a greater effort to get
competent treatment' (emphasis mine). The words 'very real consequences' are
important here, especially when, as omniscient readers, we know what is coming:
HIV and AIDS. Cancer, Sontag notes (104), loses some of its metaphorical punch
with the emergence of AIDS: 'And not least among the reasons that cancer is
now treated less phobically, certainly with less secrecy, than a decade ago is that
it is no longer the most feared disease'.

   After Sontag tallies the various ways that the AIDS epidemic has been used to
push political and religious platforms to the foreground, she elucidates that even
'[w]ith the most up-to-date biomedical testing, it is possible to create a new class
of lifetime pariahs, the future ill' (120–121). The very real consequences reveal
themselves more clearly here as Sontag (120) points out: 'Testing positive for HIV
(which usually means having been tested for the presence not of the virus but of
antibodies to the virus) is increasingly equated with being ill'. Put another way,
the 'infected but not ill' backlash 'reviv[es] the antiscientific logic of defilement,
and make infected-but-healthy a contradiction in terms', also creating a 'social
death that precedes the physical one'. And this 'social death' is enhanced by further
consequences in terms of finding and/or keeping a job, housing, medical care,
and so forth. More harshly, Sontag (160) notes that AIDS, or becoming infected,
'obliges people to think of sex as having, possibly, the direst consequences: suicide.
Or murder' (160). The 'murder' Sontag refers to is the reaction of some carriers to
continue having unprotected sex and not informing their partner of their positive
HIV status. In the last pages, Sontag (181) adds,

> But it is highly desirable for a specific dreaded illness to come to seem
> ordinary. Even the disease most fraught with meaning can become just an

illness. … It is bound to happen with AIDS, when the illness is much better understood and, above all, treatable.

It is within this last quote that two questions are raised: first, is AIDS 'just an
illness', and second, should it be considered 'ordinary'? Sarah Schulman addresses
these questions, 30 years after the start of the epidemic; however, for now,
Sontag's narrative serves as an overarching metanarrative that encompasses large
swaths of individuals who have, or might have, HIV and AIDS.

Schulman writes her text quite a bit later than Sontag; however, this delay does
not mean she is not invested or writing during the beginnings of the epidemic.
As Schulman begins to recount her experiences with the epidemic, the reader
senses immediately that she is experiencing this epidemic in a much different
manner than Sontag. She describes (25–26):

It is not a conspiracy, but simply a tragic fact of historic coincidence that in
the middle of this process of converting low-income housing into housing
for the wealthy, in 1981 to be precise, the AIDS epidemic began.

There are absolutely no metaphors in this sentence; in other words, while Sontag
writes her metaphorical analysis of AIDS, Schulman takes more of a boots-to-
the-ground retelling. She continues (26):

In my neighborhood … over the course of the 1980s, real estate conversion
was already dramatically underway when the epidemic peaked and large
numbers of my neighbors started dying, turning over their apartments
literally to market rate at an unnatural speed … The process of replacement
was so mechanical I could literally sit on my stoop and watch it unfurl.

Clearly, Schulman writes from an entirely different place than Sontag; she
writes from a place where, like myself, she does not experience HIV or AIDS
personally, but she experiences them nonetheless. This more personal narrative
causes the reader to react viscerally to Schulman's text, whereas Sontag's, while
still important, encourages a more philosophical reaction.

The reason Schulman writes *Gentrification* is expressly translucent from page 1:
as Schulman listens to an NPR interview in which the announcer proclaims, '[a]t
first America had trouble with People with AIDS … But then, they came around'
(2), Schulman's reaction was swift: 'I almost crashed the car' (2); she is furious at
this historicization of the AIDS epidemic, thinking '*Oh no … Now this … Now,
they're going to pretend that naturally, normally things just happened to get better …
This? This is going to be the official history of AIDS?*' (2–3). From there, Schulman
walks the reader through the basement level of the beginning struggles to get
something, *anything*, started to help those affected by the epidemic. She declares
that 'We cannot let the committed battle of thousands of people, many to their
deaths, be falsely naturalized into America "coming around",' noting that '[n]o

one with power … "comes around". They always have to be forced into positive change. But, in this case, many of the people who forced them are dead' (3).

This fact is made even more transparent as Schulman begins working as the director of ACT UP:

> All these years of conducting interviews, we had been focused on conveying the heroism of ACT UP. *But we had not succeeded at conveying the suffering.* We had conveyed how profoundly oppressed we had been … And we certainly had not addressed the consequences of AIDS on the living. No one had. Something had happened between A and B. Something had been erased. Some truth had been forgotten and replaced.
>
> *(emphasis mine; 11)*

For Schulman, what happened at the start of the epidemic should no longer be the focus; rather, the *consequences* of what happened must be moved to the foreground. Here, we hear a whispering of Sontag's 'very real consequences' noted above. Once they realize this misstep, Schulman and her cohort add both the birth date *and* the death date to each activist in their project to emphasize that all of the leaders in the early activism of HIV were no longer living. Here, we see another very real consequence and one that speaks to the power of the personal narrative of HIV and AIDS when compared to the more overarching metanarrative. Treichler (2012, 256) points out another key difference between Sontag and Schulman: '[o]ne does not really see Sontag, the quintessentially elite intellectual of the twentieth century, hanging out at street fairs, gay and lesbian parades, and vegan potlucks', whereas, 'Schulman was intimately involved in the New York queer community's response to the mysterious syndrome that came to be known as HIV/AIDS'. Given these elemental differences, it is not surprising that, on the surface, these texts appear radically different. However, this observation should not be taken as a way to diminish Sontag's work.

Analytical discussion 3

The positive boon and destructive curse of blood

Fröhlich and Davidson (2016, 262) ask a crucial question when considering the cultural and medical influence of blood: 'Why blood? Once noticed, blood seems to flow, trickle, and ooze everywhere, its presence filling works on history, theology, politics, medicine, social criticism, and creative texts'. Only with HIV and AIDS, blood does not 'flow, trickle', or 'ooze', it floods, gushes, and coagulates into systemic and long-term discrimination, especially where blood transfusions and donation restrictions are concerned. During the earliest years of the crisis, this systemic discrimination is directed at anyone who gives (or receives) blood, including those who depend on it to exist.

Michael Davidson (2008, 35) describes how advances in the late 1970s for the treatment of haemophilia allow for an easier, more cost-effective way of receiving treatment. However, these purported life savers soon turned deadly: Although receiving blood products that might contain other viruses, such as hepatitis, is always a risk, the advent of HIV and AIDS presented an even deadlier contamination. As early as 1982, the CDC and the Food and Drug Administration (FDA) began receiving death reports of haemophiliac patients but, instead of fully investigating the distributive blood centres, the FDA 'did nothing, fearing a panic that would severely diminish the blood supply' (2008, 36). The results of these deaths and the FDA's reluctance to mandate any distributive restrictions led not only to multiple lawsuits and the National Hemophilia Foundation (NHF) insisting that blood centres institute screening procedures, but also the transmission of HIV to a significant percentage of the nation's (then) 20,000 haemophiliacs.

Even though the NHF's request is put forth in 1983, it is not until 1985 and the appearance of the AIDS antibody screening tests that the blood screening actually began, screening procedures that demanded a lifelong ban for gay men. The ban lasted from 1985 to 2015 and has only recently been relaxed amongst much protest, fear, and prejudice. When I started drafting this chapter, the restrictions towards gay and trans men, referred to as MSM – men who have sex with men – by the American Red Cross (ARC), included a deferment of 12 months 'from the most recent sexual contact' (ARC 2017). To be clear, this restriction applied to *monogamous* relationships as well; in other words, a man who wishes to donate blood and is in a monogamous relationship must abstain from sex with their life partner *for 12 months*. The abstinence policy also applies to trans men whose assigned birth sex is female. Despite the organization's assertions that 'We believe all potential blood donors should be treated with fairness, equality and respect' (ARC 2017), this restriction is clearly discriminatory towards gay and trans men. Put another way, one would not expect a heterosexual couple to abstain from sex for *any* number of months in order for one or both partners to donate blood.

Ironically, it is the appearance of COVID-19 that encouraged the FDA to decrease the deferment time to three months in April 2020. The *American Journal of Managed Care* (@2020) reports,

> The FDA has announced a relaxing of its restrictions on gay men being allowed to donate blood, in light of the coronavirus disease 2019 pandemic. Instead of 1 year, if a male has had sex with another male, he need only wait 3 months to donate blood.

The words 'he need only wait 3 months' prove problematic; in this context, it seems as though gay and trans men should be *grateful* that their deferral is only three months. Moreover, it is only the impetus of cancelled blood drives and a 'drop-off of 86,000 fewer blood donations' (Shaw, 2020) that gay and trans men are 'allowed' to donate blood. To me, this shortened deferral time, which appears outwardly progressive, still reeks of prejudice and a subtle hint that, should things go back to normal in terms of blood donations, gay and trans men would, once again, be the target of an increased deferral time.

Concluding discussion

In 1996, a mere 15 years into the crisis, Andrew Sullivan famously declared the AIDS epidemic to be nearing an end. Retrospectively, this declaration seems a bit hurried; however, there is a plethora of activity in the epidemic's course between 1995 and 1996, which leads to Sullivan's declaration. To name a few (KFF@2018), the advent of medication regimes such as HAART and, as a result, a significant, and first, decrease in new AIDS diagnoses (in the United States) since the beginning of the crisis. Alongside of this, HIV falls off the top of the cause-of-death list for all (white) Americans from 25 to 44 – though, in this same age group in African-Americans, there is no change – and the US FDA approves several HIV testing methods, including the viral load, urine, and home test kits. In short, there is a reason for Sullivan to risk making this bold statement. Alas, Sullivan's aspirations faltered.

More recently, the impact of COVID-19 on individuals experiencing HIV or AIDS has, for the most part, gone unrecognized. This misstep represents yet another way that HIV and AIDS *personal* narratives are in jeopardy: They are not only superseded by the overarching metanarrative of HIV and AIDS, but they are also now at risk to be consumed by the metanarrative of COVID-19. As mentioned above, the terminology of how we identify AIDS and HIV as an epidemic and COVID-19 as a pandemic certainly plays into this perception; however, it is crucial to consider the 'very real consequences' (Sontag 1989, 102) that this displacement has on individuals experiencing HIV and AIDS. In a recent *NPR* interview, Ukrainian AIDS advocate Anton Besenko (Brink, 2020) observes that 'For people with HIV, it's double, triple the crisis since the start of the lockdown … I have a bad feeling that organizations and governments are so concerned on COVID that they are completely forgetting about HIV. For marginalized people, it's a question of life and death'. If the reduction of deferral for gay and trans men to donate blood is any indication, it would seem that Besenko's concerns are real. And, this concern is not expressed just in the global arena; in the United States, researchers and physicians express worry that 'AIDS is already being set back by COVID-19' (Brink, 2020). Put another way, the metanarrative of HIV and AIDS, if we are not careful, is about to be consumed by the metanarrative of COVID-19.

What is at stake if the COVID-19 metanarrative overtakes the HIV and AIDS metanarrative or, if we assume that, because of recent advances in research and medical management, we are on the brink of curing HIV and AIDS? The statistical data provided by Whiteside (2016, 4) speaks to this conundrum: 'At the end of 2015, more than thirty years after the virus was identified, an estimated eighty-two million people have been infected with

HIV, and of them over forty-one million have died from AIDS-related causes'. Preventing the transmission of HIV (with daily medicine like PrEP) is certainly making an impact; however, this prevention does not equate to an automatic resolution to those living with AIDS. With the addition of COVID-19 to this already turbulent landscape, the aforementioned population will feel the brunt as quarantines and transportation across borders delay much needed medical supplies. Moreover, something as simple as proper nutrition effects the progression of the virus, as Whiteside (28–29) posits that basic needs such as a healthy diet and drinkable water can actually increase the virus's advance in these individuals. In sum, as Weinstock (1997, 96) rightly reminds us: 'The danger is not forgetting what a virus is, but what it does. As society isolates certain segments of the population, splintering and blaming, society macroscopically recapitulates the action of the infection with the body itself'. Schulman (42) adds,

> We still have to work every day to assert the obvious, that in fact there are two distinctly different kinds of AIDS that are not over: there is AIDS of the past; there is ongoing AIDS. Neither is over, although they are treated quite differently in the present moment.

By rejecting the all-encompassing metanarrative of HIV and AIDS and, now, COVID-19 and embracing more personal narratives like Schulman's (and, perhaps, mine), the incredible impact of the HIV and AIDS crisis will be remembered and curated.

References

Altman, L. K. (1981) Rare Cancer Seen in 41 Homosexuals. *The New York Times* [online]. 3 July. [Accessed 7 July 2020]. Available from: https://www.nytimes.com/1981/07/03/us/rare-cancer-seen-in-41-homosexuals.html/.

American Red Cross (2017) Blood Donation Eligibility for LGBTQ. [Viewed 6 July 2020]. Available from: https://www.redcrossblood.org/donate-blood/how-to-donate/eligibility-requirements.html.

Brink, S. (2020) What Happens When A Pandemic and An Epidemic Collide. NPR [online]. 14 July. [Accessed 17 August 2020]. Available from: https://www.npr.org/sections/goatsandsoda/2020/07/14/890492472/what-happens-when-a-pandemic-and-an-epidemic-collide.

Centers for Disease Control. (2012) Principles of Epidemiology. [Accessed 27 July 2020]. Available from: https://www.cdc.gov/csels/dsepd/ss1978/lesson1/section11.html.

Davidson, M. (2008) *Concerto for the Left hand: Disability and the Defamiliar Body.* Ann Arbor: University of Michigan Press.

Fröhlich, S. and Davidson, M. (2016) Introduction: Blood bound. *Journal of Literary and Cultural Disability Studies* 10 (3): 261–269.

Gibson, W. (1993) *Virtual Light.* New York: Bantam Books.

Kafer, A. (2013) *Feminist, Queer, Crip.* Bloomington: Indiana University Press.

Kaiser Family Foundation (KFF) (2018) *Henry J. Kaiser Global HIV/AIDS Timeline.* [Accessed 6 July 2020]. Available from: https://www.kff.org/global-health-policy/timeline/global-hivaids-timeline.

Johnson, M. and McRuer, R. (2014) Cripistemologies: Introduction. *Journal of Literary and Cultural Disability Studies* 8 (2): 127–147.

Lynch, L. (2001) 'Not a virus, but an upgrade': The ethics of epidemic evolution in Greg Bear's Darwin's radio. *Literature and Medicine* 20 (1): 71–93.

McRuer, R. (2006) *Crip Theory: Cultural Signs of Queerness and Disability.* New York: NYU Press.

Price, J. and Shildrik, M. (2002). Bodies together: Touch, ethics and disability. In M. Corker and T. Shakespeare (Eds.), *Disability/Postmodernity: Embodying Disability.* New York: Bloomsbury, 62–75.

Price, M. (2009) Access imagined: The construction of disability in conference policy documents. *Disability Studies Quarterly* 29 (1): 6.

Schulman, S. (2012) *The Gentrification of the Mind: Witness of a Lost Imagination.* Berkeley: University of California Press.

Shaw, M. (2020) FDA's Revised Blood Donation Guidance for Gay Men Still Courts Controversy. American Journal of Managed Care [online]. 4 April. [Accessed 17 August 2020]. Available from: https://www.ajmc.com/view/fdas-revised-blood-donation-guidance-for-gay-men-still-courts-controversy.

Spinrad, N. (1995) *Journals of the Plague Years.* New York: Bantam Books.

Sontag, S. (1989) *Illness as Metaphor and AIDS and Its Metaphors.* New York: Picador.

Sullivan, A. (1996) When Plagues End. *The New York Times.* 10 November. [Accessed 7 July 2020]. Available from: https://www.nytimes.com/1996/11/10/magazine/when-plagues-end.html.

Thomas, A. M. (2000) To devour and transform: Viral metaphors in science fiction by women. *Extrapolation* 41 (2): 143–160.

Treichler, P. (1999) *How to Have Theory in an Epidemic: Cultural Chronicles of AIDS.* Durham: Duke University Press.

Treichler, P. A. (2012) Collectivity in trouble: Writing on HIV/AIDS by Susan Sontag and Sarah Schulman. *Amerikastudien/American Studies* 57 (2): 245–270.

Weinstock, J. (1997) Virus culture. *Studies in Popular Culture* 20 (1): 83–84.

Whiteside, A. (2016) *HIV and AIDS: A Very Short Introduction.* Oxford: Oxford University Press.

14

THE METANARRATIVE OF SARCOIDOSIS

Life in liminality

Dana Combs Leigh

Preliminary discussion

It has long since been argued that illness and disability are not synonymous. Indeed, one can exist without the other, and the lived experiences of each, critically, are full of complexities and nuance, each unique. However, they share many important similarities, namely the objectification by the normate subject, and the common notion from said subject position that they, the object, are 'deviant', somehow defective, and should be fixed and cured (Clare, 2017; Garland-Thomson, 1997). As a result of the power inequities such positions inherently demand, it is from an assumed authority that the metanarratives of the ill and disabled are dictated, often silencing the individual voices of those who have actually lived the experience in question. This can result in ongoing under-representation in all facets of society from film to politics, and lead to further inequalities and oppression.

Sarcoidosis itself, strictly but simply speaking, is a *disease*, an immune-mediated inflammatory condition with an incidence of 5–40 people for every 100,000 per year (British Lung Foundation, 2020). It often presents as possible lymphoma or lung cancer, and sarcoidosis patients become all too familiar with the words 'at least it's not cancer' (Weltin, 2020). It is true that for many this comes as a huge relief; their sarcoidosis comes and goes, and leaves little to no experience of illness. It is also true that for others, sarcoidosis results in significant morbidity and impairment, which leads to lower quality of life and disability (Drent, Strookappe, Hoitsma, and De Vries, 2015), and also death.

In this chapter, I contextualize sarcoidosis within the spectrums of disease/illness/impairment/disability. By exploring the differences and similarities in the experiences of these bodymind conditions and the models used by medical and social scientists alike, we can begin to evaluate the effects on those living with the conditions. This includes their resulting ongoing representation in media, culture, and politics, and their treatment by social authorities and society in general (Garland-Thomson, 2002).

Though somewhat limited in its direct examinability, due to the relative rarity of sarcoidosis (NHS, 2020) and subsequent lack of portrayal, the metanarrative of the condition offers, first, a significant chance to analyze the metanarrative of chronic, invisible illness as a whole. Its metanarrative's effect on those who live with sarcoidosis (and similar illness and disability) is not diminished by the specific condition's scarcity. Reducing the sarcoidosis experience to a generalized one of chronic illness could risk the very validity of our insistence that recognition of the individual narrative is vital. However, in this case, it simply shows that regardless of our exact diagnoses, we are similarly excluded and often reduced to tropes and stereotypes when included in narratives at all.

I begin my analysis by examining potential explanations for such lack of literary and cultural representations of chronic illness in narrative, looking at audience satisfaction, how we cope and make sense of ourselves and the world by telling stories (Broyard, 1992; Frank, 1995; Storr, 2019), and how disease is related to the 'art' of narrative. Focusing on popular culture, I then analyze the fleeting representations of sarcoidosis in two award-winning, American prime-time dramas: *House, M.D.* (Shore, 2004–2012) and *NCIS* (Bellisario and McGill, 2003–), both watched by millions, and both reducing sarcoidosis to simple tropes and convenient conclusions. Finally, I explore the 'true story' of sarcoidosis: analyzing the language used in information sources, which are generally deemed trustworthy. I examine the prolific rise of the medical and illness non-fiction and the potential impact of memoir on the future of chronic illness in narrative.

Underpinning all of this is my personal 15-year experience of living with sarcoidosis in multiple countries under vastly different health and social care systems. As a creative writer myself, I also briefly critique my own part in the ongoing metanarrative of sarcoidosis and chronic illness, and the social responsibility we all possess as scholars, policymakers, medical and creative practitioners, and simply fellow human beings.

I would like to note my intentional use of the metaphors most easily available to me when discussing what is so commonly called an 'invisible illness'. This means that some language could seem ocularnormative (Bolt, 2014), but it is my hope that in a volume like this, it would be obvious that this act is an intentional one, used to further illustrate the power of any normate subject position and its reductive nature.

Methodological discussion

Critical discourse analysis (CDA) offers an appropriate starting point when setting out to analyze the cultural representations of chronic illness. By focusing on the language that society uses to communicate within and throughout its hierarchies, how everything is represented, how each story is told, by whom, and under what conditions, we can analyze the stories around us. However, the more we begin to examine such discourse of ourselves, the more we change what we're examining. Autoethnography itself recognizes the impossibility of the complete and total objectivity of human observation (Adams, Ellis, and Holman Jones, 2015). This is true in formal observational settings and in everyday social interaction. Such subjectivity is inevitable when coexisting in society, even within confining constructs.

'Disability Studies' has, in recent decades and particularly in the United Kingdom (Shakespeare and Watson, 2002), focused intently on the shift from the medical to the social model in its vital efforts for change. No longer do disabled people need to be 'fixed' or 'cured' (Clare, 2017); it is instead societal attitudes and policies that need to be altered. Though successful in raising awareness and removing some barriers, it has had the unfortunate effect of neglecting the true embodiment of disability, creating a divide between the 'healthy' and 'unhealthy' disabled (Wendell, 2001). For the 'unhealthy' disabled, there is often a required medicalization to maintain quality of life. This complicates the cure debate due to the obvious desire of many ill people to be, at the very least, acknowledged in their suffering and treated for their symptoms.

Another hierarchy seemed to emerge, excluding and oppressing at times (Shakespeare and Watson, 2002), just as social structures tend to do. Those of us with invisible conditions, chronic pain, and other 'non-traditional' disabilities have been left wondering where and how we fit into society at all. Though there are undeniably more power inequities in certain societal relationships, we can all take turns being object or subject, being observed or doing the observing (and the judging). It is, therefore, the normate's *or* fellow disabled person's expectations alike that can create 'additional disability by making it harder for … individuals to feel good about themselves' (Goering, 2015). A large part of feeling good about ourselves is a sense of identity and belonging. We look to society to find such things, analysing and evaluating how we all fit together. If we are lucky, society will acknowledge and even reflect our identities. But many of us are not always so fortunate. Either way, it should not end there, as 'all analysis and evaluation has political implications' (Hall, 2019). Surely then, we must continue to re-evaluate and re-analyse, on a constant quest for representation that recognizes disability in all its manifestations, including the more bodily focused experience of illness, pain, and suffering.

Consequently, a complementary approach should be embraced, one which does not just ask questions of and examine the power structures it initially seeks to disrupt, but that continuously critically examines itself and the hierarchies which naturally continue to be created within (Minich, 2016; Schalk, 2017). Through a truly holistic and humanistic biopsychosocial model (Petasis, 2019; Shakespeare, Watson, and Abu Alghaib, 2016; Wade, 2017) of illness and disability and the approach afforded by 'reframing disability studies as methodology' (Minich, 2016), we can begin to establish a new 'critical disability studies' (CDS). CDS 'responds to the traditional disability studies project by pointing to its limits … including … downplay of pain and suffering' (Hall, 2019), and we can at once examine the cultural and philosophical studies of illness as disability in all its realities. Although nomenclature can get messy, and clearly cross meanings through disciplines, I suggest that in this chapter, I primarily utilize the present volume's autocritical discourse analysis method in a sub-field of CDS that can be termed 'illness studies'. I almost prefer the even messier, 'critical illness studies', but this obviously invites certain assumptions that I am getting busy with scientific studies of so-called critical illnesses.

A phenomenological methodology can also be beneficial in our studies of disability and illness (Hall, 2019). One method in particular, life-writing, has become a massive market in modern publishing (Walker, 2019) and therefore contributes significantly to current culture. Through a phenomenological approach, my own lived experiences as observed by myself contribute to my authority over my own illness narrative. However, my own authority is often overridden by the assumed authority afforded through the power inequities that are initiated by the 'clinical gaze' (Foucault, 1973). While in hospital, I am reminded by red letters stamped across my files that I do not have the authority to read notes written about me. If I wish to access them, I must formally request to do so (Davies, 2012). Weeks of my own complex hospital experiences are reduced to a couple of short paragraphs in the 'medical narrative' section of my discharge papers, which often include inaccuracies and language, which reduces me to a dehumanized object. I am not even Dana, I am simply, 'the patient'. Through life-writing, blogs and memoirs, many of us who are ill and disabled are reclaiming our narratives, our authority, and authorial voices.

My experiences of sarcoidosis (and the constellation of conditions which often orbit a chronically ill person) have been rife with pain and suffering and resulted in multiple disabilities. The disease has impacted virtually my entire body at one time or another. Due to its effects on my lungs, I spent two years wearing oxygen every time I moved. I felt my disease, illness, impairment, and disability acutely every time I wound those plastic tubes behind my ears and across my upper lip, adjusted the dial to my prescribed litres per minute. On the rare occasions I ventured out in public, my appearance invited curious, awkward, and lingering glances, but also consistent offerings of other people's seats.

When I was 26 years old, I received my first implanted defibrillator when the sarcoidosis was discovered in my heart. This can be relatively well hidden, but simply knowing you have a computerized machine inside you can be unnerving, especially when it alarms. I have experienced transient visual and neurological impairments, including a cranial nerve palsy which gave me severe double vision for several months, leaving me unable to see or walk down a hall without intense headaches and nausea. I have also suffered from reversible cerebral vasoconstriction syndrome (RCVS), causing hypertensive crises and thunderclap headaches, which are known as one of the most painful conditions that exist (Ogden, 2017; Singhal, 2019). Additionally, I had a tonic-clonic (previously known as grand mal) seizure, and had to give up driving for a minimum of a year.

Scarring in my small intestine has led to several obstructions, requiring urgent surgery to remove parts of me, though not yet resulting in an ileostomy bag. My recurrent pain and nausea from this often leave me unable to participate in daily life. I also live with postural orthostatic tachycardia syndrome (PoTS), which is an autonomic nervous system disorder, leaving my body malfunctioning when I stand up, my heart racing, blood pressure unstable. At times, I black out. It is not dangerous in itself but is certainly debilitating when at its worst. I also enjoy the 'bonus' of a permanently dislocated coccyx, which causes significant, at times severe, chronic pain. All of these experiences have increased my already present anxiety and depression, and I have been left traumatized.

There is much more, of course, but I suspect this quick list of some of my illness experiences could qualify me to some level of authority on living with what I do. This should bestow upon me some 'credentials' which my doctors treating me, however well-educated and experienced in their observations they may be, will never have. As a creative writer, my writing forms part of my own phenomenological practice and potentially contributes to the cultural representation of illness and disability. I am, therefore, also conscious and critical of my own authority as expressed through my authorship of creative output, particularly in the form of fiction.

Analytical discussion 1

An invisible condition lived in the in-between

Sarcoidosis results in a specific type of inflammation called granulomas: growths of white blood cells. Though not malignant in themselves, granulomas and the scar tissue they can leave behind are capable of impairing the functioning of virtually any organ or body part. With a predilection for the lungs and lymphatic system, it can also wreak havoc on the heart, liver, eyes, brain, spinal cord, bones, spleen, and more. Notably, one of its more outwardly damaging manifestations is on the skin. Indeed, it was not until 1877, when sarcoidosis was first recognized as a 'dermatological curiosity' (Sharma, 2020), that it was first identified and given a name at all, which, originating from Greek, essentially means 'fleshy'. This itself illustrates the way in which the visibility of a disease or disability can potentially impact its awareness and recognition.

In many ways, it is no wonder that the metanarrative of sarcoidosis as a chronic illness is stripped away of its myriad manifestations and often true chronic nature. Western society has been conditioned to expect certain narrative arcs and conclusions since classical antiquity, in the face of illness or otherwise. From Aristotle's *Poetics* (350 BCE) to Freytag's *Technique of the Drama* (1863) and Campbell's 'Hero's Journey' (The Hero with a Thousand Faces, 1949), we have come to expect certain things from our stories and their protagonists. This includes, of course, fiction or real life, in any one of the infinite stories that swarm around us. What then, is it that we expect from a narrative and its protagonist? We expect a journey and to be moved, persuaded. Authors (of any type) do this through rhetoric, and in the case of illness narratives, primarily pathos. The 'rhetoric of sympathy' (Garland-Thomson, 1997, 17) is often employed in stories of illness and disability to achieve the desired outcome (new policies or simply satisfaction of an ending, a sense of catharsis). Pathos is indeed an interesting notion to examine. Not only do we find its derivative, 'path', as the root word of sympathy, but we can also trace its evolution of meaning from emotion to suffering, and finally, to disease, seen in modern words such as *pathogen*.

It is also interesting to highlight the link between disease and the narrative in general in the ancient Greek word, *krisis*, which meant judgement (seen now in the word *critic*) and evolving by several hundred years ago, into the English, *crisis*, which was at that time used literally to denote the turning point in a disease where the ill would either heal (and be cured) or die. Currently, the word *crisis* is hard to escape, as it has come to encompass so many critical moments of both judgement and disease. The 'critical disease' process mirrors the common expectations of an audience, but 'chronic illness' does not. It appears far too convenient to rest on the crisis of disease itself when telling stories of illness, ignoring the complexities. The true experiences of chronic illness do not often result in imminent tragic, even romantic, death or the 'happily ever after' of a cure.

It is natural for humans to form our experiences into stories (Storr, 2019) and it can be beneficial for us when trying to make sense of illness or disability (Frank, 1995). Anatole Broyard speaks in *Intoxicated By My Illness* (1992) of his experience of prostate cancer, how he wished to bring it 'under control by turning it into a narrative' (1992, 19). When we turn experiences into narratives, we often turn to metaphor in a bid to make sense of things we do not understand, to try to glean meaning from our emotions, from pain and suffering, that of ourselves and others. Susan Sontag famously both recognized and cautioned against using '*Illness as Metaphor*' (1979). Though Broyard might believe that Sontag is 'too hard on metaphor' (1991, 18), I cannot help but be swayed by his apparent obsession with the 'critical' nature of his illness (indeed he mentions it in such terms no less than thirteen times, in addition to his references to being a literary critic himself) and his wish to find 'style', how his friends found his '*performance* courageous' (1992, 42, my emphasis). It is, of course, his own narrative to find, to experience, to witness, to share, and I certainly do not blame him for framing his experience in whatever way worked for him. However, he admits that he is an older man, one who has avoided illness until later in his life and that

> Illness is primarily a drama, and it should be possible to enjoy it as well as to suffer it. I see now why the Romantics were so fond of illness – the sick man sees everything as metaphor.
>
> *(Broyard, 1992, 10)*

It is here that he draws the clear line between 'drama' and the everyday, the incessant, even monotonous, experience that is that of chronic illness. Audiences tend to get bored of monotony that lacks drama, an existence that simply is, without a satisfying ending with which they can neatly tie up a story.

Sontag, though dubious of the overuse of metaphor, referred to a kingdom of the sick (Sontag, 1979), and this is certainly a metaphor that is helpful for this discussion. Due to its invisibility and reduction of personal experience, those with sarcoidosis are often refused entry at the border to the kingdom of the sick. Sometimes, we are deported at a later date, told by doctors and loved ones alike that 'at least it's not cancer' (Weltin, 2020; White, 2016). This so-called consolation is a common strand of the metanarrative of sarcoidosis, offered through assumed authority and implying we are not really that ill at all. However, since we are ill, despite the assumptions of others, we cannot simply return to the kingdom of the well either. We often become stateless citizens of nowhere. We may find some comfort in the shared experiences of disabled people of all variety, and yet, we are often denied entry to the 'kingdom of the disabled' as well. There is an assumed authority that often patrols such borders. We are often, quite literally, questioned when accessing areas such as disabled toilets or parking spaces (O'Malley, 2019; Williams, 2019) if we do not appear obviously disabled. Laurie Edwards reflects upon her experience through reference to the kingdom metaphor in her own book, noting that she is 'literally ... crossing Sontag's threshold' (Edwards, 2013, 30) simply by entering a hospital as a patient. Though she also acknowledges that 'chronic illness is somewhere in the middle', and that it is 'confounding and unfamiliar' (Edwards, 2013, 10). Accordingly, we are often left with little sense of permanent residency, and of any resulting identity.

Ill and disabled people are often used as spectacles (Bolt, 2014; Garland-Thomson, 1997), whether or not the protagonist. As Mitchell and Snyder tell us:

> while stories rely upon the potency of disability as a symbolic figure, they rarely take up disability as an experience of social or political dimensions.
> *(2000)*

Though our illness and disability experiences are often filled with ongoing crises, sometimes of a 'critical' nature in the pathological sense, but also, crises of identity, of representation, of belonging, of access, those very 'social or political dimensions' (Mitchell and Snyder, 2000) that structure reality and our ongoing experiences, they are still often relegated to the side-lines (Garland-Thomson, 1997). Similarly, if we are 'lucky' enough to be recognized as either sick or disabled, we may be reduced again to metaphor, but still stuck on the peripheral. Either way, whether in fiction or not, the established expectations set out by the metanarrative convinces the audience (who is observing in judgement) to reject the more complex experiences in favour of their preconceived ideas and prejudices.

Analytical discussion 2

As seen on TV (fiction as reality with audiences of millions)

Television is a medium of communication and entertainment that for several decades has pervaded the lifestyles of most Western households and can therefore have massive impacts on the metanarratives of anything they portray. Studies show television's effects on social identity (Harwood and Roy, 2002), and that 'minorities on television can help increase social tolerance, but differences in the substance and quality of these portrayals likely condition this link' (Garretson, 2015). Thus, the portrayal of chronic illness in general and sarcoidosis specifically, not only affects how ill people think of themselves but also contributes to their treatment in society.

Shows like *Grey's Anatomy* (Rhimes, 2005-) and *CSI: Crime Scene Investigation* (Zulker, 2000–2015) have been incredibly popular despite, or perhaps due to, their formulaic structure and predictability. *CSI: Crime Scene Investigation* (Zulker, 2000–2015) in particular is known for its inaccurate portrayal of forensic science. However, it appears most viewers believe what they see on such shows to be true (Druckman and Bolsen, 2011).

House, M.D. (Shore, 2004–2012) was a massive success, attracting tens of millions of viewers in over 50 countries, and once being dubbed, 'the world's most popular TV show' (*Huffington Post*, 2009). Its protagonist, Dr. Gregory House, is an opiate addict who suffers from chronic pain, walking with a limp and a cane. Additionally, it seems possible that his 'genius' diagnostic abilities matched with his *dis*-abilities (physical and mental) are not only evidence of the trope of bestowing disabled characters with special powers, but also an attempt to compensate for the reduction and objectification of people that is necessary for the show to function as it does. The show revolves around illness and its disabling effects, thrives off of presenting the oddities, rarities, and complexities of disease. However, it is still a medical drama from the perspective of a doctor, in this case where each episode serves as a mystery to be solved. Each one features the 'critical' patient, with House coming to the rescue in the nick of time with a diagnosis and cure.

Sarcoidosis and lupus are amongst the characters' favourite differential diagnoses (Martin, 2009). In fact, it has become such a common joke among the sarcoidosis community and beyond that some even playfully suggest to 'drink every time they say sarcoidosis' (Robertson, 2008).

It is finally in the 5th season that the correct diagnosis is indeed sarcoidosis. In 'House Divided' (Yaitanes, 2009), a teenage boy, Seth, suffers a debilitating headache and falls suddenly to the ground. Seth's story involves a debate on 'curing' impairments, how his social identity is closely linked to his deafness. It is worth noting, but not directly relevant to this chapter, as it does not create the 'crisis' on which this narrative relies. Seth is struck with sudden blindness and House and his team find lesions in his brain, briefly entertaining the diagnosis of brain cancer. Predictably, as the metanarrative dictates, it is not cancer. Seth continues to experience severe symptoms, including incontinence and deadly arrhythmia before the team confirm the diagnosis. The whole sequence of Seth's story is not completely medically accurate or immediately believable. However, considering this volume argues in favour of acknowledging the individual experiences of illness and disability, perhaps I can accept that Seth's experience of sarcoidosis was simply not of a typical sort. Perhaps we can even forgive the show's ongoing use of tropes and reliance on 'crises to be cured' in the name of entertainment.

The major problem with the portrayal of sarcoidosis in *House, M.D.* (Yaitanes, 2009) is how quickly the notion of any lasting impact of the disease is dismissed. When Seth's mother asks the doctors if her son's newly diagnosed sarcoidosis is treatable, one of House's team, Thirteen, replies, nodding and seemingly pleased: 'usually responds to corticosteroids and methotrexate. I'll start the meds' (Yaitanes, 2009). Seth is then shown in his hospital bed, no longer appearing to be experiencing a single ailment, symptom, or impairment. He appears *totally* cured. In actuality, it usually takes weeks to notice an improvement from sarcoidosis with such medications, particularly methotrexate, which can take up to 12 weeks to work (NHS, 2020). High-dose intravenous corticosteroids can work much faster but often bring severe side effects. Regardless, Seth is shown just hours later, with no IV, apparently experiencing no side effects. He is never shown discussing the long-term implications of such a diagnosis or its treatments. He simply chats happily to his mother from his bed, without a hint of anything that has just occurred.

The last thing we hear of him is when House's boss, Cuddy, tells House that his patient is 'doing fine' (Yaitanes, 2009). The audience is left with the impression that sarcoidosis has made no lasting impact on Seth's quality of life and that no disabilities will continue to result from the illness, despite the dramatic nature of his apparently transient disabilities earlier. The audience is effectively offered the satisfaction of a cure, left to move on to watch and enjoy House's next Holmesian medical mystery.

NCIS (Bellisario and McGill, 2003–) falls into a similar metanarrative trap. The show misses an opportunity to represent sarcoidosis as the chronic and disabling illness it too often is. A main character, Vance, the Director of NCIS in the show, has 'a major health scare' (CBS, 2020), which turns out to 'just' be sarcoidosis. A discussion among Vance's family and colleagues, including friend, Dr 'Ducky' Mallard, goes as follows:

Dr. Mallard (laughing). He's going to be fine.
Kayla. Really? There's nothing wrong with him?
Dr. Mallard. No, Kayla, nothing serious.
Lara. What is it?
Dr. Mallard. Well, the biopsy revealed the spots on your father's lungs are not lymphoma, but rather, sarcoidosis. It's a viral condition that mimics cancer on CAT scans and X-rays.
Gibbs. So, it's not cancer?

Dr. Mallard. No.
Lara. Thank God.
Gibbs. Does it require treatment?
Dr. Mallard. In most cases, no. (Bellisario and McGill, 2003–)

In this example, sarcoidosis is not only entirely miscast as a viral condition, but they also utilize the 'at least it's not cancer' (Weltin, 2020) trope and, once again, reduce sarcoidosis to its metanarrative. Vance does not have symptoms, does not require treatment, and the disease is never mentioned again. Both shows rely on the drama of disease (or in Vance's case the potential diagnosis) with a neat and tidy conclusion, both effectively offering a 'cure' for a disease which has none.

Analytical discussion 3

Based on a true story

It seems very reasonable that trusted organizations, sources which people wanting information would commonly look to first, these days online, would want to reassure the newly diagnosed sarcoidosis patient that they will most likely not experience the more extreme and deadly variations of the disease. Though most websites mention the possibility of more severe impacts from the disease, the language used is often reductive and limiting, nearly to the point of excluding such possibility at all.

Though it is not inaccurate to say 'most people with sarcoidosis do not need treatment' (NHS, 2020) or that 'if your sarcoidosis is causing you pain … a pain-killer such as ibuprofen or paracetamol can help' (British Lung Foundation, 2020), such statements reduce sarcoidosis to something of little significance and imply that it can be treated by over-the-counter medications. These are often the first things a person reads about sarcoidosis, and could be what they continue to believe.

This is especially problematic when it comes to friends and family who have looked it up, and continue to insist it is nothing serious. Interpretations can often rely on the precise use of words. When Harvard Medical School says, 'a few develop more serious illness' (2020), this can leave us having to convince those people, loved ones, strangers, or doctors alike, that maybe, just maybe, we are some of the supposed 'few'. Unfortunately, the assumed authority of the metan-arrative can make this practically impossible.

Other organizations appear, however, to recognize the myriad realities, using language which is not so restrictive and reductive:

> Each patient's sarcoidosis is unique. It can affect any organ and, while some sarcoidosis patients are able to live reasonably normal lives, many others endure chronic pain, organ damage and a very poor quality of life.
>
> *(University of Hull, 2019)*

Though science loves to be specific in its methods and results, focusing on its numbers, quantifying everything, the way this information is relayed (to themselves and the public) often fails to recognize or represent the minority, and, again, unintentionally generalizes each illness experience it seeks to understand, undermining some particular efforts of the biopsychosocial model of illness (Wade, 2017) and the recognition of the importance of individuality and inclusion. It often feels like we chronically ill folks are trying to persuade doctors and society alike with 'the fallacy of anecdotal evidence' to convince others that what we experience is true. However, we are not ignoring scientific evidence; we are simply asking not to be generalized by said evidence and numbers, the very kind of 'hasty generalizations' (Groarke, 2001) the anecdotes are said to create in the first place. Perhaps it is finally time to 'integrate scientific evidence with people's experiences' (Karvonen, Kestila, and Mäki-Opas, 2018). It is possible, and I argue preferable, to combine the quantifiable with the qualitative when interpreting such complex bodymind experiences, and how best to approach them as an integrated society.

Though it can prove difficult to find fiction that represents or portrays the indefinite and complex nature of chronic illness at all, specifically sarcoidosis, there is a wave of medical and illness nonfiction sweeping through the literary world. From Porochista Khakpour's *Sick: A Memoir* (2018) to former junior doctor, Adam Kay's *This is Going to Hurt* (2017) and to doctor-come-patient, Paul Kalanithi's, posthumously published memoir, *When Breath Becomes Air* (2019), there is an obvious interest in the realities and representations of illness and health. And yet, fictional protagonists with chronic illness and disability remain elusive.

Memoirs are the beginning of a narrative. They are the stories we tell ourselves about our own lives, the phenomena we observe, a first level of mimetic representation. It is my suggestion that the surge of the illness memoir is, like 'the first wave of any struggle' (Davis in Bolt, 2014, 134), a step towards equal and accurate representation in cultural output and media, and ultimately, to becoming authors (and authorities) of our own illness experiences, captured in all their complexities, no longer limited to the memoir, but represented in fiction as well.

I have, so far in my research, been unable to find a work of literary fiction that portrays sarcoidosis. There are, however, several memoirs. It seems that even within memoir, we are too often prone to turning illness into metaphor. *Model Patient: My Life as an Incurable Wise-Ass* (2000), by self-confessed C-list celebrity, Karen Duffy, seems to look for meaning behind the illness that stops her in her career as a model. Though perhaps self-deprecatingly, she blames herself for her disease. Amidst ongoing celebrity name-dropping, which seems to sensationalize and dramatize her story, she finds advantages to being sick, lessons to be learned, and she has a 'big fat happy' (Duffy, 2000, Chapter 20) ending. Again, I cannot blame anyone for finding reason or meaning behind their own illness experience, but I fear that this approach perpetuates potentially damaging tropes and stereotypes we are all expected to fulfil in our illnesses.

Nora Gallagher's *Moonlight Sonata at the Mayo Clinc* (2013), though vastly different to Duffy's, and a beautifully observed story, similarly relies on expectations. This memoir is framed in a traditional linear structure, where her crisis, somewhat like that of a *House, M.D.* (Shore, 2004–2012) episode, is framed as a mystery, with the final diagnosis acting nearly as the 'cure'. Sarcoidosis is not even mentioned until the last several pages, when she is finally, after nearly two years, given the long-awaited diagnosis which might offer hopeful options for treatment. For Gallagher, her sarcoidosis experience is primarily with optic neuritis, an inflammation of the optic nerve, which impairs her vision and threatens blindness. There are lyrical passages and Gallagher spends a great deal of her time exploring faith and meaning, questioning the nature of suffering. But mainly she relies on the idea of, the metaphor of, the journey, so much so that she uses literal maps as narrative tools and compares her illness to falling into 'Oz'. Like Broyard (1992), Edwards (2013), myself, and so many more, Gallagher revisits Sontag's (1991) kingdom metaphors. For Gallagher, these kingdoms may be even more metaphorical, allegorical perhaps, existing in spiritual planes in relation to her faith. As if to illustrate the liminal nature of sarcoidosis, Gallagher names the middle section of her book, 'Limbo'. As expected though, she does not remain there. In the final part, entitled, 'Recalled to Life', a labyrinth is used to symbolize how, by finding her diagnosis at last, she has found her way out of the maze, finally back home (much like any good hero's return), a place in which she knows how to identify herself.

Memoirs are the anecdotes, but they are also the evidence, even when moulded into metaphor and squeezed for meaning. It is hopeful that there is currently so much more representation of illness and disability in life-writing and I hope it is a step towards the 'normalizing' of such conditions. Though it is refreshing to see a protagonist that is ill or disabled, and to be moved by their 'inspirational journey', or their 'courageous battle', I, myself, will find much more satisfaction when we can simply be part of the everyday social fabric, when we can exist as we are, somewhere and someone in between, and it is not only our illness or disability that makes us worthy of such representation.

Concluding discussion

The stories we observe, the stories we tell, the ones that get repeated, over and over, are often the ones told through the assumed authority gained by power inequities of the social structures and ongoing lack of representation. This will keep us in a cycle where the metanarratives of disability and illness ignore the individual experiences so many of us live through, stripping us of some of our identity along the way. Living with sarcoidosis can often mean a life of straddling the threshold, of being stuck in liminal space between ill and well, disabled and non-disabled. When the very limited portrayals and representations of the condition seem to either dramatize or dismiss our experiences, it can impose an artificial identity, one dictated by the assumed authority and not one found for ourselves.

This assumed authority not only affects the day-to-day social interactions of disabled people but also bleeds through to the actual authority of governmental policymaking. Even the supposedly more inclusive biopsychosocial model can be used to create barriers by blaming ill and disabled people for their conditions and attempting to restrict their access to the very things designed to give them equality, such as the United Kingdom's Personal Independence Payment (Shakespeare, Watson, and Abu Alghaib, 2016). The social model of disability focused intently on removing barriers and gaining in 'accessibility'. However, it becomes evident that even the more holistic biopsychosocial model as it stands today, which can encompass the experiences of chronic illness and pain, fails to address fully the barriers that already exist and those that the various models themselves also create. I contend it is the very notion of place and access which continues to affect disabled people and that the barrier to access reaches far into the identity politics of disability. The extant social structures can leave us with both little access to identity (via the places and spaces, both literal and figurative, which could afford us so) and identities which continue to limit our access to our own authority and adequate representation. It is by breaking down the metanarratives of disability and reclaiming our individual authority that we can begin to claim our space in society.

References

Adams, T., Ellis, C., and Holman Jones, S. (2015). *Autoethnography*. New York: Oxford University Press.

Aristotle (350 BCE). *Poetics*.

Bellisario, D. and McGill, D. (2003–). NCIS. S. *12, E. 2. 'Kill the Messenger'*.

Bolt, D. (2014). *The Metanarrative of Blindness: A Re-Reading of Twentieth-Century Anglophone Writing*. Ann Arbor: University of Michigan Press.

British Lung Foundation (2020). *Sarcoidosis Statistics*. Retrieved July 2020, from Lung Disease in the UK: https://statistics.blf.org.uk/sarcoidosis.

Broyard, A. (1992). *Intoxicated by My Illness*. New York: Fawcett Columbine.

Campbell, J. (1949). *The Hero with a Thousand Faces*. New York: Pantheon Books.

CBS (2020). *Everything You Need to Know About this Season of NCIS*, CBS. Retrieved August 2020 from: https://www.cbs.com/shows/recommended/photos/1004050/everything-you-need-to-know-from-this-season-of-ncis/.

Clare, E. (2017). *Brilliant Imperfection: Grappling with Cure*. London: Duke University Press.

Davies, P. (2012). Should patients be able to control their own records? *British Medical Journal*, 345 (Patient Centred Care): 24–25. Accessed at https://www.bmj.com/bmj/section-pdf/187619?path=/bmj/345/7871/Feature.full.pdf.

Drent, M., Strookappe, B., Hoitsma, E., and De Vries, J. (2015). Consequences of sarcoidosis. *Clinics in Chest Medicine* 36 (4): 727–737.

Druckman, J. N. and Bolsen, T. (2011). Framing, motivated reasoning, and opinions about emerging technologies. *Journal of Communication* 61: 659–688.

Duffy, K. (2000). *Model Patient*. London: Harper Collins.

Edwards, L. (2013). *In the Kingdom of the Sick*. New York: Bloomsbury.

Foucault, M. (1973). *The Birth of the Clinic*. Abington: Routledge.

Frank, A. (1995). *The Wounded Storyteller*. Chicago: University of Chicago Press.

Freytag, G. (1863). *Technique of the Drama*. Chicago: Scott, Foresman.

Gallagher, N. (2013). *Moonlight Sonata at the Mayo Clinic*. New York: Vintage Books.

Garland-Thomson, R. (1997). *Extraordinary Bodies*. New York: Columbia University Press.

Garland-Thomson, R. (2002) Integrating disability, transforming feminist theory. *Feminist Formations* 13 (3): 1–32.

Garretson, J. (2015). Does change in minority and women's representation on television matter?: a 30-year study of television portrayals and social tolerance. *Politics, Groups, and Identities* 3 (4): 615–632.

Goering, S. (2015). Rethinking disability: The social model of disability and chronic disease. *Current Reviews in Musculoskeletal Medicine* 8 (2): 134–138.

Groarke, L. (2001). Anecdotal Reasoning. OSSA Conference Archive, University of Windsor, Windsor.

Hall, M. C. (2019, September). *Critical Disability Theory*, The Stanford Encyclopedia of Psychology. Retrieved July 2020 from: https://plato.stanford.edu/cgi-bin/encyclopedia/archinfo.cgi?entry=disability-critical.

Harvard Medical School (2020). *Harvard Health Publishing*, Sarcoidosis. Retrieved from: https://www.health.harvard.edu/diseases-and-conditions/sarcoidosis-a-to-z.

Harwood, J. and Roy, A. (2002). Social identity theory and mass Communication research. In J. Harwood and H. Giles, *Language as Social Action. Intergroup Communication: Multiple Perspectives* (pp. 189–211). Bern: Peter Lang.

Huffington Post (2009). Retrieved July 2020 from: https://www.huffingtonpost.co.uk/entry/house-becomes-worlds-most_n_214704?ri18n=true.

Kalanithi, P. (2019). *When Breath Becomes Air*. New York: Random House.

Karvonen, S., Kestila, L., and Mäki-Opas, T. (2018). Who needs the sociology of health and illness? A new agenda for responsive and interdisciplinary sociology of health and medicine. *Frontiers in Sociology* 3 (1): 1–4.

Kay, A. (2017). *This is Going to Hurt*. London: Picador.

Khakpour, P. (2018). *Sick: A Memoir*. New York: Harper Collins.

Martin, R. (2009). *For House, It's Either Lupus or Sarcoidosis*, Global Comment. Retrieved from: http://globalcomment.com/for-house-its-either-lupus-or-sarcoidosis/.

Minich, J. A. (2016). Enabling whom? Critical disability studies now. *Lateral* 5 (1).

Mitchell, D. and Snyder, S. (2000). *Narrative Prosthesis: Disability and the Dependencies of Discourse*. Ann Arbor: University of Michigan Press.

NHS (2020). *Methotrexate*, NHS. Retrieved from: https://www.nhs.uk/medicines/methotrexate/.

NHS (2020). *Sarcoidosis*, NHS. Retrieved from: https://www.nhs.uk/conditions/sarcoidosis/.

Ogden, G. (2017). *The NHS has Revealed the 20 Worst Pains Known to Man*, ShortList. Retrieved August 2020, from: https://www.shortlist.com/news/the-nhs-has-revealed-the-worst-ten-pains-known-to-humans.

O'Malley, K. (2019). *90% of People Think They're Helping Society By Challenging People Who Don't 'Look Disabled', Says Study*, Independent. Retrieved July 2020 from: https://www.independent.co.uk/life-style/health-and-families/hidden-disabilities-crohns-colitis-abuse-disabled-toilets-a8871111.html.

Petasis, A. (2019). Discrepancies of the medical, social and biopsychosocial models of disability; A comprehensive theoretical framework. *International Journal of Business Management and Technology* 3 (4): 42–54.

Rhimes, S. (Director). (2005). *Grey's Anatomy* [Television Series].

Robertson, L. (2008). *The 5 Most Ridiculous Things About 'House M.D.'*, Stereogum. Retrieved July 2020 from: https://www.stereogum.com/1777630/the_five_most_ri diculous_thing/vg-loc/videogum/.

Schalk, S. (2017). Critical disability studies as methodology. *Lateral* 6 (1).

Shakespeare, T. and Watson, N. (2002). The social model of disability: An outdated ideology? *Research in Social Science and Disability* 2: 9–28.

Shakespeare, T., Watson, N., and Abu Alghaib, O. (2016). Blaming the victim, all over again: Waddell and Aylward's biopsychosocial (BPS) model of disability. *Critical Social Policy* 1 (37): 1–36.

Sharma, O. (2020). *Definition and History of Sarcoidosis*, ILD. Retrieved from: http://www .ildcare.nl/Downloads/artseninfo/Sarcoidosis/Chapter%201%20Definition%20and %20history%20of%20sarcoidosis.pdf.

Shore, D. (2004–2012). House, M.D.

Singhal, A. (2019). *Thunderclap Headache: The "Worst Headache of My Life"*, Harvard Health Publishing. Retrieved August 2020 from: https://www.health.harvard.edu/ blog/thunderclap-headache-the-worst-headache-of-my-life-2019062516939.

Sontag, S. (1991). *Illness as Metaphor and Aids and its Metaphors.* London: Penguin.

Sontag, S. (1979) *Illness as Metaphor.* New York: Random House.

Storr, W. (2019). *The Science of Storytelling: Why Stories Make Us Human and How to Tell Them Better.* London: William Collins.

University of Hull (2019). *University of Hull and SarcoidosisUK Unite for Clinical Trial That Aims to Halt Killer Disease.* Retrieved from: https://www.hull.ac.uk/work-with-us/ more/media-centre/news/2019/sarcoidosis-clinical-trial.

Wade, D. H. (2017). The biopsychosocial model of illness: A model whose time has come. *Clinical Rehabilitation* 31 (8): 995–1004.

Walker, R. (2019). *Doctor, Teacher, Bestseller: Why Real-Life Memoirs Are Such a Hit*, The Guardian. Retrieved July 2020 from: https://www.theguardian.com/books/2019/m ay/04/real-life-memoirs-are-a-hit-with-readers.

Weltin, P. (2020). *At Least it's not Cancer*, The Epic Foundation. Retrieved July 2020 from: https://epictogether.org/at-least-its-not-cancer/.

Wendell, S. (2001). Unhealthy disabled: Treating chronic illnesses as disabilities. *Hypatia* 16 (4): 17–33.

White, C. (2016). *At Least It's Not Cancer – A Prejudice That Harms Patients*, HuffPost. Retrieved July 2020 from: https://www.huffpost.com/entry/at-least-its-not-cancer- ---a-prejudice-that-harms-patients_b_9278690?guccounter=1andguce_referrer =aHR0cHM6Ly93d3cuZ29vZ2xlLmNvbS8andguce_referrer_sig=AQAAAN5Kl AzfGq61a3VGU3axG__CGtd6rn29CXuGci9uFJwZdnzMqcXmTZfe0yb2nApKH yIRg_8WmF.

Williams, I. (2019). *Paddy McGuinness hits back as man claims his family 'don't look disabled' after parking in disabled bay*, Metro. Retrieved July 2020 from: https://metro.co.uk/ 2019/11/04/paddy-mcguiness-hits-back-as-man-claims-his-family-dont-look-dis abled-after-parking-in-disabled-bay-11036964/.

Yaitanes, G. (Director) (2009). House Divided. *House, M.D.*, 5 (22).

Zulker, A. (Creator). (2000–2015). *CSI: Crime Scene Investigation* [Television Series].

15

THE METANARRATIVE OF ARTHRITIS

Playing and betraying the endgame

David Bolt

Preliminary discussion

Arthritis can hardly be thought of as an obscure medical term. From an etymological perspective alone, given that the prefix *arthr-* means joint and the suffix *-itis* means inflammation, it is quite easy to infer that the term denotes joint inflammation. This being so, arthritis is widely recognized as a medical condition that affects one joint or multiple joints and causes swelling, stiffness, and significant pain. These facts are common to the numerous types of arthritis (e.g. ankylosing spondylitis, gout, rheumatoid arthritis, and osteoarthritis). The trouble is that there are also overarching assumptions, tropes, and stereotypes about the condition that constitute yet another problematic metanarrative of disability: the metanarrative of arthritis.

Although not usually prominent, the metanarrative of arthritis can be found in a number of Anglo-American cultural texts published since the mid-twentieth century. One such text is John Steinbeck's classic American novel *East of Eden* (1952), wherein Cathy is initially characterized as very beautiful but soon emerges as monstrous and twisted in her morality, identified in literary studies as the most evil of all fictional American women (Gladstein, 1991). The key point here is that with age Cathy's hands become disfigured by arthritis. The associated pain, moreover, is such that it renders her reliant on a comparably deceitful ex-convict, Joe Valery, with whom she runs a brothel. Whether crassly interpreted as karmic justice for evil acts or an outward manifestation of the twisted person within, Cathy's characterization illustrates multiple strands of the metanarrative of arthritis.

According to the metanarrative, the definition of someone who has arthritis is an aged, twisted, painful, moaning figure. This sociocultural construct is considered here in relation to three diverse texts published since the mid-twentieth century. First, Samuel Beckett's play *Endgame* was staged in 1957 and remains popular today. Second, Noah Baumbach's film *While We're Young* was released in 2014. Third, Godfrey Baseley's radio soap opera *The Archers* has been broadcast since 1951, although the episodes on which the chapter focuses are far more recent. The texts are considered in this order so as to explore representations of arthritis in the final stages of life, where it is something of an expectation, but also in midlife and youth, where it is unlikely to be featured at all. These factors all add detail to the metanarrative by which people who have arthritis are often defined.

Methodological discussion

When conducting research on the metanarrative of arthritis, one useful method is Critical Discourse Analysis (CDA), which enables ethical explorations of disability via multiple levels and forms of textual representation (Price, 2009; Cowley, 2012; Penketh, 2014; Grue, 2015; Houston, 2015; Mapley, 2015; Burch, 2018; Priyanti, 2018). With ethical approval from the School of Social Science at Liverpool Hope University, the research presented in this chapter is predominantly textual because of concerns about the potential impact on the lives of 'over-researched populations' (BERA, 2018, 20). The rationale is that textual methods centre on disability experience without adding to the exhaustion associated with people-based alternatives; that researchers alone are inconvenienced by the process (Snyder and Mitchell, 2006). It is, however, from this very concern that further ethical tensions arise, given that much work in disability studies asserts the necessity for the voice (broadly conceived) of disabled people in disability research (Finkelstein, 1980; Charlton, 1998; Cook, Swain, and French, 2001; Barnes, 2003; Crowther, 2007; Caslin, 2014). In an endeavour to address these ethical tensions, CDA can be combined with autoethnography, the result of which is a hybrid research method hereby termed autocritical discourse analysis.

If the coinage of autocritical discourse analysis is led by ethics, it also pertains to profound epistemology. Beyond ethical concerns, a reason for choosing a textual method is to 'contribute to the community spirit of critical analysis and constructive criticism that generates improvement in practice and enhancement of knowledge' (BERA, 2018, 29). When underpinned by autoethnography, this enhancement can illustrate what, via a double special issue of the *Journal of Literary and Cultural Disability Studies*, Lisa Johnson, Robert Mcruer, and other disability scholars in the United States term cripistemology – a contraction of the appropriated offensive words *cripple* and *epistemology*. Cripistemology is said to speak to, and through, a notion of 'disability justice that connects us on an important level', it represents 'new ways of thinking, knowing, and communicating across difference' (Johnson and Mcruer, 2014, 247, 254). These new ways of thinking may involve the 'turning over of failed capacities into productive incapacities' (Mitchell, Snyder, and Ware, 2014, 296), one example being the recognition of impairment and disability as the bases for profound epistemology.

Autocritical discourse analysis is introduced on the understanding that, when researching social attitudes and encounters, cripistemology is a new variant of epistemology that truly values personal narratives. A particular concern in the present chapter, and indeed the volume more broadly, is that the personal narratives of disabled people are often overshadowed by ubiquitous metanarratives of disability. The premise of autocritical discourse analysis is that due consideration of these personal narratives can help to disrupt the overarching assumptions and generalizations by which social encounters are frequently influenced. For this reason, prior to engaging in the textual analysis of various representations of arthritis, I must begin with a brief personal narrative about my own recent and, crucially, not so recent experiences of the chronic condition.

A few years ago, at the end of 2014, when I was in my late 40s, I registered with my local medical centre in order to make an appointment with the General Practitioner (GP). The trouble was that my hands had become a bit stiff, very inflamed, and quite painful. I probably should say that, having been in academia for about 15 years at that point, I had spent much time using a computer keyboard, which (because of my visual impairment) I used for both writing and reading. Before that, moreover, I had spent many long days and nights in cold recording studios, playing guitar, bass, synthesizer, percussion, and so on, trying desperately to make the numerous mediocre demos of my songs sound great. As such, I thought I had worked my hands too hard for too long, an inference with which the GP neither agreed nor disagreed. I was, however, promptly directed to have various blood tests and then referred to a specialist.

Very soon after my initial visit to the local medical centre I received a letter about a hospital appointment with a rheumatologist. I anticipated a brief consultation in which I would be advised to avoid working so much with my hands, to include more oily fish in my diet, to take better care of my joints – a proverbial rap on the increasingly tender knuckles. In actual fact it was a pretty intense session, where I was required to strip down to my underwear for a thorough examination, not to mention more tests and numerous X-rays. Although I have been registered as blind since my teenage years, owing to the untreatable nature of my eye condition, I had been neither an inpatient nor an outpatient for decades and so, for the purpose of this autocritical discourse analysis, must admit to finding the whole experience rather unnerving. Little was I to know that I would soon become quite accustomed to hospital appointments with not only the rheumatologist but also the rheumatology nurses, physiotherapist, occupational therapist, podiatrist, surgeon, and so on.

It turned out that the trouble with my hands was symptomatic of an autoimmune disease called psoriatic arthritis, 'where symptoms are unpredictable or not immediately visible' (Barnes and Mercer, 2003, 73). This diagnosis combined with that of retinitis pigmentosa (i.e. the cause of my visual impairment) and meant that I was thereafter classed as having comorbidity (Centers for Disease

Control and Prevention, 2011). In fact, as a result of the numerous hospital appointments, it soon became apparent that, more than trouble with my hands, I had pretty clear signs of related pain and/or inflammation in my jaw, feet, neck, spine, wrists, and elbows. The trouble with my hands was just far more obvious because, having no vision, I had come to rely on haptic means of perception, which is perhaps why some of the joints in my fingers had already become permanently damaged (i.e. eroded and disfigured).

Treatment for psoriatic arthritis is varied, so I have discovered, but the main aims are to relieve the symptoms and slow down the overall progression of the disease. To this end I was prescribed what is known in the medical profession as a disease-modifying anti-rheumatic drug called Methotrexate, which would serve to deaden what can be loosely understood as the overactivity of my immune system. The logic of this prescription made some sense to me, insofar as I had been diagnosed with an autoimmune disease, but I was nonetheless concerned about becoming prone to other things while taking the medication. It was carefully explained to me that this was indeed one of several side effects, along with nausea, diarrhoea, and mouth ulcers, not to mention an increased vulnerability to liver problems, sensitivity to sunlight, and so on. In time, all of these things proved relevant to me, to varied extents, but I must admit that back then I was most struck by the prospect of having to stop drinking alcohol – I had enjoyed a dozen or so bottles of lager across each weekend for many years. Ultimately, though, being part of the high-risk group when the global pandemic hit the United Kingdom in 2020 was the lowest point in these unintended consequences, for the requisite self-isolation proved that bit more difficult for someone who has long since acknowledged the importance of interdependency and community.

For all that, as well as the ongoing hassle of regular medical appointments and the sometimes negative impact of chronic pain, among other things, again for the purpose of this autocritical discourse analysis I must say that my treatment for arthritis has proven worthwhile. Methotrexate has been around for decades, so there might well be (or at least should be) better drugs available, but it does seem to have hindered the progression of the disease; it has certainly made a massive difference to my manual dexterity. For example, within a few months of starting the weekly dose I was able to play the guitar again. Indeed, now, some five years on, I am touch-typing these words, meaning I am still able to use all of my fingers, although some do work far better than others, given the irreversible damage incurred prior to the commencement of the treatment. In addition, I now have a couple of pints of albeit weak lager most weeks and my liver count has been fine for a long time. That is to say, the disease has resulted in physical impairment, complicated by the fact that I do not perceive by visual means, and the pain and side effects of the medication are unpleasant, but thus far my situation is manageable.

While this personal narrative could continue for many pages and take various negative and positive turns, there are a few points that must be raised in the epistemic contextualization of the chapter (i.e. in this foundational stage of the autocritical discourse analysis). Some of the pain and inflammation in my hands, among other places, dates back to when I was in my 20s. Indeed, I mentioned these things to more than one GP at the time. Neither they nor I were overly concerned, partly because I found that if I waited long enough, the symptoms would fade and not return for quite some time. More significantly, I know that I for one was distracted by an age-related strand of the metanarrative of arthritis. On one occasion, for example, I can remember sitting in a cafe waiting to be served and overhearing two women talking. One woman said that her hand was stiff and painful, that it was arthritis, probably flaring up because of the bad weather. The other woman retorted, with assumed authority, that it was age-related. It was this very same assumption that convinced me that when in my twenties, I was far too young for arthritis. When I was in my 30s and early 40s, moreover, although increasingly concerned by the protracting rhythm of relapses over remissions I remained mindful that the trouble started when I was much younger. Indeed, to my shame, when I did finally go to the rheumatologist, at the end of the consultation I was quick to put the arthritis leaflets away for fear of being assumed older than I was by anyone who may have noticed me carrying them.

Paving the way for what some people might at this juncture deem my midlife crisis, arthritis was linked to ageing even within the British disability studies books I was reading and re-reading when in my late 30s and early 40s. For instance, it was in considering the situation of 'individuals who acquire an impairment in later life' that Colin Barnes and Geof Mercer cited arthritis as a condition that forced some into a 'sudden and substantial re-evaluation of their identity, perhaps reinforced within a short time period by downward economic and social mobility' (Barnes and Mercer, 2003, 63). Likewise, when considering the principle of cure, Tom Shakespeare illustrated the diversity of ways in which impairment was experienced. A few groups of disabled people were thereby identified, one being those who became impaired as part of the ageing process and the operative thing to note here is that arthritis was the first condition mentioned (Shakespeare, 2006). Thus, if these influential leaders of disability studies were not always in agreement with each other, they did align when it came to positing examples of age-related impairments.

It almost goes without saying that I have since come to learn that, although longevity surely raises the odds, in fact, people experience arthritis at all ages. In the United Kingdom, for example, approximately 15,000 young people, including children, have some form of the condition (National Health Service, 2018). Accordingly, I have sat in hospital waiting rooms alongside people far younger than I was even when my pain and inflammation first started. What is more, I have been educated by some of my own students who have had the condition since childhood. I have also started to recall and notice the cultural artefacts that reinforce the metanarrative of arthritis on which this chapter focuses. Most often, although arthritis 'strikes people of every age, from infants to adults' (Canadian Arthritis Society, 2020), it tends to be portrayed as an aspect of the ultimate stage of life; as an element of what is sometimes dramatically termed the endgame.

Analytical discussion 1

Endgame

The prolific and highly influential Irish writer Samuel Beckett – who, like Steinbeck, received the Nobel Prize for literature – is best remembered for works defined by both the reduction of context to minimal details and the existential contemplations of an ageing figure. One such work is *Endgame* (1957), a one-act play set in a bare room with the main focus on Hamm and Clov, two of only four characters named in the dramatis personae. Hamm has no sight and cannot walk, while Clov has poor sight and cannot sit down. The play's other two characters, Nagg and Nell, have both lost limbs and live in a pair of ashbins. These details contextualize the bleak scene for this definitive drama of the absurd; they sketch out what is often deemed an exemplary model of theatre that disrupts character and plot conventions to explore the idea of life in a meaningless universe.

The play's very title, *Endgame*, implies figurative meanings, given the invocation of the final stage of the board game chess, where only a few pieces remain. From this titular metaphor comes an easy comparison with the 'winding down of the characters' lives, when everything is coming to an end' (Quayson, 2007, 66), for what is 'universal in life, if there are universals, is the experience of the limitations of the body' (Davis, 2002, 32). On an expansive level, moreover, the ending for Hamm is also an ending for humanity (Ware, 2015), which seems troublingly pertinent in present times. These implicit yet nonetheless prioritized comparisons invite many complex interpretations. In one such reading, for example, Hamm is 'not simply an imperial oppressor, but a metaphor for the enlightened, ex-imperial figure whose modes of writing and interpreting relationships with his various others perpetually fall back on binary and hierarchical perceptions of those relationships' (Pearson, 2001, 229). This example illustrates something of the fact that the play's mode of expression initiates not only multiple but also multilayered figurative readings.

The multiplicity of readings notwithstanding, the dominant literary discourse around *Endgame* is illustrative of critical avoidance – that is, the conspicuous lack of academic engagement with disability studies, despite the abundance of representations of disabled people in primary texts (Bolt, 2019). More generally, the critical avoidance of disability in Beckett 'coincides with concerns around saleable narratives and emphasizes an individualism – in spite of the interdependent behaviour of his characters – that precludes inclusivity of a wider range of embodiments and experiences' (Ewart, 2016, 164). After all, 'despite the many obvious referents to the body's deterioration', the phenomenology of pain is absent from most interpretations (Quayson, 2007, 56). This absence places the numerous impaired bodies 'on the boundary between comedy and tragedy', for 'because pain is not a central part of their characterization, the phenomeno-logical specificity of their impairments gets blurred and thus easily assimilable to philosophical categories' (Quayson, 2007, 84). That is to say, the discursive absence around pain has allowed Beckett's characters not to be considered disa-bled (Quayson, 2007), as the tenor of metaphorical meanings has been exhumed and explicated to the detriment of literal embodiments.

When critical avoidance is addressed, the metaphorical comparison between the ending of a chess game and that of humanity might well be recognized, but particular attention must be paid to the intermediate line of meaning, the embodied experiences of the four characters. A notable commonality in these interrelated experiences is pain. Most directly, Nell and Nagg, in the ashbins to which they are confined, are said to 'turn painfully towards each other' (Beckett, 1964, 18). A little later, Clov, having been pacing back and forth, staring at the ground with his hands behind his back, comes to an expressive halt: 'The pains in my legs! It's unbelievable! Soon I won't be able to think any more' (Beckett, 1964, 33). This direct reference to overwhelming pain is echoed when Hamm, during his monologue, 'pushes himself painfully off his seat' and then 'falls back again' (Beckett, 1964, 45). Illustrative of the 'indeterminate relationship between pain and being' (Gould, 2017, 179), the endgame for Nell, Nagg, Clov, and Hamm is manifestly painful to play.

Although pain is a factor in the endgame of all four characters, this is espe-cially true of Hamm. Specific medical reasons are not given in the play, but for the purpose of this chapter it is perhaps worth noting the biographical detail that Cissie Sinclair, Beckett's aunty, had arthritis, used a wheelchair, and has been named as the model for Hamm (Knowlson 1996; Quayson, 2007). Certainly, it is the case that the one-act play contains more than a dozen direct and indirect references to pain and it is to Hamm that most of them pertain. For instance, in an exchange about whether or not he has brought too much suffering to Clov, Hamm asks, 'Is it not time for my pain-killer?' (Beckett, 1964, 14), a question repeated verbatim throughout the play (Beckett, 1964, 16, 28, 34, 46). The refer-ent of this pain-killer refrain is Hamm's pain, the significance of which increases with each repetition and beyond.

In a key contribution to the foundational work on cripistemology, it is posited that pain is never experienced in isolation, yet its context is likely to neither value nor acknowledge interdependence (Patsavas, 2014). It is therefore notable that, on the contrary, for the bulk of *Endgame*, the representation of pain is not defined by isolation but does involve interdependence. When Hamm asks if it is not time for his pain-killer, he reveals the feelings of pain he nonetheless avoids asserting. The pain becomes apparent via a repeated enquiry that, unlike the alternative of a direct assertion, overtly includes his interlocutor, Clov. In keeping with what has become something of a 'tradition' in disability studies, that 'values interde-pendence over independence and seeks to situate experiences within frameworks of relationality', such critical emphasis on the 'discursive processes of isolation paves the way for recognizing pain as an experience that exceeds the boundaries of individual bodies' (Patsavas, 2014, 213). Like other works by Beckett, then, *Endgame* may be said to represent disability in the context of a dialectic of dependency, as explored in another special issue of the *Journal of Literary and Cultural Disability Studies*, guest edited in the United States by Michael Davidson. In these terms, the audience is presented with a post-apocalypse world at the centre of which is the relationship between the two disabled characters: Hamm, who imitates a fallen king, and Clov, who imitates his son and servant (Davidson, 2007). Pain indirectly connects the two characters amid the ultimate life experience – that is, during their eponymous endgame.

The repeated invocations of the pain-killer grow in complexity as the play progresses. Hamm comes to expand on the refrain in an aggressive mode, whereby the enquiry becomes a demand: 'Give me my pain-killer' (Beckett, 1964, 23). Clov retorts that it is too soon after the tonic has been taken. Temporarily dissuaded, Hamm reasons that in the morning the pain-killers stimulate and in the evening they sedate but admits that in fact it might be the reverse. Pain is still represented indirectly, via the analgesic antithesis whose effectiveness nonetheless starts to become uncertain. At this point in the play, the chain of signification (i.e. pain, age, endgame, death) is shaken if not broken by confusion about the very purpose of the pain-killer.

By the end of the play, the human connections have all but broken down. In the vein of negativity, Hamm and Clov function in accordance with an ableist ideology that regards dependency as weakness, whereby reliance on an assistant is emasculating and a caregiver's benefits simply do not register (Davidson, 2007). As such, resonant with Steinbeck's *East of Eden*, specifically the productive-destructive relationship between Cathy and Joe, Beckett's *Endgame* represents a 'seemingly perpetual co-dependency that paralyzes Hamm and Clov' (Pearson, 2001, 235). Like dependency, paralysis is rendered totally negative, from which it follows that, juxtaposed with Clov, Hamm is disabled and burdensome, if not parasitic.

In the final analysis, from the play's burgeoning normative perspective, Hamm's pain-killer refrain is repeated ad nauseam. Clov's annoyance becomes increasingly apparent as, over and over again, he answers the question in the negative. But broken for both characters is the growing frustration when Clov finally affirms that it is indeed time for Hamm's pain-killer and the relief is climactic: 'Ah! At last! Give it to me! Quick!' (Beckett, 1964, 46). After all that, the assumed authority of the excuses and hesitations becomes evident as Clov admits that, in fact, the final pain-killer has gone:

Clov. No more pain-killer. You'll never get any more pain-killer.
Hamm. But the little round box. It was full!
Clov. Yes. But now it's empty. (Beckett, 1964, 46)

Hamm despairs, if only momentarily, at what he will do without the pain-killer. This being so, a charge of disability dramatics might seem fitting, whereby exaggerated representations obscure the real issues, complexities, subtleties, and joys of disability (Bolt, 2019). However, a pivotal point is that pain itself is still not defined by isolation. Rather, it is the end of the pain-killer refrain that marks the end of the discursive connection, which constitutes the ultimate crisis, a finale in terms of dependency and thus community.

Analytical section 2

Midlife crisis

More than half a century on from the first staging of Beckett's *Endgame*, film director Noah Baumbach's *While We're Young* (2014) is a comedy that centres on the midlife crisis of Josh Schrebnick (played by Ben Stiller). Josh works at a college, makes documentary films, and lives in New York with his wife Cornelia (played by Naomi Watts). In more than one aspect of his life he has started to become uncertain if not unsuccessful and, as such, finds some solace when seemingly befriended by a vibrant young couple, Jamie and Darby Massey (played by Adam Driver and Amanda Seyfried respectively). The midlife crisis on which the film centres is said to be 'more exquisitely horrible' than might be expected, for Josh makes a fool of himself with a younger man rather than a younger woman, not in a 'sexual relationship, but something more painfully intimate: a matter of self-esteem and social status' (Bradshaw, 2015). While Josh and Cornelia are in their 40s, the younger couple are in their 20s, and this chronological juxtaposition underscores attitudes towards age as a thematic focus of the film. Defined by disappointment, Josh's midlife crisis is manifest in his endeavours to behave and, where possible, become more like his young friends.

If a midlife crisis is an endeavour to redefine the present by the possibilities and pleasures of the past, it also means avoiding the real prospects of the future. This being so, *While We're Young* contains significant moments of foreboding. In one such moment, Josh injures his leg and as a result attends a medical appointment with Dr Nagato (played by James Saito). It transpires that the actual reason for the visit is nothing to worry about, just the pain of a pulled muscle, but that Josh has arthritis in his knee. This diagnosis is received with some confusion, whereby Josh asks if *arthritis* is an umbrella term for miscellaneous injuries. The manifest incredulity spreads from patient to doctor as the humour of the scene builds:

Dr Nagato. No, arthritis is a degradation of the joints.
Josh. I know what traditional arthritis is.
Dr Nagato. I'm not sure what you mean by 'traditional', but this is arthritis.
Josh. Arthritis arthritis?
Dr Nagato. Yes, I usually just say it once.
Josh. At my age? (*While We're Young*, 2014)

In keeping with the age-related strand of the metanarrative of arthritis, Josh simply cannot imagine having the chronic condition at his time of life. The doctor demonstrates some criticality insofar as he guesses Josh's age is 42, which is hastily amended to 44, and then makes the point that in any case arthritis occurs in people of both these ages. However, the doctor does not make the much stronger medical point, that in fact the condition is experienced across the lifespan, from youth to old age (Canadian Arthritis Society, 2020; National Health Service, 2018). What is more, the doctor implicitly if sardonically reinforces the link between arthritis and ageing, for as Josh squints at his prescription for pain-killers, he is probed about when he last had his eyes tested and jibed about maturity. The doctor thereby maps the direction of the very future against which Josh is trying to turn his back, for arthritis serves to signpost the kind of endgame characterized by Beckett's Hamm.

A little later in the film, the midlife crisis begins to dissipate as the present is tentatively opened to the prospects of the future. At one point, owing partly to unwanted and unanticipated childlessness, Josh is having marital difficulties and ends up staying at the apartment of old friends Fletcher and Marina (played by Adam Horovitz and Maria Dizzia, respectively). Fletcher and Marina have a newborn baby, Willow, who completes a familial unit about which Josh confesses to having been jealous, but it becomes apparent that parenthood is not all it is said or meant to be; that it is not necessarily the answer to everyone's quest for existential fulfilment. In this reflective mood Josh smiles as he notices the sleeve of an album by Wilco – an alternative rock band formed in the United States a couple of decades earlier, when he, like his new friends, would himself have been in his 20s – and Fletcher pours a drink of whiskey for them both. The conversation becomes more embodied when Fletcher sits down, winces, explains that he has a herniated disk, and adds that he is due to have an epidural. Josh laughs and enters into the confessional spirit with an assertion that he has arthritis in his knee. They thereby connect, like Beckett's Hamm and Clov, via the expression of pain and, by extension, an implicit invocation of disability community, and reflect on what 'is happening' to them (*While We're Young*, 2014). In other words, they start to define the present with allusion to the prospects of their future.

Analytical discussion 3

Salad days

Remarkably contemporaneous with both Beckett's *Endgame* and Baumbach's *While We're Young*, not to mention Steinbeck's *East of Eden*, Godfrey Baseley's dramatic creation, *The Archers*, has been Broadcast by BBC Radio 4 for seven decades, since 1951. Widely enjoyed as a celebration of the ordinary (Taylor, 1999), a microcosm of British society (Runswick-Cole, 2016), it is set in a fictional village called Ambridge, home to families such as the Aldridges, the Carters, the Grundys, the Pargetters, and the Snells, as well as the eponymous

Archers. The original objective was to disseminate information that would help farmers improve productivity in post-war Britain but, also billed as an everyday tale of rural folk, it went on to become what is now, all credit to Baseley and subsequent producers, the world's longest-running soap opera.

In general terms, Daniel Hebden-Lloyd (played by Will Howard) is a significant character insofar as his namesake and great grandfather was the original Dan Archer (played by Harry Oakes). In the context of the present chapter, though, Daniel is relevant because he is diagnosed with arthritis. As such, his characterization has already been critiqued from within the field of British disability studies (Runswick-Cole, 2016), for the diagnosis primarily facilitates a brief affair between his mother, Shula Hebden-Lloyd, and the family GP, Richard Locke (played by Judy Bennett and William Gaminara respectively), after which the arthritis seems to somehow clear up. In other words, the condition appears fleetingly, only to prop up the main storyline (Runswick-Cole, 2016), and thereby provides an all-too-familiar illustration of the classic critical concept coined in the United States, narrative prosthesis (Mitchell and Snyder, 2000). This illustration becomes still more explicit when Daniel subsequently decides on a career in the armed forces, enlists at Sandhurst, and rises through the ranks to Second Lieutenant.

In relation to the metanarrative of arthritis, the salient point about Daniel's characterization is that his diagnosis comes during childhood. This detail makes the illustration of narrative prosthesis a bit more complex. The scriptwriters do indeed miss an 'opportunity to explore the wider social-political contexts of disability' (Runswick-Cole, 2016), which is all the more notable because *The Archers* has been elsewhere criticized for imparting left-wing, subversive, revolutionary attitudes (Hitchens, 1999; Taylor, 1999). Furthermore, in harsh contrast with the sustained breakdown in relationships impacted by Shula and Richard's affair, the rapidity and very matter of Daniel's recovery defy medical science (Smith, 2011), where the expectation is that arthritis 'stays for life' (Canadian Arthritis Society, 2020). However, contrary to the Shakespearean notion of salad days that define youth by greenness (i.e. inexperience), Daniel remains a significant character because he is one of very few who disrupt the metanarrative and represent arthritis without linking it to old age.

Concluding discussion

In this exploration of the metanarrative of arthritis, not only the interpretations but also the rationale behind the selection of primary texts are indicative of autocritical discourse analysis. First, consciously or unconsciously, it is no doubt because of my own multiple impairments that, for decades, I have been drawn to the work of Beckett. At the start of the century my visual impairment led me to investigate representations of blindness for my doctorate, so *Waiting for Godot* (1953), as well as *Endgame*, was of obvious interest, and as my physical impairment became increasingly apparent, my mind wandered back to the so-called comorbid figure of Hamm. Second, during the first year of my treatment for arthritis, Baumbach's *While We're Young* was the representation that caught my attention for, as tends to be the way with these things, it seemed to be on in the background every few days. Third, as I began to realize that I have had the condition since I was a very young man, I started to recall late-twentieth-century episodes of the Radio 4 soap opera, *The Archers*, where Daniel had arthritis as a child. This rationale is restricted by my woefully limited knowledge of culture but the emergent structure of endgame, midlife crisis, and salad days serves well to illustrate the dominance of age in the metanarrative of arthritis.

Many ramifications of the age-related strand of the metanarrative become apparent when consideration is given to the value of community uncovered here. In terms of the tripartite model of disability (Bolt, 2019), as well as non-normative negativisms (i.e. difficulties), there are non-normative positivisms (i.e. qualities) attached to arthritis, as illustrated by the historian Mary Felstiner, who started to notice her symptoms in her mid-20s and in time identified positively with the disability community (Felstiner, 2005). However, obscured by normative positivisms (i.e. indifference to disability), precisely because many people who have arthritis regard it as an aspect of so-called normal ageing, they are less likely to make this identification (Shakespeare, 2006). Accordingly, the poet Josephine Miles had the condition from an early age but 'did not identify as disabled or with the disability rights movement' (Davidson, 2008, 242). That is to say, more than rendering someone unlikely to recognize arthritis until later in life, and thus reducing the efficacy of available treatments, the age-related strand of the metanarrative identifies the condition in terms of isolation rather than community.

Some values of disability community are in the creation, recognition, critique, and expansion of related epistemology. After all, classic feminist disability studies in the United States observes that disabled people's knowledge tends to be trivialized and thought of as 'complaining' (Wendell, 1989, 104), non-normative negativisms that resonate with the metanarrative of arthritis from which emerges the aged, twisted, painful, moaning figure invoked in, among other works, Steinbeck's *East of Eden*. It is, therefore, worth revisiting Hamm's refrain in Beckett's *Endgame*, from a perspective enhanced by cripistemology, where it is understood that ableism makes pain feel unshareable (Patsavas, 2014). The question – 'Is it not time for my pain-killer?' – provides Hamm a means of expressing pain indirectly. He does not say that he is in great pain, which in reality is a difficult assertion to make – an admission almost, a submission somehow, and in practice an intimate expression that nonetheless adds fire to the flames – although it is implied by the repetition of the question. Indeed, Amber DiPietra is a poet who has arthritis and whose collaborative work with Denise Leto suggests that a direct assertion of pain seems dishonest insofar as it is more likely to appear in representation than reality (Gould, 2017). Their contention, though, is that even if, in the day-to-day, arthritic pain tends not to be disclosed on account of its constancy, its unremarkableness, this is no reason for it to be 'erased from the text' (Gould, 2017, 179). One hope for the recognition of cripistemology is that it permits people to '*think pain otherwise*, to produce painful new knowledge, but also to construct analyses about pain that are less painful, and less dangerous to those of us in pain, and, in doing so, to re-imagine our (shared, pained) futures' (Patsavas, 2014, 216). In this chapter's autocritical discourse analysis, the indirect representation of pain – much like putting medical leaflets out of sight at the end of a rheumatology appointment – illustrates reluctance to key oneself to the metanarrative that defines arthritis as, at best, a harbinger or, at worst, an indicator of decrepitude. The thing is that, with a tug on the age-related strand, the metanarrative unravels and there is recognition of values and vitality underpinned by pain, disfigurement, and tricky medication, but countless other things too, not least the non-normative enhancement of epistemology from which everyone may benefit.

References

Barnes, C. (2003) What a difference a decade makes: Reflections on doing emancipatory disability research. *Disability and Society* 18 (1): 3–17.

Barnes, C. and Mercer, G. (2003) *Disability*, Cambridge: Polity Press.

Baseley, G. (1951) *The Archers*, BBC Radio 4.

Beckett, S. (1964) *Endgame*, London: Faber and Faber.

BERA. (2018) Ethical Guidelines for Educational Research [online]. *YUDU*. Available from: https://www.bera.ac.uk/wp-content/uploads/2018/06/BERA-Ethical-Gu idelines-for-Educational-Research_4thEdn_2018.pdf?noredirect=1 [accessed 23 November 2018].

Bolt, D. (2019) *Cultural Disability Studies in Education: Interdisciplinary Navigations of the Normative Divide*, Abingdon: Routledge.

Burch, L. (2018) 'You are a parasite on the productive classes': Online disablist hate speech in austere times, *Disability and Society* 33 (3): 392–415.

Bradshaw, P. (2015) While We're Young Review: A Fine Bromance, *The Guardian*. Available from: https://www.theguardian.com/film/2015/apr/02/while-were-youn g-review-baumbach-stiller-watts. [accessed 9 March 2020].

Canadian Arthritis Society (2020) About Arthritis. Available from: https://arthritis.ca/ about-arthritis [Accessed 9 March 2020].

Caslin, M. (2014) Behaviour, emotion, and social attitudes: The education of 'challenging' pupils, in D. Bolt (ed.) *Changing Social Attitudes Toward Disability: Perspectives from Historical, Cultural, and Educational Studies*, Abingdon: Routledge.

Centers for Disease Control and Prevention (2011) Comorbidities [online]. Available from: http://www.hope.ac.uk/media/liverpoolhope/contentassets/documents/libr ary/media,44088,en.pdf [accessed 17 April 2015].

Charlton, J. (1998) *Nothing About Us Without Us: Disability Oppression and Empowerment*, Berkeley: University of California Press.

Cook, T., Swain, J., and French, S. (2001) Voices from segregated schooling: Towards an inclusive education system. *Disability and Society* 16 (2): 293–310.

Cowley, D. (2012) Life writing, resistance, and the politics of representation: A critical discourse analysis of Eli Clare's 'learning to speak'. *Journal of Literary and Cultural Disability Studies* 6 (1): 85–95.

Crowther, N. (2007) Nothing without us or nothing about us? *Disability and Society* 22 (7): 791–794.

Davidson, M. (2008) *Concerto for the Left Hand: Disability and the Defamiliar Body*, Ann Arbor: University of Michigan Press.

Davidson, M. (2007) 'Every man his specialty': Beckett, disability, and dependence. *Journal of Literary and Cultural Disability Studies* 1 (2): i–vi.

Davis, L. J. (2002) *Bending Over Backwards: Disability, Dismodernism and Other Difficult Positions*, New York: New York University Press.

Ewart, C. (2016) How I can go on: Embracing modernity's displeasure with Beckett's *Murphy*, in D. Bolt and C. Penketh (eds.), *Disability, Avoidance, and the Academy: Challenging Resistance*, Abingdon: Routledge.

Felstiner, M. (2005) *Out of Joint: A Private and Public Story of Arthritis*, London: University of Nebraska Press.

Finkelstein, V. (1980) *Attitudes and Disabled People*, Washington DC: World Rehabilitation Fund.

Gladstein, M. (1991) The strong female principle of good – or evil: Women in *East of Eden*. *Steinbeck Quarterly* 24 (Winter-Spring): 30–40.

Gould, D. (2017) 'I am/in pain': The form of suffering in David Wolach's *Hospitalogy* and Amber DiPietra and Denise Leto's *Waveform*. *Journal of Literary and Cultural Disability Studies* 11 (2): 169–185.

Grue, J. (2015) *Disability and Discourse Analysis*, Surrey: Ashgate.

Hitchens, P. (1999) *The Abolition of Britain: From Lady Chatterley to Tony Blair*, London: Bloomsbury.

Houston, E. (2015) 'Mabel is unstable': A feminist disability studies perspective on early-twentieth-century representations of disabled women in advertisements. *Considering Disability Journal* 1 (1): 21–29.

Johnson, M. L. and McRuer, R. (2014) Introduction: Cripistemologies and the masturbating girl. *Journal of Literary and Cultural Disability Studies* 8 (3): 245–256.

Knowlson, J. (1996) *Damned to Fame: The Life of Samuel Beckett*, New York: Touchstone.

Mapley, H. (2015) 'In search of disability: A critical discourse analysis of a Key Stage 1 guided reading scheme. *Disability and Society* 30 (6): 896–909.

Mitchell, D. T. and Snyder, S. L. (2000) *Narrative Prosthesis: Disability and the Dependencies of Discourse*, Ann Arbor: University of Michigan Press.

Mitchell, D. T., Snyder, S. L., and Ware, L. (2014) '[Every] child left behind': Curricular cripistemologies and the crip/queer art of failure. *Journal of Literary and Cultural Disability Studies* 8 (3): 295–314.

National Health Service (2018) Arthritis. Available from: https://www.nhs.uk/conditions/arthritis/ [Accessed 9 March 2020].

Patsavas, A. (2014) Recovering a cripistemology of pain: Leaky bodies, connective tissue, and feeling discourse. *Journal of Literary and Cultural Disability Studies* 8 (2): 203–218.

Pearson, N. C. (2001) Outside of here it's death: Co-dependency and the Ghosts of Decolonization in Beckett's *Endgame*, *ELH* 68 (1): 215–239.

Penketh, C. (2014) Putting disability studies to work in art education. *International Journal of Art and Design Education* 33 (3): 291–300.

Price, M. (2009) 'Her pronouns wax and wane': Psychosocial disability, autobiography, and counter-diagnosis. *Journal of Literary and Cultural Disability Studies* 3 (1): 11–33.

Priyanti, N. (2018) Representations of people with disabilities in an Indonesian newspaper: A critical discourse analysis. *Disability Studies Quarterly* 38 (4).

Quayson, A. (2007) *Aesthetic Nervousness: Disability and the Crisis of Representation*, New York: Columbia University Press.

Runswick-Cole, K. (2016) Why the Archers Needs More Disabled Characters, *The Independent*, 6 March. Available from: https://www.independent.co.uk/arts-enter tainment/tv/news/why-the-archers-needs-more-disabled-characters-a6915471.html [Last accessed 9 March 2020]

Shakespeare, T. (2006) *Disability Rights and Wrongs*, Abingdon: Routledge.

Smith, R. (2011) Archers Characters More Likely to Die in Accidents, *The Telegraph*, 16 December. Available from: https://www.telegraph.co.uk/culture/tvandradio /8958384/Archers-characters-more-likely-to-die-in-accidents.html [Last Accessed 9 March 2020].

Snyder, S. L. and Mitchell, D. T. (2006) *Cultural Locations of Disability*, Chicago: University of Chicago Press.

Steinbeck, J. (1952) *East of Eden*, St Ives: Penguin.

Taylor, D. S. (1999) An everyday tale of rural folk? *The Spectator*, 283 (8917): 36–37.

Ware, B. (2015) Tragic-dialectical-perfectionism: On the ethics of Beckett's *Endgame*, *College Literature* 42 (1): 3–21.

Wendell, S. (1989) Toward a feminist theory of disability. *Hypatia* 4 (2): 104–24.

While We're Young (2014) Film Directed by Noah Baumbach, Scott Rudin Productions.

EPILOGUE

This volume was something of an achievement to complete. An edited volume, by definition, involves the bringing together of many contributors, which is obviously a salient strength, a meeting of minds, a mixture of approaches, even a microcosm of community, but all these things can multiply individual issues around deadlines and guidelines. These are basic considerations in the editorship of any volume of new work. However, it was no such issue that made the timely completion of this volume such an achievement.

It is surely fair to assert that when the volume was conceived, proposed, reviewed, and contracted for publication, the world seemed a very different place from the one in which we now find ourselves. Everyone commenced work on the project with drive and focus that, to different degrees, was soon impacted by the COVID-19 pandemic that, while devastatingly global, was especially dangerous to certain groups, one of which was disabled people. Implicit from the outset (in the Track and Trace artwork), given that most of the authors are close to the conditions under discussion, it follows that the writing here has been profoundly affected and thus informed by COVID-19. In the case of some chapters, for instance, the authors were writing in a lockdown extended or otherwise worsened precisely because of matters related to the conditions under discussion. In any case, the contributors might well have started work in offices equipped and designed for the job but almost certainly completed the research and writing at home, against a backdrop of distraction, at best, or isolation, fear, and multiple levels of loss, at worst.

The volume was largely written and edited in the first lockdown, a period of transformation, from the historical context before the COVID-19 pandemic to the present one of uncertainty and varied but widespread loss of personal liberties. This intense period of change rendered people, disabled and otherwise, powerless as to if and when they could leave their homes. For a poignant moment, in some parts of the world, it may have seemed like coronavirus would mark the end of disability history. Considered decades ago in critical theory, the end of history is a provocation made about the triumph of equality over prestige, governmental democracy over communism and fascism (Kojeve, 1947; Fukuyama, 1992; Derrida, 1994). The end of disability history, then, for the sake of this analogous provocation, would be the triumph of equality over the dominance of normative positivisms (i.e. indifference to disability would be displaced in favour of appreciation). Indeed, when approaching the first peak of the pandemic, in the United Kingdom, for example, a number of disabled people were given airtime and column inches to provide personal narratives of isolation and social limitations with which they were only too familiar (e.g. Pritchard, 2020a; Pritchard, 2020b). This appreciation of personal narratives of disability disrupted the normative divide as many people, disabled and non-disabled, sought and shared such survival strategies.

As the first lockdown was considered to be nearing its end; however, the apparent appreciation of personal narratives of disability soon began to fade. Rather than turning to non-normative positivisms, the normative positivisms were to be replaced by what amounted to neonormative positivisms. Everyone was talking about the new normal, a term by which our present historical context has now become known. Unfortunately, then, the world into which we started to move still accorded with the normative social order, for connotations of assumed authority were attached to every COVID-19 death whose documentation was somehow softened by that now familiar qualifying note about underlying conditions.

The new normal notwithstanding, this edited volume unapologetically prioritizes non-normative personal narratives over the metanarratives of disability that continue to define the normative social order and thereby enable assumed authority. Blindness, mental illness, OCD, learning disability, autism, Down syndrome, dwarfism, chronic pain, diabetes, cancer, HIV and AIDS, sarcoidosis, and arthritis, among many other conditions, oddly provoke opinions from many people who have neither direct nor even intimate experience of them. Indeed, authority is often assumed on that very basis, one of normative positivisms, whereby not being disabled renders people vocal and ostensibly knowledgeable about disability. Thus, the 15 chapters of variously embodied textual analyses and reflections in this edited volume disrupt many of the foundations upon which the social phenomenon of assumed authority is built. This is not to suggest that only disabled people can contribute to autocritical disability theory, nor autocritical disability studies more broadly, but it is to state that non-disabled colleagues must be truly comfortable being led by non-normative principles (not to mention professors, directors, editors, managers, chairs, and so on). The new normal is just another myth, which is to say a lie, belief in which amounts to denial of the very lived reality of disability that, in fact, defines the truth of all humanity.

References

Kojeve, Alexandre (1947) *Introduction: A la Lecture de Hegel*, Paris: Gallimard.

Derrida, J. (1994) *Specters of Marx*, London: Routledge.

Fukuyama, Francis. (1992) *The End of History and the Last Man*, London: Hamish Hamilton.

Pritchard, E. (2020a) How the pandemic is eroding disability access, British Sociological Association [online] Available from: https://es.britsoc.co.uk/how-the-pandemic-is-eroding-disability-access/

Pritchard, E. (2020b) The impact of social distancing for disabled people, who are just not disabled enough, British Sociological Association [online] Available from: https://es.britsoc.co.uk/the-impact-of-social-distancing-for-disabled-people-who-are-just-not-disabled-enough/

INDEX

Made in the USA
Coppell, TX
03 June 2022

78440159R00142